TREATING AFFECT PHOBIA

TREATING AFFECT PHOBIA

A Manual for Short-Term Dynamic Psychotherapy

Leigh McCullough
Nat Kuhn
Stuart Andrews
Amelia Kaplan
Jonathan Wolf
Cara Lanza Hurley

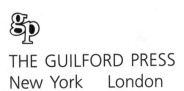

THE GUILFORD PRESS
New York   London

© 2003 Leigh McCullough
Published by The Guilford Press
A Division of Guilford Publications, Inc.
72 Spring Street, New York, NY 10012
www.guilford.com

Printed in the United States of America

This book is printed on acid-free paper.

Last digit is print number: 9 8 7 6 5 4 3 2 1

Library of Congress Cataloging-in-Publication Data

Treating affect phobia : a manual for short-term dynamic psychotherapy / Leigh
   McCullough ... [et al.].
      p. cm.
   Includes bibliographical references and index.
   ISBN 1-57230-810-9
   1. Brief psychotherapy. 2. Affect (Psychology). 3. Phobias. 4. Psychodynamic
psychotherapy. I. McCullough, Leigh.
RC480.55.T735 2003
616.89′14–dc21

                                                                    2002155163

To our patients and our mentors

About the Authors

Leigh McCullough, PhD, is an Associate Clinical Professor and Director of the Psychotherapy Research Program at Harvard Medical School (Boston, Massachusetts), and a visiting professor at the Norwegian University of Science and Technology (Trondheim, Norway). She was the 1996 Voorhees Distinguished Professor at the Menninger Clinic and received the 1996 Michael Franz Basch Award from the Silvan Tomkins Institute for her contributions to the exploration of affect in psychotherapy. Dr. McCullough is on the editorial board of the journal *Psychotherapy Research* and of the *Journal of Brief Therapy,* and conducts training seminars in Short-Term Dynamic Psychotherapy (STDP) worldwide. She is in private practice in Dedham, Massachusetts.

Nat (Nathaniel S.) Kuhn, MD, PhD, is a Clinical Instructor in Psychiatry and an Assistant Director of the Psychotherapy Research Program at Harvard Medical School. He teaches STDP and supervises at the Cambridge Hospital and elsewhere. Dr. Kuhn has a private psychotherapy and psychiatry practice in the Boston area, and a Web site, www.natkuhn.com. Before going to medical school he was a mathematician.

Stuart Andrews, LMHC, NCC, is a psychotherapist in private practice in Brookline, Massachusetts, and an Assistant Director of the Psychotherapy Research Program at Harvard Medical School. He has presented at international conferences and conducted training seminars on STDP. He has taught and supervised clinicians and students, and published articles on psychotherapy integration and short-term therapy. Mr. Andrews is also the Director of the Center for Families in Transition, where his program, "For the Sake of the Children," is mandated in a number of communities in Massachusetts for parents going through divorce. He is a PhD candidate in clinical psychology at the Fielding Graduate Institute.

Amelia Kaplan graduated from Harvard University with a BA in history and literature of America. While there, she was editor of *Let's Go: USA and Canada 1995*. Since then, she has worked in organizational psychology with the Social Capital Group, and engaged in cognitive neuroscience research at Columbia University. She is currently a graduate student in clinical psychology at the Graduate School of Applied and Professional Psychology, Rutgers University, where she pursues interests in mind–body psychology, STDP, group therapy, and human sexuality. Ms. Kaplan recently coauthored a chapter on short-term therapy. She travels spiritedly in her free time.

Jonathan Wolf was a member of the Psychotherapy Research Program for three years and is currently pursuing an MD at Boston University School of Medicine.

Cara Lanza Hurley graduated from Boston College in 1996 with a BA in psychology. She is in her fourth year as a PhD student in clinical psychology at Loyola University of Chicago, having earned her MA in 2002. Clinically, she has held practica at Loyola University Counseling Center, Loyola University Medical Center–Cardinal Bernardin Cancer Center, and the Rehabilitation Institute of Chicago Chronic Pain Care Center. She maintains clinical and research interests in adult health psychology, stress, and emotion.

Preface
and Acknowledgments

Paul Wachtel's (1977) classic book entitled *Psychoanalysis and Behavior Therapy* was an early inspiration for the integrative style of this treatment. Leigh McCullough was a graduate student when her behavior therapist supervisor, Joe Cautela, recommended Wachtel's book to her.

Cautela was a progressive behavior therapist who pioneered bringing learning theory principles into our inner life, with his methods of covert conditioning (Cautela, 1966, 1973). This treatment approach used imagery to apply reinforcement principles to modify behavior. Influenced by both Cautela (e.g., Cautela & McCullough, 1978) and Wachtel, Leigh began to note the similarities between covert conditioning principles and psychodynamic principles. Wachtel's book was a reference text during this process and was formative in much of Leigh's thinking.

From the late 1970s until the present, David Malan (1979), one of the pioneers in brief psychotherapy, has been tremendously formative in Leigh's thinking. Words cannot fully express the gratitude we all have for his contributions; his Two Triangle schema forms the basis of our teaching and his influence will be found on almost every page of this book.

Another inspiring figure in the evolution of this work is Habib Davanloo (1980). The main focus of this book is on affect, and it was Davanloo who taught Leigh the tremendous value of breaking through defenses to the depth of feeling. His influence can also be found throughout.

In the early 1990s, while viewing thousands of hours of videotape, Leigh began to notice that psychodynamic conflict parallels the behavioral concept of phobias—except that these phobias are about internal feeling states. She coined the term **Affect Phobia** and discussed the concept briefly in her book *Changing Character* (McCullough Vaillant, 1997). In 1998, Nat Kuhn and Stuart Andrews saw the power in this concept and pushed Leigh to make Affect Phobia a central focus of treatment. Then, in early 2001,

Stuart found the mention of "phobias about feelings" in Wachtel's book. Leigh deduced that, although she had no explicit memory of this passage, she probably had read it almost 25 years ago in Wachtel's book and had had the concept of "phobias about feelings" tucked somewhere in the back of her mind since then. It is really true that we can see so far because we stand on the shoulders of giants.

In addition to giants, there have been comrades-in-arms over the past two decades that have greatly contributed to understanding what makes therapy more efficient and effective. Space does not permit a full listing, but there are now a number of books that have emerged from this group, offering valuable and complementary ways of learning STDP. To name a few: *Psychodynamics, Training, and Outcome in Brief Psychotherapy* (Malan & Osimo, 1992), *Intensive Short-Term Dynamic Psychotherapy* (Della Selva, 1996), *The Transforming Power of Affect* (Fosha, 2000), *0 Futuro da Integracao: Desenvolvimentos em Psicoterapia Breve* (Lemgruber, 2000), *Short-Term Therapy for Long-Term Change* (Solomon, Neborsky, McCullough, Alpert, Shapiro, & Malan, 2001), *Parole, Emozionie Videotape: Manuale di Psicoterapia Breve Dinamico-Esperienziale* (PBD-E) (Osimo, 2001), and the *Handbook of Integrated Short-Term Psychotherapy* (Winston & Winston, 2002). Our book is richer for the long and fertile sharing that has taken place among these colleagues and ourselves.

A special acknowledgment must be given to the fourth author, Amelia Kaplan, who got the writing of this book off the ground. Leigh had started the manuscript, and then, with Nat and Stuart, had been planning to "get to it" for over a year. However, they were all involved in an extensive reliability study on the Achievement of Therapeutic Objectives (ATOS) rating scale—the research tool for evaluating this treatment (available on our Web site, www.affectphobia.org). So the book was placed on the back burner. When Amelia joined the research program, she heard about the treatment manual and immediately became interested. She insisted that this manual was too important to put off, and she offered to devote four months to getting the first draft of the manuscript ready. She did so with tremendous zeal—and then left for graduate school at Rutgers. Four years and countless revisions later, Leigh, Nat, and Stuart completed the final draft. But without Amelia's initial push, and a significant amount of denial on our parts (for believing it would be a breeze), this book would not have seen the light of day for many more years.

In the arduous process of writing this book, we learned that making very complex concepts simple was a far, far more difficult task than we ever anticipated. A book that we thought would take less than one year to write has taken more than four. We were blessed to have readers who, over the years, read and reread, and then read again our many iterations of the chapters and the exercises.

For example, we were honored to have as readers the mothers of two of our authors, who are themselves accomplished and senior medical professionals: Amelia's mother, Annette Hollander, MD (University of Medicine and Dentistry of New Jersey), and Jonathan's mother, Katherine Wolf, MD (Harvard Medical School). Annette Hollander is a psychiatry training director and urged us to make a videotape to accompany this book. We wish we could have done that, and still hope to do so someday. Martha Sweezy and Lisa Freden have been faithful readers from start to finish, going through many versions and making many helpful suggestions. The exercises evolved greatly as a result of Martha and Lisa's nudging us toward making them more user-friendly. Dan Brenner gave us many useful and, shall we say, challenging suggestions; even better, he gave us a lot of encouragement. Jane Mortimer commented on the manuscript from Adelaide, Australia, and Julie Felty did so from Belmont, Massachusetts.

Elke Schlager has been helpful in catching last-minute inconsistencies, and reading the very final copies when Nat, Stuart, and Leigh were bleary-eyed. Martha Stark must be thanked for helping polish the title. Allen Larsen from Stavanger, Norway, and Elisabeth Schanche from the University of Bergen, Norway, spent four months with Leigh in the summer of 2000; during that time they read and commented on the entire treatment manual, and also carefully evaluated and suggested revisions for the exercises. We are all grateful to Nancy Sowell for her patience with and steadfast support of Nat.

And last, but definitely not least, is our editor extraordinaire, Barbara Watkins, who taught us with her brilliant early suggestions for revisions that this book was not going to be the walk in the park that we had anticipated. Her contributions have been consistently so exceptional that from here on we will refer to her as the Maxwell Perkins of mental health editing, recalling Thomas Wolfe's legendary editor. We don't pretend to compare ourselves to Wolfe—either in brilliance or in alcohol tolerance—but Barbara is definitely as good as Max.

Contents

Introduction

STDP and Affect Phobias

The aim of this book is to teach you how to do **Short-Term Dynamic Psychotherapy (STDP)** by focusing on **Affect Phobias**. STDP is an active, time-efficient, focused, integrative form of treatment that has resulted in significant and lasting character change for many patients, even ones who have failed to benefit from extended therapies of other types.

Skills Focus

Although "step-by-step" instructions are too rigid for a process as rich as STDP, this book will help you acquire a set of skills that will make your therapy more powerful and effective. Most readers will find that some of these skills seem comfortable and familiar, while other skills may seem alien and challenging. There is a growing body of research evidence and clinical experience indicating that, taken together, these skills constitute a highly effective model of psychotherapy.

Exercises Enhance Procedural Knowledge

We believe that doing therapy—as opposed to talking about it—is based more on skills (i.e., **procedural knowledge**) than on ideas (i.e., **declarative knowledge**). To help you acquire those skills, we have included exercises at the ends of the first 10 chapters, which we strongly encourage you to do. However, exercises are not to everyone's taste, and if these aren't to yours, you can skip some or all of them. You won't be missing any "new concepts," but some of the material is clarified, and there are opportunities to build skills.

Changing Character

This book originated as a companion volume to *Changing Character: Short-Term Anxiety-Regulating Psychotherapy for Restructuring Defenses, Affects, and Attachment* (McCullough Vaillant, 1997; referred to from now on as *Changing Character* or just CC). Our aim here is to help the reader acquire the skills necessary to do the therapy that is discussed in more theoretical depth in the earlier work. To that end, there are extensive references to *Changing Character* throughout this book, and readers who are looking for a fuller discussion of many points here will be able to pursue them in that volume. In addition, our thinking has evolved since *Changing Character* was written, particularly in bringing the concept of Affect Phobia—which is present but not emphasized in CC—to the forefront.

Research Evidence

This treatment model has been developed and repeatedly revised on the basis of both clinical observations and research findings. The work of Malan and his colleagues, has provided us with a 50-year careful study of "the science of psychodynamics" as applied to brief psychotherapy. More recently, there have been two clinical trials that have demonstrated the efficacy of STDP for patients with Axis II, Cluster C, diagnoses. The first took place at Beth Israel Medical Center in New York City from 1982 to 1990 (Winston et al., 1991, 1994). The second trial, conducted at the Norweigan University of Science and Technology (NTNU) in Trondheim, Norway, from 1988 to 1999, compared this model of STDP with a cognitive therapy model (Svartberg, Stiles, & Seltzer, in press). There are also many process studies showing the importance of the affect and defense work covered in this book (for a summary, see Ch. 12 of CC). Research on this therapy continues at Harvard Medical School and NTNU.

Integration of Psychodynamic Theory and Learning Theory

This therapy is based on the idea that much psychopathology is rooted in **Affect Phobia**—a fear of feelings. The concept of Affect Phobia is a recasting of the concept of psychodynamic conflict into the language of learning theory and behavioral therapy. The result is that the well-established techniques and concepts of phobia treatment (e.g., systematic desensitization) can be brought to bear on psychodynamic issues in a way that helps to focus STDP and avoid common pitfalls.

Affect Phobias Extend the Freudian Dual-Drive Model

Most patients will have one or more central Affect Phobias (which we also refer to as **core psychodynamic conflicts**), which lead them into the difficulties they experience. These Affect Phobias can be centered around not only sex and aggression (as classical Freudian conflict theory would suggest), but around any of the fundamental human affects. In clinical practice, the vast majority of Affect Phobias center around a few basic feeling categories—for example, grief, anger (which includes healthy assertion), closeness, and positive feelings toward the self.

Part I of the Book: Introductory Material

Part I of this book consists of four chapters of introductory material. We introduce affect and list the basic affects in Chapter 1. These include activating affects such as grief or anger/assertion, and inhibitory affects such as anxiety or shame. We then go on to introduce Affect Phobia and the central concept of **anxiety regulation**—the key to keeping an active, focused therapy from feeling too "confrontational" to the patient.

Chapter 2 shows how Affect Phobia can be viewed, in psychodynamic terms, as a triangular constellation of defenses and inhibitory affects that block adaptive feelings. Defensive behaviors (e.g., passivity, avoidance, self-attack) allow the patient to avoid the conscious experience of conflict between an adaptive affect (e.g., assertion/anger) and the inhibitory affect that goes with it (e.g., anxiety or shame over being rejected). One of the critical skills for doing this therapy is to be able to identify these key components of Affect Phobias **as the patient is speaking**. The exercises at the end of Chapter 2 should help you start to acquire this ability.

The central **therapeutic** implication of the Affect Phobia schema is that psychodynamic conflict can be treated in a way that is analogous to standard phobia treatment: by **systematic desensitization**. This means helping patients gradually to experience more and more adaptive affect, while helping them keep their anxiety or other inhibitory affects at a manageable level.

Chapter 3 introduces the assessment process and shows how the *Diagnostic and Statistical Manual of Mental Disorders* (DSM) multiaxial diagnostic system—particularly the Global Assessment of Functioning (GAF) Scale—helps in deciding whether short-term treatment of Affect Phobia is appropriate for the particular patient sitting in your office.

Part I closes with Chapter 4, which will teach you the nuts and bolts of how to make an Affect Phobia **formulation**—that is, how to work with the patient to identify the triangles of defense, adaptive affect, and inhibitory affect introduced in Chapter 2.

Case Example

We believe that the best—perhaps the only—way to learn psychotherapy is through specific examples. In that spirit, we will illustrate these concepts and introduce the remainder of the book by using the example of a fictional patient, a 37-year-old woman who works as an administrative assistant.

The therapy starts from a specific problem:

Starting from a Specific Problem

THERAPIST: Could you tell me what's the main problem that brought you into therapy?

PATIENT: I don't know. I just seem to be depressed all the time.

THERAPIST: Can you give me an example of something that depresses you?

PATIENT: I don't know, there are so many . . . well, my boss came in yesterday and gave me a whole new stack of work. I still haven't finished the last stack he gave me. I'm working like a dog, but he never seems to notice, and I just feel like I'll never even catch up.

Identifying the Underlying Affect Phobia

Even after an exchange as brief as the one above, the therapist will begin tentatively formulating an Affect Phobia underlying the patient's problem. In this case, the patient's immediate association is to feeling overwhelmed by her boss's expectations. Perhaps she experiences a phobia that centers around assertion and setting limits with her boss on how much she can be expected to do. Her depression may then be an Affect Phobia about assertion that results in "anger turned inward." The therapist can test this hypothesis:

Checking Out the Phobic Response

THERAPIST: Have you told him that you can't start something new if he wants you to finish up the work he's already given you?

PATIENT: Oh, I couldn't do that . . . he's really been good to me. I thought about doing that, and that's when I started to feel really bad, like I'm lazy and won't amount to anything. I couldn't bear to disappoint him.

By asking these questions about assertion, the therapist starts to see how phobic the patient is of this healthy, adaptive response. The therapist has also started to elicit examples of behaviors on the patient's part that may serve as defenses against assertion. In this case, the patient is using a number of defenses: She's being passive, she's idealizing her boss, and she's attacking herself.

Exploring Anxieties Causing the Affect Phobia

The therapist can also start to explore the Affect Phobia—that is, the inhibitory affects (anxieties) centering around assertion:

THERAPIST: What would be the hardest thing about just telling him he that needs to choose between finishing up or starting something new?

PATIENT: I'd be afraid that he would get angry at me.

Of course, this fear may be justified or it may be a projection, and more exploration will be needed. Nevertheless, the therapist is beginning to uncover some anxieties.

Parts II and III of the Book: Treating Affect Phobia

Parts II and III (Chapters 5–10) are devoted to the treatment of Affect Phobia. To organize the treatment, it has been broken down into three primary treatment objectives, each of which has two components. Each of these six components is covered in a separate chapter.

- **Defense Restructuring** (Defense Recognition, Chapter 5, and Defense Relinquishing, Chapter 6): identifying and giving up phobic behavior.
- **Affect Restructuring** (Affect Experiencing, Chapter 7, and Affect Expression, Chapter 8): reducing the fear about experiencing and expressing conflicted affect.
- **Self- and Other-Restructuring** (Self-Restructuring, Chapter 9, and Other-Restructuring, Chapter 10): changing the view of self and others.

Part II (Chapters 5–8) covers Defense Restructuring and Affect Restructuring, which can be thought of as "the basics" in STDP. With patients who are more impaired, there may be a need to start almost exclusively with Self- and Other-Restructuring, as covered in Part III (Chapters 9 and 10).

Defense Recognition: Identifying the Affect Phobia

Defense Recognition, covered in Chapter 5, helps patients recognize their phobic avoidance of adaptive feeling. Let us return to our example:

THERAPIST: You've told me a couple stories where people want burdensome things from you and you go along with them [defense of passivity], because it made you too anxious [inhibitory feeling] to set any kind of limits [activating feeling: assertion/anger]. Is that a general pattern with you?

PATIENT: Oh, boy, is it ever!

Chapter 5 explores a number of techniques for helping patients to recognize their defensive behaviors on their own. Many techniques from this chapter will be familiar to psychodynamic therapists: clarification, interpretation, and others.

Defense Relinquishing: Giving Up the Maladaptive Response

As any psychodynamic therapist can tell you, intellectual insight into defenses and the desire and readiness to change them are quite separate issues. Defense Relinquishing, the topic of Chapter 6, aims to help increase the patient's motivation to give up their defenses. Its chief tool is anxiety regulation, already introduced in Chapter 1. The idea is to help reduce the need for defenses by reducing the anxiety that the warded-off affect brings up, and cognitive therapists will find much of this material familiar.

Building Motivation to Give Up the Affect Phobia

THERAPIST: What would be the hardest thing about setting a limit with some of these people?

PATIENT: I like being a nice person. It makes me uncomfortable to say no to people [anxiety that assertion will cause others to think ill of her].

THERAPIST: Saying no means that you're not a nice person?

PATIENT: I'm just generous by nature.

THERAPIST: That's wonderful. The world really needs generous people. But think of all the generous people you know. Do they always say yes when people ask them something?

PATIENT: Yeah, pretty much.

THERAPIST: Really? Even when they're already busy doing 10 other generous things at the same time, like you are? They always say yes when you ask them for something?

PATIENT: Well, maybe not always . . .

THERAPIST: OK, think of a time when one of these people said no to you. Did you think that they weren't nice?

Affect Experiencing: Desensitizing the Affect Phobia

The treatment objective of Affect Experiencing, covered in Chapter 7, is the heart of systematic desensitization: **Exposing** the patient to the physiological experience of the conflicted affect (while at the same time lowering the level of the associated anxiety) will heal the patient's conflict. Gestalt therapists are likely to feel at home with this material.

Exposure to Phobic Affect

THERAPIST: If you imagine your boss coming in with more work and expecting you to get it all done, how does it make you feel?

PATIENT: Like I'll never get it done [defends against anger with self-attack].

THERAPIST: So you would attack yourself again. But how would you feel **to-ward him**?

PATIENT: I don't know.

THERAPIST: Well, try to imagine the situation. What do you feel in your body?

PATIENT: I don't know, kind of an energy . . .

THERAPIST: What does your body want to do?

PATIENT: I . . . (*surprised*) it wants to hit him! That's terrible, isn't it? [Shame]

Regulating Anxiety during Exposure

THERAPIST: Well, if you **actually** hit him, that **would** be terrible—for both of you. We're never talking about actually hitting anyone; we're talking about freeing you up to have your feelings in your imagination. This way, you'll hurt no one, and it can help empower you to act more effectively. I will encourage you to experience your emotions in a safe place—here in this office—so that you can learn to understand them, bear them, and **always** control them. Later, this will help put your feelings in perspective and help you decide on the best course of action. But now let's go over that scary feeling once again, until you're feeling comfortable with the internal experience of anger [repeated exposure].

Affect Expression: Adaptive Expression of Feelings, Wants, and Needs in Relationships

Patients with Affect Phobias often will not have acquired skills for handling affect adaptively in interpersonal situations. After the conflict is reduced by repeated exposure, such skill acquisition is a relatively straightforward but terribly important part of the therapeutic work. The objective of Affect Expression, covered in Chapter 8, has a skill focus that many behavior therapists will find familiar.

PATIENT: Well, now I feel angry, but what good does it do? He's the boss, I can't do anything.

THERAPIST: Well, what are some ways you could use that new angry energy within you to make a firm but appropriate response to your boss and take better care of yourself?

Self-Image and Relationship with Others

Many of the conflicts that patients bring into therapy are accompanied by distorted views of themselves or others, and this is the focus of Chapters 9 and 10. This material will seem most familiar to those who focus on object relations. Work may focus on a balanced, compassionate view of the self and others:

PATIENT: But how can I ever find someone to love me if I'm just thinking about me, me, me all the time?

THERAPIST: Does saying no to people mean that you just think about "me, me, me"?

PATIENT: Yeah, it kind of feels that way. I mean, intellectually, I know it's not true, but that's how it seems to me.

THERAPIST: Of course, it's not doing someone else a favor to let yourself get overwhelmed by their desires. So where was it that you got that message that saying no meant you were selfish?

Therapy can also focus on a more integrated, balanced view of others:

PATIENT: He's been so good to me. I can't just say no to him.

THERAPIST: You've told me about a number of things that he's done that have been generous to you, it's true. But, actually, the behavior you've described around this—piling work onto you, and then pouting when you don't do the impossible—doesn't sound to me like he's being good to you.

PATIENT: Oh, he's a wonderful man.

THERAPIST: You know, he may be in many ways. But suppose your friend Beth told you that her boss was completely wonderful, even though he acted hurt when she didn't get five things all done at the same time?

PATIENT: Actually, a friend did tell me something like that—it wasn't Beth, it was someone else—and I got really mad. [Thus her perspective is changed, and she begins to see that it's all right to have angry feelings. She does not need to idealize her boss.]

As noted above, more impaired patients may need a heavy focus on this Self- and Other-Restructuring work, but small doses of it are important in many short-term therapies.

Part IV: Final Chapters

The book concludes with Part IV. Chapter 11 discusses how to apply this therapy in the context of specific DSM-IV diagnoses, and Chapter 12 covers termination.

Discussion of Main Terms

The full title of our companion volume, *Changing Character: Short-Term Anxiety-Regulating Psychotherapy for Restructuring Defenses, Affects, and Attachments* (McCullough Vaillant, 1997) contains a number of terms which appear repeatedly throughout this book. Below we discuss how each phrase in that title reflects an aspect of STDP.

Changing Character: . . .

Defenses, at their inception, generally represent a person's best attempt to cope. They may even have been adaptive, given the situation at that time. As years pass, however, defenses can generalize to situations in which they are increasingly less adaptive. At best, rigidly entrenched defenses block the fullness of experience; at worst, they lead to **character disorders**—long-standing maladaptive patterns of thoughts, feelings, and behavior.

Viewing psychodynamic conflict as Affect Phobia allows the application of the behavioral principles of learning theory to resolve psychodynamic conflict and therefore to **change character** or **personality** (i.e., to eliminate or greatly reduce these long-standing maladaptive patterns).

Short-Term . . .

This therapy has brought lasting helpful change in as little time as a single 3-hour evaluation for high-functioning, motivated patients who are ready for change. Other successful treatments have taken as many as 50 or more sessions. The goal is to be as time-efficient as possible, while allowing enough time for adaptive change. This necessitates a focus on specific treatment objectives related to the patient's core psychodynamic conflicts (Affect Phobias). The goal is not to complete all aspects of character change, but to start the process and put the tools of treatment into the patient's hands as soon as possible, so that change can continue in the ongoing context of the patient's life.

Fifty sessions or more is clearly not "short-term" as the managed care industry might define it. However, resolving many decades of character pathology in 12–18 months of therapy can certainly be considered time-efficient! The goal is to reduce the patient's suffering as much as possible as rapidly as possible. In addition to striving for lasting character change, this goal means that we must offer such change as rapidly as we can. There is often an economic benefit to the patient and society as a by-product; although this is important, it is a secondary consideration. This therapy is not offered as a "second-rate quick fix," but as a "first-rate, in-depth healing process." If it is also "quick"—in relative terms—we see that as enhancing its value to the patient.

Anxiety-Regulating . . .

Anxiety regulation is one of the fundamental techniques of this therapy. Patients' anxieties (or other maladaptive inhibitory affects) are repeatedly elicited, explored, and reduced in the process of systematic desensitization of Affect Phobia. This is in contrast to **anxiety-provoking** therapies (analogous to the behavior therapy technique of flooding). Although these therapies are effective for patients who can tolerate a high level of anxiety provocation, we believe that anxiety regulation can bring these benefits to a much broader group of patients.

Psychotherapy . . .

This therapy is fundamentally psychodynamic, but it differs from classical psychoanalysis and some traditional long-term psychodynamic psychotherapy in important ways. One fundamental difference is that the therapist is not "neutral," but actively engaged:

- **The therapist maintains a goal-directed treatment focus.** Otherwise, the therapist might collude with the patient's defenses in avoiding conflicted affect and avoiding change.
- **The treatment style is active and collaborative.** Interpretations are generated almost immediately and developed in an active therapeutic collaboration between patient and therapist.

- **The treatment can be directive.** The therapist is willing to teach or guide the patient when appropriate.
- **A full transference neurosis is not allowed to develop.** Transference issues are generally identified immediately, so that they can be worked through as they arise.

for Restructuring . . .

Restructuring can be thought of as reorganizing the way people view, experience, and remember the world. It is achieved primarily through the process of systematic desensitization, but the treatment objectives outlined above help the therapist focus on several aspects of restructuring. In this process, defenses become more flexible, affects are freed up, anxieties are reduced to adaptive levels, and self-image and attachments to others are altered.

Defenses, Affects, . . .

The overarching goal is the resolution of the psychodynamic conflicts underlying the patient's difficulties by systematic desensitization of their Affect Phobias. To do this, the patient first needs to give up defenses—the behaviors used to avoid conflicted adaptive affects. When the defenses are less firmly entrenched, the patient is better able to experience the adaptive affects with a reduced level of anxiety.

and Attachment

Healthy attachment means having a balance between autonomy and interdependence, with relationships that are intimate and authentic, and that also allow for healthy (rather than need-based) dependence. In addition, attachment to others is intimately intertwined with what can be thought of as "attachment to self." We all need affirmation from others throughout our lives. But we also need to do what healthy early attachment enables people to do: hold onto and contain in our memories a "reservoir" of the love and support of others, so that we are not quickly depleted when others are absent or less affirming than we would like. Although transference distortions are readily pointed out, this therapy emphasizes the real relationship between patient and therapist to help build a new capacity for healthy attachment.

Conclusion

Our intention in this book is to offer a coherent "package" of STDP theory and technique—one that leads to effective, time-efficient therapy. Of course, every therapist assimilates new information and techniques through and then into his or her individual style. We recognize that aspects of this therapy may not be to everyone's taste, and if that's the case for you, we invite you to "take what you like and leave the rest." In any case, our hope is that the point of view and techniques in this book will help you as they have helped us: to do more effective and time-efficient therapy for our patients.

PART I | **THEORY, EVALUATION, AND FORMULATION**

Affect and Affect Phobia in Short-Term Treatment

Chapter Objective To describe the basic concept of Affect Phobia and its importance for psychotherapy.

Topics Covered

I. WHAT IS AN AFFECT PHOBIA?

This model of Short-Term Dynamic Psychotherapy (STDP) is based on the premise that conflicts about our feelings—what we call **Affect Phobias**—underlie most psychologically based disorders.

"External" Phobias

Phobias are a familiar concept to most therapists. People with phobias may fear a wide variety of external stimuli: bridges, spiders, open spaces, heights, or social situations, for example. To minimize anxiety, patients will use various behaviors to avoid them. Because these phobic stimuli are external, the phobias can be thought of as "external" phobias.

"Internal" (Affect) Phobias

Surprisingly, similar patterns can be observed in psychodynamic therapy. After watching many hours of videotape of short-term dynamic psychotherapy, it became clear to Leigh McCullough that what was conceptualized as "psychodynamic conflict" could equally well be viewed in learning theory terms as **Affect Phobia**—a phobia about feelings (McCullough, 1991, 1993,

1994, 1998). Since these phobias concern internal feeling states, she thought of them as "internal" phobias.

Patients Use Defenses to Avoid Affects

Just as someone with a phobia may drive miles out of the way to avoid a bridge, patients often phobically avoid the experience and expression of certain affects (feelings). One patient may avoid grief, another may avoid anger, and a third may avoid closeness. And, like patients with external phobias, patients with Affect Phobias avoid feelings by developing certain avoidant thoughts, feelings, and behaviors—referred to as **defenses** in psychodynamic language. A principal way that avoidant responses—or defenses—help patients avoid conflicted feelings is by keeping the feelings unconscious or outside of awareness. (However, feelings continue to have powerful effects even when they are unconscious. For example, anger, sadness, or tenderness can be building within us long before we realize it.)

Examples of Affect Phobias

A person who is phobic of being **angry or assertive** may instead act defensively by being silent, crying, feeling depressed, acting compliantly—or, when pushed to the limit, losing control and lashing out inappropriately. Because of the Affect Phobia, this person may be unable to respond more adaptively to their feelings of anger or assertion by setting appropriate limits.

If **grief** is the feared feeling, the person may choke back tears, chuckle to lighten up, or become numb and unfeeling rather than sob and get relief. People who are phobic about **tenderness or caring** often act tough, stay busy, or devalue others rather than open to closeness. These are just a few examples of Affect Phobias; there are many ways to defend against adaptive feelings.

To support our position that these many ways of avoiding feared affects lead to most of the problems that we encounter in outpatient psychotherapy, we turn to the subject of affect itself.

II. WHY THIS THERAPY FOCUSES ON AFFECT

Feelings Are Important Signals

Feelings carry extremely important information about people's reactions to life experiences. To dismiss this "feeling information" is to cut off an essential part of the self. Because of the importance that we place on affect, this therapy teaches patients to ask,

"**What** are my feelings telling me?"

Patients should treat all feelings as vital signals—not necessarily to be acted on, but always to be attended to.

Affect Has Received Less Attention Than Cognition

Both the psychodynamic and cognitive traditions have focused heavily on cognitions (thoughts), intellectual insight, and interpretation; there has been relatively little emphasis on the actual **experience** of affect. This is surprising, since so many patients come to therapy with problems of depression and anxiety. Indeed it may be easier to focus on cognitions because they are more consciously available. In this therapy, we attempt to shift the cognitive–affective balance by emphasizing the central and crucial role of the experience of adaptive affect in therapeutic change.

We emphasize that it is not our intent to say, "An affect focus is good, while a cognitive focus is bad." Cognition is, and always will be, a fundamental agent in therapeutic change. Furthermore, many cognitive therapists work effectively with affect (e.g., with the theory of "hot cognitions"), while many psychodynamic therapists help patients **talk about** affect without helping them to **experience** affect.

Of course, a great many patients come to therapy because of problems directly related to affect, such as depression or anxiety. But there are numerous other reasons why therapy should focus on affect.

Affect Is a Primary Motivator

In addition to symptoms such as depression or anxiety, much of the work in therapy focuses on changing patients' **behavior**. According to affect theorist Silvan Tomkins (1962, Vol. 1, pp. 28–87), there are three motivational systems—inner bodily sensations or feelings—that move us to act or spur specific action tendencies:

1. Biological drives (hunger, thirst, sex, etc.).
2. Physical pain.
3. Affects (anger, grief, sadness, excitement, fear, shame, joy, etc.).

As Tomkins pointed out, **affects are the primary motivators of behavior**, because affects amplify or intensify whatever experience they are associated with. Excitement enlivens an experience, whereas fear, shame, or disgust inhibits it. Joy will encourage participation in a task while shame can all too easily thwart it. Even though drives (e.g., hunger, thirst, sex) motivate behavior, affects can be more powerful. Consider, for example, how easily the affect shame can inhibit the sexual drive, or how the affect disgust (about being fat) can lead some individuals to refuse to eat. (See Tomkins, 1984, 1992).

If affect is the fundamental motivational force in human nature, then affect needs to be central in our clinical theory and practice, in order to have a strong impact on changing patients' behavior.

Affective Connections Can Be Changed

Tomkins also pointed out that, unlike drives, affective connections can be changed (1992, pp. 23–27). We cannot change our drives; we need to eat food and drink liquids—and our sexual orientation is fairly well fixed. But we can change what we have learned to feel ashamed or afraid of. We can learn to be proud of ourselves rather than ashamed, to be joyful about social relationships rather than anxiety-ridden, or to be interested in a task rather than angry or disgusted. We can also learn to become less afraid or less ashamed to experience our sorrow, anger, tenderness, or sexual feelings. In addition to the sense of emotional comfort or pain that affects bring, these inner signals also guide, determine, and motivate behaviors. So, to help patients understand, predict, and control behavior, it is essential to understand and alter the affective connections that lead to maladaptive or adaptive responses. **Affective connections that have been "learned" can be unlearned and relearned.**

Of course, "learning" means more than cognitive book learning, declarative knowledge, or intellectual insight. For behavior change, patients must experience procedural learning, or learning by doing. Patients' feelings, thoughts, and behaviors must be grounded in **physically felt, bodily experience.** The goal of this therapy is to give patients visceral affective experiences that will lead to "relearning"or change in maladaptive behaviors.

The fact that affective connections are learned through experience—and can be changed—makes an affect focus particularly useful and powerful for the psychotherapeutic process of changing unwanted behaviors.

Affects Are Difficult to Identify

Although affects are bodily signals that direct people's actions, they are often outside of their awareness (i.e., unconscious). Affects are therefore difficult for both patients and therapists to identify. For example, patients often say that they are unaware of increasing anger, sadness, or tenderness until it suddenly bursts forth. Thus, if inner affective signals are not sought out, brought into consciousness, and attended to, then unseen affective forces will be directing and/or maintaining patients' behaviors. Missing the presence of core motivating affects will mean that crucial therapeutic opportunities for change may be missed.

Affects Are Feared and Avoided

Feelings can often seem difficult to face, bear, or control. Not only do patients have fears of affect and tend to avoid it, but therapists often do as well. Explicitly focusing on affect in therapy can curb both patients' and therapists' tendency to move away from it. A focus on affect can also help to shape training programs to prepare therapist trainees for this extremely challenging endeavor of focusing on feelings.

Affect Has Neurological Primacy

The limbic and midbrain areas evolved before the neocortex and have been preserved relatively intact through evolutionary development. Affect appears to be generated predominantly in the limbic system and midbrain, whereas language-based thought and the modulation of affect are apparently processed predominantly in the cerebral neocortex. Although affect and cognition eventually become highly interconnected, the possibility that affect may play a more fundamental or preliminary role needs to be taken into account.

Although the limbic and midbrain systems are often devalued as "primitive," they have been preserved so well by evolution precisely because emotional processing is critical to life. A good example of this is the "conditioned fear" response (LeDoux, 1996). For survival, sensory input regarding possible threats needs to be processed as quickly as possible—a job that falls to the limbic system's amygdala. The price of this speed is accuracy: The amygdala may mistake a stick for a snake and initiate the "fight-or-flight" response. The cortex takes a few extra milliseconds to process the information more discriminately, and can inhibit the amygdala's response after the fact if the snake does turn out to be a stick.

By analogy, we can speculate that interventions targeting the experience of affect will have more effect on the limbic and lower brain systems, while interventions targeting cognition will have more effect on the cortex. More purely cognitive (cortical) interventions such as coping skills may be able to inhibit immediate affective (limbic) responses, but to get to the root of the problem will require dealing with the limbic and midbrain systems, where the experience of affect is mediated.

Affect Precedes Language-Based Cognition

Just as affect preceded language-based cognition (thought) in evolution, affect and motivation emerge before language-based cognition in the development of the infant. Although cognition and affect become thoroughly interwoven as development proceeds, affect is present and predominant in the infant at birth and precedes the development of language. Stern (1985, Ch. 4) points out the significance of affective experiences in the development of the "core" self in the infant. Since affects are fundamental forces in motivating the infant and in the development of the sense of self, these profound and early affective learning experiences need to be taken into account in clinical work.

Affect Is Interwoven with Cognition

Because affect and cognition become deeply intertwined during development, both become major motivators of behavior in adulthood. Cognition plays a vital role in guiding, controlling, and selecting affect, and maladaptive cognitions are strong contributors to pathology. In addition, because of the strong relationship between affect and cognition, cognitive interventions are very effective in modifying affect and behavior. However, attending to cognition without also attending to affective experience is ignoring a fundamental motivator of behavior. In addition, we believe that a substantial portion of the effect of cognitive interventions on behavior can be attributed to **the interventions' impact on underlying affect.**

Throughout this book, our emphasis is on affective experience, but we also stress always attending to (1) **maladaptive cognitions** that block affective change, as well as (2) **adaptive cognitions** that help guide, support, and control adaptive affective responses.

Affect Focus Has Research Support

Finally, an increasing body of research and clinical experience shows that systematic pursuit of conflicted feelings relieves patients' suffering. Two clinical trials have demonstrated the efficacy of this therapy with Axis II Cluster C disorders and many Axis I mood disorders (Winston et al., 1991, 1994; Svartberg & Stiles, 2003). In addition, the efficacy of a focus on affect has been demonstrated in a number of process studies (reviewed in McCullough, 1998, 2000).

Summary

Although cognition (thought) has generally received more attention than the experience of affect, this model of STDP focuses on affect, for these reasons:

- Affect is the primary system for motivation and therefore for change.
- Affective connections that have been learned can be unlearned and re-learned.
- Affect is not always conscious, and thus can be easy to miss.
- Affect can be difficult to face and bear, and thus is easily sidestepped if it's not addressed systematically.
- Affect emerged before cognition in the process of evolution, and is processed separately and often before cognition in the brain.
- Affect emerges before cognition in the development of the infant.
- Focus on affect has demonstrated effectiveness in two clinical trials of STDP.

III. THE DEFINITION AND CLASSIFICATION OF AFFECT

Problems with Definitions of Emotions

Emotions are intangible and unseen, and thus harder to label than are concrete external objects. There is very poor consistency about words that denote feeling, both in languages worldwide and in writing about emotions. Given the lack of clarity and the enormous variation in definitions of emotion words, we offer below the definitions of feeling, emotion, and affect that we follow in this book.

Definition of Affect

An **affect** is a biologically endowed set of psychological, bodily/physiological, facial, and hormonal responses that motivate us or move us to act. Affects include interest, joy, anger, sorrow, fear, shame, and contempt. These affect labels are not discrete entities, but different families of feelings. For example, the category of fear includes a range of responses, such as worry, anxiety, fright, or terror; similarly, anger includes a range of forms, such as irritation, assertion, or rage.

Although many authors have proposed distinctions between emotion words (e.g., Tomkins, 1962, 1963, 1991, 1992; Basch, 1976; Damasio, 1994, 1999; Frijda, 2001; Lazarus, 1991; Oatley & Jenkins, 1996, Watson & Clark, 1995), the definitions vary widely and are used inconsistently in the literature. For example, Tomkins uses the word **emotion** as a synonym for affect, while other theorists define emotion as including biography or memory combined with affect (e.g., Basch, 1976; Nathanson, 1992). Given the many conflicting definitions, it seems unlikely that any one proposed set of distinctions will prevail. For this reason, we, like Tomkins, generally use the words **affect**, **emotion**, and **feeling** interchangeably.

The Definition of Feeling

The word **feeling** is often not given a formal definition, though many emotion theorists reserve this term for the conscious experience of emotion or affect. In the practice of STDP, the therapist frequently identifies "feelings" that are outside of the patient's conscious awareness, as in this example:

THERAPIST: Your face looks like you're feeling sad right now. What do you think?

PATIENT: Yes, now that you mention it, I am. I hadn't realized it.

Therefore in our clinical practice and in this book, we do not limit the term **feeling** to conscious experience, but also use it to include the preconscious and unconscious experience of affect.

Furthermore, the verb **feel** has a somewhat broader meaning, because people not only can "feel their feelings," but can feel other sensations as well: external sensations, such as texture or movement in space. Because of this, **feeling** can have broader use than **affect** or **emotion**.

Basic Affects

Though the terminology can be confusing, fortunately the basic affect categories are few in number. Although experts debate the fine points of classification, the four most widely agreed-upon affects are:

Sorrow   Anger   Joy   Fear
(Easily remembered as Sad, Mad, Glad, Scared)

The second four most agreed-upon affects are

Excitement   Shame   Contempt/Disgust   Tenderness/Care

Because each of these affect words represents a "family" of closely related feelings, covering a range of intensities, we follow Tomkins in using dual terms for affect families, such as **enjoyment/joy** or **fear/terror**.

Two Groups of Affects

In clinical work, when changing behavior is a main focus, it is helpful to separate these affect families into two groups:

1. **Activating affects** (e.g., anger), moving us to open up, engage, or approach.

2. **Inhibitory affects** (e.g., shame), moving us to close down, withdraw, or avoid.

Most affects fall into one group or the other, but a few (fear and disgust) can both activate and inhibit. The following is a list of the primary affect families, with a list of related affect terms for each one. These affect categories are derived from the work of Tomkins, but have been modified for clinical use.

Activating Affects

The activating affects move us to become energized and initiate action, to approach rather than avoid, to open rather than shut down, to run rather than freeze. Each of these affects can be used in either adaptive or maladaptive ways (see Section IV below). However, this therapy guides patients toward the adaptive, constructive versions of the activating affects. The eight categories of activating affects are as follows:

ANGER/ASSERTION: ANNOYANCE, IRRITATION, IRE, WRATH, FURY, RAGE.

Function: Activation to assert needs, set limits, push back, or stop an undesired action or boundary violation. Note that while Tomkins refers to **anger/rage**, we always refer to **anger** in combination with **assertion** to emphasize the importance of the adaptive expression of anger.

SADNESS/GRIEF: SORROW, WEEPING, CRYING, SOBBING, MOURNING.

Function: Activation to cry, to engage social support, to relieve pain, and to accept the fact of loss. Tomkins calls this category **distress/anguish**. We refer to it as **sadness/grief** to emphasize the major goal in clinical work—"grief work"—and to distinguish it from emotional pain, an inhibitory form of feeling that often involves maladaptive forms of distress or anguish.

FEAR/TERROR: ALARM, FRIGHT, TREPIDATION, PANIC.

Function: Activation to run away. Fear can also inhibit action (as in anxiety), and we discuss this below in the section on inhibitory affects.

ENJOYMENT/JOY: HAPPINESS, CONTENTMENT, TRANQUILITY, CALMNESS, PLEASURE, ACCEPTANCE, MASTERY, PEACE, AWE, WONDER, RAPTURE, GRACE.

Function: To calm and soothe the mind and body and to repeat pleasurable actions. Activation of relaxing muscles and letting go, accepting with equanimity.

INTEREST/EXCITEMENT: ATTRACTION, CURIOSITY, ENTHUSIASM, HOPE, EAGERNESS, EXUBERANCE, ZEST.

Function: Activation of focused attention, approach, or exploratory behaviors.

CLOSENESS/TENDERNESS: CARE, COMPASSION, LOVE, ATTACHMENT, DEVOTION, PRIDE OR JOY IN OTHERS, TRUST, VULNERABILITY.

Function: Activation of nurturant response to others' needs, as well as openness and trust in others. Activation to embrace, touch, hold, and care for others, and to be receptive, open, and vulnerable to them. Because of the importance of attachment and object relations in clinical work, we separate out this blend of Tomkins's positive affects as they are experienced with others: **interest/excitement** (the basis of attraction and romantic love) versus **enjoyment/joy** (the basis of bonding or committed love). Please note that we often use the term **closeness** to refer to the blend of tenderness, care, and trust.

POSITIVE FEELINGS TOWARD THE SELF: SELF-COMPASSION, SELF-CARE, SELF-ESTEEM, [healthy] PRIDE OR JOY IN SELF, SELF-CONFIDENCE, SELF-WORTH.

Function: Like the previous category, this is a blend of Tomkins's basic affects, but this time directed toward the self. The function of positive feelings for the self is the maintenance of positive self-esteem and the protection of the integrity of the self or self-care. Because of the significance of sense-of-self issues to mental health, this category is very important in clinical work.

SEXUAL DESIRE: AROUSAL, AMOROUSNESS, LUST, SEXUAL PASSION.

Function: Activation to engage in sexual behavior. According to Tomkins, this category is technically a drive rather than an affect. It is included here because phobias of sexual feeling are important in clinical work and can be treated in exactly the same manner as affects.

Inhibitory Affects

The inhibitory affects move us to cease action, to withdraw rather than advance, to tighten rather than loosen. They rein us in and modulate our responses. Inhibitory affects can be extremely helpful when used in moderation, but pathology can result when they are used either too much or too little. The five categories of inhibitory affects are as follows:

ANXIETY/PANIC: FEAR/TERROR THAT PARALYZES, APPREHENSION, WORRY, NERVOUSNESS, VIGILANCE, DREAD, HORROR.

Function: Inhibits behaviors that would put the person in danger.

SHAME/HUMILIATION: SELF-CONSCIOUSNESS, EMBARRASSMENT, MORTIFICATION.

Function: Inhibits behavior that is unacceptable to one's sense of self.

GUILT: CULPABILITY, BLAME, SELF-REPROACH.

Function: Inhibits behavior that is unacceptable to a cultural or societal rule or law. According to Tomkins, this is a derivative of shame/humiliation.

EMOTIONAL PAIN/ANGUISH: HURT, UPSET, DEPRESSION, TORMENT, SUFFERING, WOE, AGONY, MISERY.

Function: Inhibits behaviors by causing discomfort or suffering. This is a response we often see in clinical work, but is not a single basic affect. It may be a mix of a number of affects (e.g., distress/anguish, guilt, shame, anger, or fear).

CONTEMPT/DISGUST: DISDAIN, SCORN, REVULSION.

Function: Inhibits closeness to others. Clinically, this affect is most often seen in sexual conflict or trauma. Although for brevity's sake we will not always include it in the list of inhibitory affects, contempt/disgust should be borne in mind when anxiety, shame, and pain do not explain an inhibition.

IV. ADAPTIVE VERSUS MALADAPTIVE EXPRESSION OF AFFECTS

Depending on how an affect is used and its consequences, an affect may be helpful (adaptive) for an individual and the individual's social milieu, or harmful (maladaptive). For example, anger can be well used to set appropriate limits, or it can be misused, as in temper outbursts, road rage, or violence.

Affect Experience versus Expression

In order to judge whether an affect is adaptive or maladaptive, it is helpful to draw a distinction between the inner (intrapsychic) **experience** of the affect and the outer (interpersonal) **expression** of the affect. Often the way an affect is expressed interpersonally determines whether it is adaptive or maladaptive. However, some affects (e.g., crippling shame about the self) can be harmful based primarily on the intensity of the internal experience.

This distinction between adaptive and maladaptive affect may be unfamiliar to many clinicians. However, to do STDP effectively, it is **crucial** to (1) **distinguish adaptive from maladaptive affects**, and (2) **guide patients toward adaptive expression of feelings and actions**.

Adaptive Expression Brings Relief

Adaptive affect is first consciously experienced within the body, then outwardly expressed interpersonally in a cognitively guided, fully controlled way. Adaptive expression of feeling is not explosive. Adaptive expression brings relief, makes things better, and can make relationships closer.

Maladaptive Expression Makes Things Worse

Maladaptive expression of feelings is interpersonally destructive, resulting in worse feelings between people—more distance, frustration, misunderstanding, loneliness and hopelessness. Here are some behavioral clues that almost always suggest maladaptive expression of affect:

Self-pity, whining, sulking, victim role

Acting out, uncontrolled behavior

Thoughtlessness

Chronic lateness

Exaggerated enthusiasm

False peacefulness, sugary sweetness

Mindless catharsis (temper tantrums, ranting and raving, hysterical sobbing)

Adaptive and Maladaptive Versions of Affects

Both activating and inhibitory feelings can have adaptive and maladaptive versions. Here are some brief examples of adaptive versus maladaptive forms of activating feelings (including inner experience and outer expression):

Activating Affects:	ADAPTIVE	MALADAPTIVE
Grief	**Grief** feels like a relief (resolves and lead to acceptance).	**Depression** feels like hopelessness, despair, futility, self-hate.
Anger	**Anger** gives relief and a solution.	**Aggression** makes things worse.
Care	**Care** brings people closer.	**Need** is addictive and cloying.

Just like activating affects, inhibitory affects can be highly adaptive. We need our anxiety, guilt, and shame to guide us in many helpful ways! Unguided expression of feelings can create havoc. Society could not function effectively if everyone wildly expressed every feeling, want, and need.

Inhibitory affects become problematic when the inhibition is so great that it is paralyzing, or when it is so little that emotional responses are not modulated.

Inhibitory Affects:	ADAPTIVE	MALADAPTIVE
Anxiety	**Anxiety** signals the need to protect self and others (e.g., softening anger expression).	Excessive or traumatic **anxiety** paralyzes, blocking adaptive action.

Shame/Guilt	**Shame and guilt** can lead to genuine healing remorse, making amends.	**Shame and guilt** leading to self-hate, self-loathing, or self-attack.
Emotional Pain	**Emotional pain** helps one avoid or leave hurtful or abusive situations.	**Emotional pain** is suffering and misery without change or relief.
Contempt/Disgust	**Contempt/disgust** is used in healthy outrage.	**Contempt/disgust** is used to inappropriately attack others or the self.

What Constitutes Adaptive Expression Is Culture-Specific

The judgment of what constitutes adaptive expression of feelings is greatly influenced by one's culture, religion, and social milieu. Although the basic affects themselves have been validated cross-culturally (e.g., Ekman, 1984, 1992; Ekman & Davidson, 1994; Izard, 1990), there can be significant cultural variations in how feelings are expressed outwardly. For example, adaptive expression of anger in China may be different from that in the United States. The examples of appropriate affect expression throughout this book are based largely on dominant North American (Western) culture. Therapists should be open to modifying these guidelines according to their patients' particular contexts and cultures, as well as their own.

We address the distinction between adaptive and maladaptive affect throughout the book. In Chapter 2 we discuss how affects can be used defensively, and thus become maladaptive—a distinction we cover in more detail in Chapter 7.

V. THE DEVELOPMENT AND TREATMENT OF AFFECT PHOBIAS: AN INTRODUCTION

Conflicts about Feelings Are Learned

Affect Phobias develop in the process of growing up. Babies do not spring from the womb burdened with inhibition and neurotic conflicts. Infants have a robust capacity to let us know what they want and don't want. They cry when wet, hungry, or tired, and don't stop crying until their often confused parents figure out what is needed. At 10 days of age infants track their mothers' eyes, and within weeks they will reach out arms to caretakers. Two-year-olds vigorously tell us, "No!" Children are naturally curious and enthusiastic about the world, exploring, touching, tasting everything in their path. Parents and other caretakers naturally use inhibitory affects, such as fear, guilt, or shame, to shape their children's behavior:

"Don't ever say you hate anybody!"

"Big girls don't cry."

"Tone it down! You're getting on our nerves!"

Problems develop when excessive inhibition is placed on a child's adaptive activating affects, such as anger, sorrow, or excitement. Children may then become phobic about feeling, and develop in ways that are excessively inhibited. A child may learn that to be loved or to escape punishment, only certain expressions are allowable. By a process of classical conditioning, the adaptive, activating affect can begin to automatically evoke the associated inhibitory affect. Just as Pavlov's dogs would salivate at the sound of the bell, a person who was overly shamed for being assertive or angry as a child will automatically feel shame when assertive or angry feelings arise and start to be felt.

Affect Phobia and Psychodynamic Conflict

Affect Phobias occur when inhibitions (such as shame) cause great distress or are too strong for activating feelings (such as anger/assertion) to be expressed adaptively. Another term that has been used to describe the same situation is **psychodynamic conflict**, which describes how activating and inhibiting affects are intrapsychic forces pushing in opposing directions. (For more on psychodynamic conflict, see Chapter 2.)

Too Little Inhibition Can Cause Phobias about the Self

There are also cases where inhibitions are insufficient. Then one of two types of problems can happen. First, without some degree of inhibition, children become impulsive and have trouble controlling their behavior. Second, because of the problems that impulsivity causes in living, shame will block positive feelings toward the self—or, in other words, Affect Phobias will develop about self-feelings (e.g., shame blocks healthy pride or self-esteem).

PATIENT: I've always been bad. I was such a bad kid. I just lost my temper all the time and drove people crazy. I don't know what is wrong with me.

Anxiety as a Catch-all Term

In a classic phobia, the feared external stimulus evokes anxiety; in an Affect Phobia, the internal stimulus (such as grief) can evoke any of the inhibitory affects: anxiety, guilt, shame, pain, or contempt. Because of the strength of the analogy to classic external phobias, we often use the word **anxiety** as a shorthand or catch-all term for any of the inhibitory affects. Thus we sometimes speak of "feared affect," even though the affect might evoke shame or pain rather than just fear or anxiety. Historically, this is how the term *anxiety* has been used in STDP (see Malan, 1979).

Resolving Affect Phobias

Conceptualizing the conflict over feeling as Affect Phobia is useful, because extensive research and clinical experience in behavior therapy have shown that the technique of **systematic desensitization** (Wolpe, 1958) can successfully treat phobias. Combining this well-tested behavioral tool within a psychodynamic framework has the potential to make treatment both more effective and more time-efficient (see Chapter 2 for further discussion).

Systematic Desensitization

Systematic desensitization includes three main (but not necessarily sequential) steps:

- **Step 1—Exposure:** Facing the feared stimulus.
- **Step 2—Response Prevention:** Discouraging the maladaptive avoidant response.
- **Step 3—Anxiety Regulation:** Decreasing anxiety in both exposure and response prevention.

Earlier "anxiety-provoking" models of short-term therapy (e.g., Davanloo, 1980; Mann, 1973; Sifneos, 1979) intentionally evoked high levels of anxiety during exposure, which is analogous to the behavioral technique of *flooding*.

Anxiety Regulation as Graded Exposure

By contrast, our model uses anxiety regulation to achieve a "systematic" or stepwise desensitization—also known as **graded exposure.** The therapist helps the patient confront the feared stimulus in stepwise fashion, by experiencing successively "closer" encounters at levels of anxiety that the patient can more easily bear. We call this model "anxiety-regulating" because if the patient's anxiety starts to get too high, the therapist uses techniques to reduce the anxiety to adaptive levels. To be successful, each encounter must continue until the patient's anxiety becomes manageable.

Graded Exposure with External Phobias

In the treatment of a typical phobia, there may be many intermediary steps, or there may be just a few. For example, a patient who is afraid of elevators may first be encouraged to think about elevators until he or she can do so with minimal anxiety. Further steps may include looking at an elevator from a safe distance, entering an elevator with the therapist, entering an elevator with the therapist standing outside, and so forth—continuing until the patient can ride the elevator up and down alone repeatedly and without fear.

The key point is that to effectively lessen the degree of phobic anxiety, each level of exposure must continue until the patient's anxiety reaches normal limits. This is because the conditioned phobic response needs to be desensitized or "deconditioned." Experiencing the phobic stimulus (in this case, the elevator) without anxiety or with successively decreasing anxiety helps break the conditioned response between stimulus and inhibitory feeling. However, it is important to note that if the exposure is terminated while the anxiety level is still high, the phobia will not be desensitized; in fact, the link between stimulus and anxiety may be **strengthened or sensitized**, making the phobia more severe.

Exposure, for Desensitizing "Internal Phobias" or Affect Phobias

The same principles that are used with typical external phobias are used to treat internal Affect Phobias. Patients with Affect Phobias are exposed to progressively higher "doses" of the feared affect (anger, grief, tenderness, etc.) in levels that they can bear, until they can experience each level of adaptive feeling with less of the inhibitory feeling (anxiety, guilt, shame, or pain) present.

Desensitization Frees Up Adaptive Affect

Desensitization does **not** mean reducing the adaptive form of the activating affect. Desensitization means using exposure to reduce or regulate inhibitory feelings—that is, freeing up the inner experience of the adaptive feeling by gradually breaking the stranglehold that anxiety, guilt, shame, or pain (the inhibitory feelings) have on the adaptive activating affect.

PATIENT: I used to feel so mortified [shame] if I even began to tear up [sadness]. Now, thank goodness, if something bad happens, I can let myself cry and feel some relief!

Response Prevention to Maintain the Exposure

Patients with typical phobias avoid the feared stimulus, so for exposure to be effective therapists must help patients prevent this maladaptive avoidant response. In a similar way, patients with Affect Phobias use many defensive tactics to avoid conflicted feelings: intellectualization, dissociation, repression, and so on. (Defenses are discussed further in Chapter 2.) For exposure to be effective, these maladaptive responses need to be reduced or eliminated (**response prevention**). We cover many strategies for response prevention in Chapters 5 and 6 on Defense Restructuring.

Anxiety Regulation Prevents Sensitization

As noted above for external phobias, terminating the exposure while the inhibition (e.g., shame or anxiety) is still high runs the risk of increasing the conflict by sensitizing the Affect Phobia. This is a risk in anxiety-provoking therapies, and is one of the reasons why anxiety regulation is so important in this therapy. For more on anxiety regulation vs. anxiety-provoking techniques, please see *Changing Character* (CC), pages 12–18 and 181–185.

VI. THE IMPORTANCE OF ANXIETY REGULATION

Provoking Anxiety Is Inevitable

When STDP is active and efficient, therapists frequently provoke inhibitory affects. As discussed in the preceding section, exposure to conflicted affect provokes anxiety (or guilt, shame, pain, or contempt), but there are also many other points at which these inhibitory affects arise. For example, simply pointing out patients' avoidant behavior (i.e., response prevention, as discussed above) often brings up anxiety or shame.

Anxiety regulation is the key to making this rapid uncovering form of treatment bearable to patients. For that reason, each chapter that focuses on treatment interventions has a special section on anxiety regulation as it pertains to that aspect of the treatment.

Expose, Regulate Anxiety, Repeat

In general, the treatment follows a simple cyclical pattern. Every kind of exposure provokes anxiety, and when a patient's anxiety starts to get too high, the therapist should use anxiety-regulating techniques to explore the fears and help reduce them. Then, as soon as possible, the focus should return to continued exposure.

From exposure and response prevention

↓

to anxiety regulation

↓

back to exposure and response prevention

This process of moving from exposure to anxiety regulation and back to exposure should be repeated again and again to desensitize conflicts until patients can free up healthy affective responses.

Keeping Anxiety within Limits

During exposure to affect, the patient's moment-to-moment experience of the conflict **must be kept within manageable limits**, so that the exposure to the feeling can continue to reduce rather than increase the Affect Phobia.

Anxiety Regulation for Graded Exposure

As long as Affective Experiencing (see Chapter 7), is proceeding (i.e., as long as the patient is proceeding through memories or reflections with bodily sensations that are affect-laden), then there is little need for anxiety regulation. However, whenever it becomes difficult for the patient to continue (e.g., visible distress, feeling overwhelmed, going "dead," etc.), then anxiety regulation is necessary. At this point, the therapist must explore the inhibition (anxiety, guilt, shame, pain) until the patient can more comfortably go back to experiencing the affect. This gentle process of exploring anxieties makes graded exposure to the feelings possible.

The cornerstone of anxiety regulation is to explore the anxiety, using a standard question from cognitive therapy: "What's the hardest [worst, scariest, most painful] thing about _____?" Many examples of patient–therapist dialogue throughout this book will contain some variant of this question, like this one:

THERAPIST: Can you see how you've just pulled away from the joy [or sadness, or anger, or tenderness] that you were feeling here with me?

PATIENT: Yes, now that you mention it . . . I guess I did.

THERAPIST: What is the hardest or most uncomfortable part of that for you? [Anxiety regulation]

PATIENT: I feel so vulnerable [anxiety] when I really let myself go and relax, I can hardly stand it!

THERAPIST: Well, before we go any further, let's talk about what feels so scary about being vulnerable. [More anxiety regulation]

Anxieties Are Never Eliminated

Anxiety regulation does not mean anxiety elimination. As we have explained, people need inhibition to guide and modulate their behavior. They need to know when they might hurt themselves or others. Healthy, cognitively balanced levels of inhibition tell people how to guide their actions without deadening their lives. So some degree of inhibition is always necessary.

Anxiety Regulation for Too Little Inhibition

Most outpatients have more problems with excessive inhibition than they do with insufficient inhibition. However, there will be some patients who act out impulsively and who thus may enter therapy with insufficient inhibition. Such uncontrolled behaviors and underlying feelings may need to be sensitized rather than desensitized. In such cases, the role of anxiety regulation is to increase rather than decrease anxiety. Thrill-seeking individuals may need more anxiety; sociopathic individuals may need more conscious guilt and shame. People who are abused will need to become more sensitized to pain to be more self-protective.

PATIENT: I always had a mean streak. In therapy, I let myself see how I'd hurt a lot of people. I learned to be more sensitive to other people's feelings and I control my tongue better now.

Some Inhibition or Conflict Always Underlies Impulsivity

But, at the same time, these impulse-ridden patients will also need to decrease their anxiety about other painful underlying feelings. As noted above in Section V, insufficient inhibition can lead to Affect Phobias about the self (e.g., shame about the self or poor self-esteem) because of the destructive results of impulsive behaviors. Furthermore, when there is poor self-esteem, other Affect Phobias may occur, such as fears of closeness, inability to grieve or longing for acceptance. Behaviors such as thrill seeking or con games may help to avoid these painful affects. Thus, even when impulses are out of control, there is always some degree of inhibition or conflict present.

PATIENT: I was so mean to so many people that I felt like a really bad person. I felt like I didn't deserve much, and I couldn't trust that people cared for me.

Summary

To summarize, this treatment model uses the following:

1. **Exposure** to stay with the experience of feeling the activating affect.
2. **Response prevention** to maintain exposure by preventing a defensive or avoidant response.
3. **Anxiety regulation** to reduce or modulate anxiety, guilt, shame, or pain linked to the activating affect.

Systematic desensitization is covered in more detail in Chapters 2 and 7.

VII. GOALS OF TREATMENT

Values in Therapy

Every therapy model is unavoidably value-laden, and its goals reflect those values. The keys are (1) to make those values explicit, and (2) to take patients' (possibly conflicting) value systems into account. In this chapter and throughout the book, we try to make explicit the central values of this therapy model, which include the following:

- Full experiencing and mature expression of feeling (authentic functioning).
- Compassion for self and others.
- A healthy balance of autonomy and interdependence.
- Therapy that is as efficient and effective as possible.

We believe that therapy based on these principles leads to an improvement in both individual and societal functioning. Of course, readers will need to weigh our values against their own and integrate them as they see fit. In addition, therapists must always remain flexible in regard to their patients' personal/cultural/relational contexts, so long as the results continue to be constructive and life-enhancing.

A good guideline for authentic expression of feeling—with profound implications—comes from a Norwegian children's story about an idyllic town called Kardemomme:

One should not bother or harm others,
One should be good and kind,
But otherwise one can do whatever one wishes.

(Man skal ikke plage andre,
Man skal vaere grei og snill,
Og for ovrig kan man gjore hva man vil.)

—Egner, 1955, p. 5; translated by Leigh
McCullough with help from Ronnaug
Leland and Roar Fosse

Authentic Functioning

Thus the goal of this therapy is to enable patients to experience affects fully and manage them intelligently, so that they are capable of adaptive, authentic functioning—but while also taking others into consideration. Affect Phobias prevent authentic functioning by blocking the affect needed to motivate healthy responses. Resolving Affect Phobias achieves this therapeutic goal by freeing up affects to motivate adaptive and interpersonally mindful responses.

Knowing and Practicing Control of Feelings

When people are not conscious of their feelings and not practiced in controlling them, the feelings are much more likely to emerge in hurtful, destructive, or embarrassing ways. Because these conflicted, maladaptive patterns are (at least in part) learned, they can be "unlearned" and more flexible and adaptive ones can be acquired. This therapy helps patients bring feelings into consciousness, tolerate them, and use them to guide effective action for themselves and in relation to others.

When affects are no longer blocked, there is no longer the phobic avoidance of honest emotional reactions. Rather than having to deny, repress, or "fake" a feeling, patients learn to experience feeling fully (inner experience), and also learn **when** and **how** it is appropriate to respond with behavior (outward expression) to others.

To Modulate, Not Obliterate Feeling

Although we advocate that feelings be cognitively guided and fully controlled, we do not mean that feelings should be squelched or thwarted. Instead, patients are helped first to experience and contain the inner experience of feelings, and then to modulate the outward expression of their feelings to others—without shutting down or obliterating them.

Optimal Balance between Autonomy and Interdependence

In Western societies, especially the United States, people often strive for "independence" and "self-sufficiency"—not needing anything other than what one can provide for oneself. Indeed, the traditional dynamic model defines maturity as autonomy and independence, achieved through the separation/individuation process and internalization of others.

In contrast, a more progressive view is that healthy **attachment** to others, not separation, is the mark of maturity. The need for others is seen as adaptive and legitimate not only in childhood, but throughout the life span. Individuals exist, grow, and develop in relation to others in a dynamic interaction, and need both autonomy and deep connection. Therefore, this therapy model helps patients develop an adaptive balance between autonomy (the ability to meet one's own needs, express what's inside, etc.) and interdependence (the ability to be receptive and responsive to feelings of others, etc.). Interventions for developing these capacities are presented in Chapters 9 and 10.

Desensitizing Affect Phobias Helps Authentic Functioning

Desensitizing Affect Phobias (i.e., resolving psychodynamic conflict) fosters authentic functioning in many ways:

• Conflicted affects become more freely and maturely expressed.
• Conflicted relationships become closer and more gratifying.
• Conflicted feelings about the self become more self-compassionate.

Examples of Authentic Functioning

Think of authentic functioning as living in the moment and responding deeply and genuinely, but always **mindfully** of others. This is exemplified by the ability to experience and express the fullest passion—the firmest, clearest anger; sobbing in grief; rapt attention in enthusiasm; the tranquility of joy—but only if such passion is used **appropriately, constructively**, and for **mature purposes**.

Authentic functioning allows people to respond in the following ways, to name a few:

Inner Affective Experience	Outward Affective Expression
When delight and surprise arise	To laugh with joy.
When waves of sorrow flood the body	To cry with sadness.
When feelings of anger build energy	To speak up and set firm limits.
When something is interesting	To pursue interests with enthusiasm.
When desire and passion arise in the body	To make love openly and freely.
When tender feelings emerge in the heart	To give and receive love wholeheartedly.

When patients have learned how and when to respond to themselves and others in affectively open, honest, and appropriate ways, they have achieved **authentic functioning**. They no longer have Affect Phobias and, in general, no longer need therapy.

CHAPTER 1 • EXERCISES

From this chapter to Chapter 10, we offer exercises at the end of each chapter. Answers can be found at the end of the book in the Appendix. We consider these "answers" to be "strong possibilities." They are not meant to be taken as absolute, and there will be many other equally good (or possibly better) answers.

EXERCISE 1A: IDENTIFY ACTIVATING VERSUS INHIBITING AFFECTS

Directions: Are the following affects activating or inhibiting? In other words, does the affect in question predominantly promote:

- Action/approach/openness/involvement (activation), or
- Restraint/withdrawal/closing off (inhibition)?

Circle the correct answer. (Also, try to think of a rationale for why the affect is either activating or inhibiting, though you need not write this down.)

Exercise 1A.1.	Shame	Activating	Inhibiting
Exercise 1A.2.	Grief	Activating	Inhibiting
Exercise 1A.3.	Healthy pride	Activating	Inhibiting

Exercise 1A.4.	Curiosity	Activating	Inhibiting
Exercise 1A.5.	Guilt	Activating	Inhibiting
Exercise 1A.6.	Self-confidence	Activating	Inhibiting
Exercise 1A.7.	Anxiety	Activating	Inhibiting
Exercise 1A.8.	Justifiable outrage	Activating	Inhibiting

EXERCISE 1B: IDENTIFY THE AFFECT

Directions: For each of the following sentences, choose what you think the speaker's affect is from the affect list in the box below, and indicate whether that affect is activating or inhibiting. More than one affect may be possible.

Affect Selection List:

Anger/assertion	Excitement
Grief	Joy
Tenderness/closeness	Sexual desire
Guilt	Shame

Positive feelings about the self (e.g., pride, self confidence, self-esteem, self-care, etc.)

Example: When I saw that cute little puppy, I just wanted to pet it!

Answer: Affect? _Tenderness/care_ (Activating) Inhibiting

Exercise 1B.1. By the time I handed in my assignment, I was so pleased with how well it came out.

Affect? _____ Activating Inhibiting

Exercise 1B.2. I heard about ethnic cleansing in Bosnia on the radio, and I almost started to cry.

Affect? _____ Activating Inhibiting

Exercise 1B.3. I finally realized I was working too hard, and I just went to bed.

Affect? _____ Activating Inhibiting

Exercise 1B.4. I told him he'd have to wait his turn.

Affect? _____ Activating Inhibiting

Exercise 1B.5.   I couldn't even look at him, I felt so bad about what I'd done.

Affect? _____   **Activating**   **Inhibiting**

EXERCISE 1C: SPOT THE AFFECT PHOBIA

Directions: In each of the following exercises, select one or more of the affects that might be blocked due to Affect Phobia. (Put another way, which affect or affects might the speaker be defending against?) Make your selections from the list of affects in the box above in Exercise 1B.

Example: A girl who loves to tap-dance dances exuberantly, but can only do so with a controlled, expressionless look on her face.

Answer: **Possible blocked affect(s):** _Excitement_____

Explanation: She might be embarrassed to show how enthusiastic she feels. She could also be feeling joy, but afraid or ashamed to show it.

Exercise 1C.1.   A man acts concerned and caring with his adolescent daughter, but refuses to give her a hug.

Possible blocked affect(s): _____

Exercise 1C.2.   A teacher complains of getting migraines at work with increasing frequency. The principal is treating him unfairly, but he has said nothing.

Possible blocked affect(s): _____

Exercise 1C.3.   A married woman finds that when she is with her husband or friends, she is unable to state her needs if they are different from the group's.

Possible blocked affect(s): _____

Exercise 1C.4.   A young woman often receives praise for her job performance, but feels that she is secretly a fraud and fears being found out.

Possible blocked affect(s): _____

Exercise 1C.5.   A young man says that he has not been able to have a girlfriend for 5 years—ever since he broke up with his fiancée, with whom he is still furious.

Possible blocked affect(s): _____

Exercise 1C.6.   A patient who has been steadily improving in therapy sits in her garden noting, for the first time in as long as she can remember, the beauty of the day. Suddenly she feels overwhelmed by anxiety.

Possible blocked affect(s): _____

Exercise 1C.7.   A young man is having a panic attack, brought on by his girlfriend's making an off-hand comment about "wanting children someday."

Possible blocked affect(s): _____

Affect Phobia, Psychodynamic Conflict, and Malan's Two Triangles

Chapter Objectives
To show how Affect Phobia and psychodynamic conflict are related, and how Malan's Two Triangles can organize treatment.

Topics Covered

I.   Reformulating Psychodynamic Conflict as Affect Phobia

II. Understanding Affect Phobias by Using Malan's Two Triangles: The Universal Principle of Psychodynamic Psychotherapy

III. Making Important Distinctions about Feelings

IV. Restructuring Affect Phobias through Systematic Desensitization: The Main Treatment Objectives

I. REFORMULATING PSYCHODYNAMIC CONFLICT AS AFFECT PHOBIA

Desensitizing Fears about Feelings

This treatment model is based on psychodynamic theory, and sees "neurotic" psychopathology as a result of conflicts about feelings. This has traditionally been called **psychodynamic conflict**. However, when psychodynamic conflict is thought of as a phobia about feeling (or Affect Phobia), therapy can harness the power of systematic desensitization, the most well-established treatment for phobias. But, as noted in Chapter 1, rather than desensitizing external phobias (e.g., elevators), we are desensitizing internal phobias, or fears about feelings—thus the term **Affect Phobia**.

Recall from Chapter 1 that Affect Phobia arises when adaptive activating affect (e.g., grief, anger, closeness/tenderness) is associated with excessive inhibitory affect (e.g., anxiety, shame, guilt, or pain). For example, a person may desire to speak up and at the same moment feel intense shame over doing so (i.e., both activation and inhibition). These opposing forces give rise to psychodynamic conflict (Affect Phobia), as in the following example:

PATIENT: I started to tell him that I didn't like what he was doing [anger/assertion], but then I just started feeling scared [anxiety] and embarrassed [shame], and I stopped myself.

Defenses Help Patients Avoid Conscious Conflict

Sometimes the connection between the activating and inhibitory affects is conscious, as in the example above. However, the process can often be unconscious, because the conflict may be so painful that patients use various avoidant thoughts, feelings, or behaviors as **defenses** to block the experience of the feeling(s) or to avoid situations that evoke the feeling(s). The purpose of defensive behavior is to limit or even eliminate from consciousness the activating affect, the inhibitory affect, or both.

PATIENT: When my boss screamed at me, I got one of my terrific headaches that I get at work, and I had to go lie down [defensive behaviors].

Note in this example that the patient reports no conscious experience of being angry at being yelled at—just the avoidant reaction of the headache and leaving to lie down. Also note that whenever we use the term **defensive behaviors**, we may be referring to thoughts, feelings, or behaviors.

In Affect Phobia (psychodynamic conflict), defenses are the "compromise responses" that reduce the level of conscious struggle between the activating and inhibitory affects. In behavioral terms, defenses represent **escape behaviors**, allowing the patient to phobically avoid the intrapsychic conflict about feeling. Consider these examples of defenses used to avoid conflicts over feeling:

PATIENT 1: I'm not [defense] mad [feeling]. I'm just confused [defense].

PATIENT 2: I won't show I'm excited [feeling]. I'll just try to play it cool [defense].

PATIENT 3: I'm not [defense] sad [feeling] over the breakup. I never really loved him [defense].

Symptoms Are Seen as Defenses

Our model views most symptomatic behavior—including the individual criteria in the definitions of the Axis I and II diagnoses (i.e., maladaptive thoughts, feelings, and behaviors)—as defenses against conflicted or phobic affects.

Anxiety and Depression as Defenses

When an inhibitory affect (e.g., anxiety or emotional pain) rises to the level of diagnosis (e.g., anxiety or depressive disorder), it is often because other defenses have failed to keep the inhibitory affect out of consciousness. At this point—even if there are significant biological contributions—the symptoms that make up the diagnosis (anxiety, pain/depression) function not only as inhibitory affects but also as defenses, because the symptoms prevent the more adaptive affects and ways of responding.

It is helpful in streamlining Short-Term Dynamic Psychotherapy (STDP) to think of each diagnostic category as the surface manifestation of one or more Affect Phobias. (See also Chapter 11.) **This is why desensitizing Affect Phobias can potentially resolve many Axis I and II diagnoses**. Resolution of symptoms and diagnoses in STDP is discussed in detail in the chapters that follow. (For further discussion of symptoms vs. source of a disorder, see *Changing Character* [CC], pp. 396–399.)

II. UNDERSTANDING AFFECT PHOBIAS BY USING MALAN'S TWO TRIANGLES: THE UNIVERSAL PRINCIPLE OF PSYCHODYNAMIC PSYCHOTHERAPY

David Malan, a renowned British psychotherapy researcher, developed a schema that is particularly useful for understanding psychodynamic conflict (or Affect Phobia). It is called the **Two Triangles** (see Figure 2.1) and includes the **Triangle of Conflict** and the **Triangle of Person** (Malan, 1979, Ch. 10). Together, the Two Triangles represent what Malan called "the universal principle of psychodynamic psychotherapy," which is that defenses and anxieties can block the expression of true feeling.

The Two Triangles Work Together

The Two Triangles schema is a clear, graphic way to organize the complexity of psychodynamic treatment and is helpful in understanding how Affect Phobias develop, are maintained, and can be resolved. The Triangle of Conflict represents defenses and anxieties that modulate or block underlying adaptive feelings. The Triangle of Person represents the relationships where the pattern of conflict is played out.

First we discuss the phobic pattern in detail as it is represented on the three poles of the Triangle of Conflict. Then we discuss the relationships represented on the Triangle of Person, where the Affect Phobias originated and are maintained.

The Triangle of Conflict: How Affect Phobias Can Be Represented in a Psychodynamic Framework

Remember, psychodynamic conflict arises when an adaptive, activating affect is blocked from being expressed by excessive inhibitory affect. Then defenses prevent or diminish the conscious experience of this conflict.

The corners of the Triangle of Conflict (which are called **Poles**) represent these three components of psychodynamic conflict. They are called the **De-**

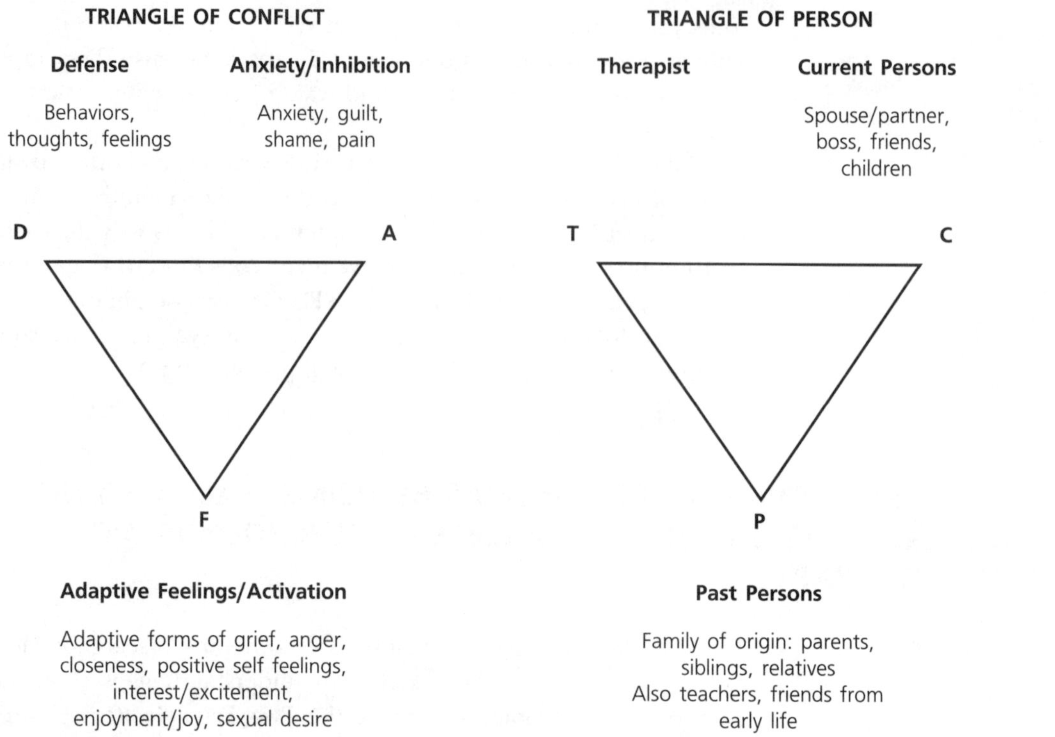

TRIANGLE OF CONFLICT   TRIANGLE OF PERSON

Defense   Anxiety/Inhibition   Therapist   Current Persons

Behaviors,   Anxiety, guilt,   Spouse/partner,
thoughts, feelings   shame, pain   boss, friends,
                                                                    children

D   A   T   C

        F   P

Adaptive Feelings/Activation   Past Persons

Adaptive forms of grief, anger,   Family of origin: parents,
closeness, positive self feelings,   siblings, relatives
interest/excitement,   Also teachers, friends from
enjoyment/joy, sexual desire   early life

FIGURE 2.1. The Two Triangles (Malan, 1979) represent what David Malan called the "universal principle of psychody-namic psychotherapy." That is, defenses (D) and anxieties (A) can block the expression of true feeling (F). These patterns began with past persons (P), are maintained with current persons (C), and are often enacted with the therapist (T).

fense Pole (abbreviated **D**), the **Anxiety Pole** (**A**), and the **Feeling Pole** (**F**). The Triangle of Conflict provides the therapist with a simple conceptual schema and visual tool with which to understand psychodynamic conflict. It can be sketched out with paper and pencil, but many therapists find that it becomes second nature to imagine or visualize the triangle during sessions as the patient is speaking.

To see the Triangle of Conflict in action, let's return to one of our earlier examples:

PATIENT: I started to tell him that I didn't like what he was doing [feeling—anger/assertion], but then I just started feeling scared [anxiety] and embarrassed [anxiety and shame], and I stopped myself [defensive behavior].

This would be represented on the Triangle of Conflict as follows:

Defense Pole (D)

"I stopped
myself."

Anxiety Pole (A)

"I started feeling
scared [anxiety]
and embarrassed
[shame]."

Feeling Pole (F)

"I started to tell him that I didn't
like what he was doing [anger/
assertion]."

**The "Normal"
Triangle of Conflict Is
Well-Balanced**

It is important to keep in mind that when the poles of the Triangle of Conflict are in balance, they describe a normal interaction of defenses, anxieties, and adaptive feelings. People always need some defenses. Anxieties or inhibitions are always needed to modulate adaptive feelings. An adaptive response to the example above might be the following:

- "I didn't like what he was doing [adaptive assertive feeling]."
- "But before I said anything, I slowed myself down and thought about it [adaptive defense of suppression]."
- "Because I didn't want to embarrass myself or him [adaptive inhibition]."
- "So when I told him what I didn't like, it came out fine, and the discussion ended well [adaptive expression of negative feeling—anger/assertion]."

**Intervention Is
Necessary When the
Poles Are Out of
Balance**

A goal in treatment is to restructure responses so that the Triangle of Conflict operates in a more adaptive manner. As therapists, we intervene when the poles are out of balance—such as when defenses or anxieties are excessive or maladaptive, and also when functioning is impaired.

Now we'll look at the poles of the Triangle of Conflict in more detail.

The Defense Pole (D)

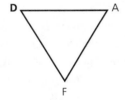

The Defense Pole ("D" in Figure 2.1) represents maladaptive or problematic responses that function to block the conflict between inhibition and activation. There are as many kinds of defensive responses as there are snowflakes or fingerprints. Defenses can be behaviors, thoughts, or even feelings used to avoid psychodynamic conflicts. At times defenses can be adaptive and useful to guide or modulate feelings. But often defenses are maladaptive or destructive—as when adaptive feelings are overly inhibited by anxiety, shame, guilt, pain, contempt, or disgust.

How Defenses Originate

Maladaptive patterns develop when children are taught that there is something frightening, shameful, or painful about their inner emotional responses. This leads them to **defend** themselves by doing, thinking, or feeling something different, as follows:

The Caretaker Evokes Inhibitory Affect	The Child Learns a Defensive Response
"What a baby you are for crying!"	"I'm not crying [D]. It doesn't bother me [D]."
"Never, say you hate anybody! It's bad."	"I don't hate anyone [D]. I'm a good girl [D]."
"Don't touch yourself. That's disgusting."	"Touching myself is nasty [D]. Ugh."
"Don't laugh, or you'll soon cry."	"I'll be quiet and not get excited [D]."

Defenses Can Be Feelings, Too

In thinking about the Defense Pole of the Triangle of Conflict, it is crucial to bear in mind that **any feeling can also function as defense**—which we call **defensive affect** (or defensive feeling). When a patient exhibits an activating affect such as anger, it is important to distinguish whether the feeling is being used maladaptively (represented on the defense pole), or adaptively (represented on the feeling pole). The following are examples of maladaptive defensive feelings and their consequences:

- Smiling—or becoming weepy—(Defensive Feeling) when one is really angry (F) lets people take advantage.
- Acting overly jubilant (Defensive Feeling) to mask sadness (F) denies needs.
- Using sexuality (Defensive Feeling) to try to find love (F) is a misguided search.
- Becoming angry or irritable (Defensive Feeling) to hide tender feeling (F) is isolating.

Another indication that an affect, thought, or behavior is being used defensively is when it is excessive, overblown, overdone, inappropriate, or regressive.

The Feeling Pole (F): The Activating Affects

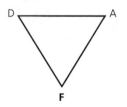

The Feeling Pole ("F" in Figure 2.1) represents affects that activate adaptive action. These true, underlying feelings are basically healthy and life-enhancing. However, patients phobically defend against them because of associated inhibitory feelings. This pole is called the Feeling Pole for historical reasons (see Malan, 1976). It's important to remember that the Feeling Pole (F) represents **only** activating affects and only in their adaptive forms. Inhibitory affects (see below) are represented on the Anxiety Pole (A), while defensive affects (see above) are represented on the Defense Pole (D).

List of Activating Feelings

The basic activating affects move us to some form of action. Recall from Chapter 1 that there are only a few categories or families of activating affects:

- Anger/assertion (irritation, annoyance, fury, rage).
- Sadness/grief (sorrow, mourning, crying).
- Fear/Terror (fright, alarm, apprehension, but **not** panic—that inhibits!).
- Enjoyment/joy (calm, tranquility, peace, wonder, awe).
- Interest/excitement (attention, curiosity, enthusiasm).
- Closeness/tenderness (care, love, concern, empathy).
- Positive feelings toward the self (self-compassion, self-esteem, pride).
- Sexual desire (passion, lust).

Some examples of patients describing these "phobic" affects are as follows:

PATIENT 1: I'm not the kind of person who gets angry [F—anger/assertion]. I hold my tongue [D].

PATIENT 2: Crying [F—sadness/grief] is for children. I keep a stiff upper lip [D].

PATIENT 3: Feeling proud of myself [F—positive feeling toward the self] is unthinkable [D]

The Anxiety Pole (A)

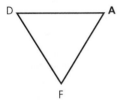

The Anxiety Pole ("A" in Figure 2.1) represents the inhibitory affects. It is the linking of excessive inhibition (A Pole) with activating feeling (F Pole) that causes Affect Phobia. As noted in Chapter 1, there are only a few main classes of inhibitory affects:

- Anxiety/fear/terror.
- Shame/guilt/humiliation.
- Emotional pain/misery/suffering.
- Contempt/disgust.

Remember that fear appears on both the activating list above and the inhibitory list, because it can be either activating (flight) or inhibitory (paralysis, freezing). Note also that we do not always include contempt/disgust in the list of inhibitory affects, because it has not been encountered as frequently as the other inhibitory affects in our clinical work. However, in certain patient population (e.g., patients who have experienced severe trauma), contempt/disgust is common and should be dealt with.

These inhibitory affects restrict, hold back, and rein in our other more action-oriented feelings, such as anger, grief, excitement, joy, and sexual desire (represented on F). Like all feelings, inhibitory feelings are natural, and can be healthy and adaptive. Too few inhibitions can be destructive. People need anxiety, guilt, shame, and pain to protect them from danger and guide them away from hurtful experiences. But excessive inhibition can destroy the joy and richness in living, and hence is the basis for neurotic psychopathology, as in these examples:

PATIENT 1: I felt so ashamed [A] when I cried [F—grief] in front of her.

PATIENT 2: I want to cuddle with my husband in the morning [F—closeness], but I get really anxious [A].

The Triangle of Person: Relationships Where Affect Phobias Occur

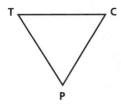

The Triangle of Person (Figure 2.1) represents the following three categories of relationships in the patient's life:

- **Past persons (P)**, with whom the Affect Phobia originated.
- **Current persons (C)**, with whom the Affect Phobia is maintained.
- **Therapist (T)**, with whom the Affect Phobia can be examined.

Identifying Affect Phobias in Relationships

The Triangle of Person is important to keep in mind, because **feelings are always associated with specific people**. Affect Phobias do not happen in isolation, but are learned and enacted in interactions with others. The therapist must consistently show the patient how conflicted feelings on the Triangle of Conflict originally began and are maintained with specific people on the Triangle of Person.

It is important for both the therapist and patient to recognize the following about the patterns of conflicted feelings:

1. How these patterns began with early life caretakers from the **past (P)**. Even when parents are still alive and the relationships are ongoing at present, we place family-of-origin relationships as "Past Persons" (P) because the past is generally where maladaptive patterns began.

    THERAPIST: Your parents [P] tended to be critical when you cried [F—sadness/grief], so of course you learned to shut down [D] that response.

2. How the patterns are maintained in **current relationships [C]**.

    THERAPIST: And even when your son [C] died, you couldn't [D] let yourself grieve [F] with your husband [C]—though you desperately needed to.

3. How the patterns are very likely to be reenacted in the relationship with or transference to the **therapist [T]**, where the Affect Phobia patterns can be examined.

THERAPIST: We see here, in therapy with me [T], how scary [A] it is to let yourself be sad [F].

Connecting Past Patterns with Current Behavior

When similarities are identified between behaviors in past and current relationships –including the relationship with the therapist - it becomes very clear how patients' maladaptive patterns have been transferred from past relationships and are maintained in current relationships. Seeing repeated patterns of conflict across several relationships gives an idea of the frequency and severity of the problem.

Autonomy and Interdependence

Remember that this model is based on healthy autonomy and interdependence of self and others. Resolution of Affect Phobias (Triangle of Conflict) happens in caring and compassionate relationships (Triangle of Person).

Malan's Two Triangles: Summary

The Mechanics of Phobic Avoidance on the Triangles

In summary, the Triangle of Conflict or Affect Phobia schema describes the mechanics of phobic avoidance (excessive inhibition) of feelings. These conflicted feelings (adaptive feelings linked with inhibitions) lead us to feel, think, and behave in ways that avoid the experience of conflict (defenses). The Triangle of Conflict (D-A-F) represents the Affect Phobia or psychodynamic conflict. The Triangle of Person (T-C-P) focuses on the interpersonal relationships where the phobic response takes place.

Examples

PATIENT 1: I just can't bear [A—pain] to think that Carol [C] cares for me [F—closeness]. I feel so embarrassed [A—shame] just talking about this that I want to run out the door [D].

PATIENT 2: We were in a dark part of the alley. I was acting tough and cool [D]—but I was really scared [F—adaptive fear] of meeting up with the other gang [C] and afraid [A—anxiety] of letting the guys [C] see that. [This is an example where fear is an adaptive response to a dangerous situation, but is inhibited by another form of fear—anxiety.]

PATIENT 3: I hate myself [D—masochism]! And I think my family [P] hates me too [possible D—projection]. I've never liked myself [F—self-esteem, self-acceptance], and I never will because I'm not worth anything [A—shame].

PATIENT 4: I feel dead [D]. There is no passion [F—interest/excitement] in my life for anything. I couldn't bear [A—pain] to get that involved. [This is represented just on the Triangle of Conflict.]

The Two Triangles as a Conceptual Schema

Keeping the Two Triangles in mind can help therapists identify the following:

- What affects are being defended against, how, and why.
- With whom these destructive patterns originated and are being maintained.

To practice STDP effectively, a therapist must be able to do these things:

1. Recognize defenses, recognize or infer the activating affects and inhibitory affects, and put them together in a psychodynamic core conflict (Affect Phobia) formulation. This is discussed in detail in Chapter 4.

2. Desensitize the conflicted affects so that the patient's feelings and defenses become more flexible and adaptive. Methods for doing this are outlined in Chapters 5–10.

III. MAKING IMPORTANT DISTINCTIONS ABOUT FEELINGS

Activating versus Inhibitory Feelings

To understand the triangles in depth, one must understand the distinction between adaptive affects that activate behavior (on the F Pole) versus inhibitory affects (on the A Pole). As we have discussed in Chapter 1,

- Activating affects motivate behavior/action, causing an appropriate outflowing of energy, movement outward, or greater openness.
- Inhibitory affects restrict or restrain behavior/action by making people cower, shrink, withdraw, gaze avert, or close off. Inhibition can be adaptive if it guides people well, or maladaptive if the inhibition is too great or too little.

Defensive, Inhibitory, and Activating Affects

In addition to the above distinction, it's important to remember that affects can be used defensively. The distinction among affects can be assessed by their function—the way each affect is used.

- Affect used to avoid another feeling or to attack the self is defensive (D Pole).
- Affect used to thwart adaptive activating responses is inhibitory (A Pole).
- Affect used to express wants and needs is adaptive and nurturing (F Pole).

As noted above in Section I, some affects can function as **both** inhibitory and defensive at the same time. For example, severe forms of depression can attack or inhibit the self as well as defensively block feelings. Anxiety can be inhibiting, as in signal anxiety that blocks feelings (A), or can function as a defensive response, as in traumatic anxiety or panic attacks (D).

Mature and authentic affective responding, such as appropriate forms of anger, grief, interest, joy, or closeness, is self-soothing, nurturing, and adaptive (F). Fear can also function adaptively if it motivates the person to avoid danger. (Also see CC, pp. 143–147.)

Not All Affect Is Helpful in Treatment

As noted above, it is crucial to be able to distinguish adaptive from maladaptive/defensive forms of affects. As therapists, we sometimes think we are doing good work when **any** affect is expressed in treatment. However, as shown in the following examples, much affect can be maladaptive—and can be detrimental to encourage:

- Raging anger can avoid the pain of grief.
- Victimized weeping can hide anger.
- Manic excitement can block sorrow and self-care.
- False calmness ("playing it cool") can mask excitement or sexual desire.

Mistaking Maladaptive for Adaptive Affects

Therapists can spend much time eliciting strong feeling from their patients, only to discover that the time has been wasted because maladaptive, defensive expressions of feeling have been mistaken for adaptive forms of feelings. In this example, helpless weepiness was mistaken for sadness:

THERAPIST: My patient howled and sobbed for weeks. I thought we were really getting somewhere, but after a while, when she felt no relief and nothing changed, I realized this was a regressive form of the feeling and wasn't helping her function more effectively in her life. She was really feeling helpless, hopeless, powerless, and frustrated.

Patients do not learn more effective ways of living by perpetuating the experience of self-defeating or "victimized" affect states. Affects of this sort are defensive and do not lead to constructive action. When such affects emerge, it is important to note them, explore them in a contained way, and help the patient bear them, so that the patient can come to understand the underlying meanings and the more adaptive feelings that need to be accessed.

Redirecting toward Adaptive Affect

PATIENT: I'm sick of this! Nothing ever goes right. I can't stand it any more!

THERAPIST: Right now, your anger is tormenting you. We are not seeing how your anger might be directed to the person you're mad at. Let's get the feeling flowing out of your body toward him—in fantasy, of course, not in reality. What would move you to respond effectively?

Maladaptive Affects Used as Defenses

Maladaptive, regressive expressions of affect are often used to avoid more painful feelings, such as anger, grief, or longing for care. When a therapist encounters an affective response that is exaggerated or nonconstructive, it can be helpful to view it as a defensive emotion. Maladaptive feelings may need some desensitizing, too, to help patients bear them enough to explore their meaning, and thereby gain greater control. **Patients need anxiety reg-**

ulation to be able to admit to, tolerate, and explore these regressive, mal-adaptive feelings—as long as it is made clear that these are *not* adaptive feelings to be put into action.

THERAPIST: We may feel and explore sadistic feelings [D] in this office, where it is safe to do so, but of course it is important not to act on them.

The exploration of these regressive affects can then point the way toward discovering what adaptive feeling the maladaptive feeling may be blocking. Consider these examples:

- **Regressive rage** (e.g., "road rage") is a helpless, frustrated form of anger that may be used to block many feelings. For instance, the adaptive form of anger (constructive assertion) may be blocked due to fear, shame, or pain of feeling inadequate or powerless.
- **Exaggerated grieving** can be a defense against replacing losses due to poor self-worth and/or lack of entitlement to move on in life (e.g., "I don't deserve a full life, since my mother lost hers"). Positive feeling about the self or healthy entitlement is needed and may be blocked by guilt or shame. Such grieving can also defend against anger.
- **Weepiness that gives no relief** can be a form of depression and self-attack (in that the person feels miserable) that can be defending against many affects (e.g., real grief, anger, or assertion).
- **Desperate longing** suggests a lack of positive feeling about the self, as opposed to a legitimate longing for closeness. The individual may be craving the love of the other as an externalized means of validating the self. In such cases, the need for validation from the other becomes exaggerated. The conflicts that need to be desensitized can be many (e.g., conflicts about feelings of self-worth, possibly blocked by shame and/or pain due to not having been adequately cared for). There may also be conflicts over grief.

IV. RESTRUCTURING AFFECT PHOBIAS THROUGH SYSTEMATIC DESENSITIZATION: THE MAIN TREATMENT OBJECTIVES

In Section VI of Chapter 1, we have talked about systematic desensitization in the context of Affect Phobias. Many therapists have been helped in formulating conflicted affect patterns by the Two Triangles, but there can be confusion about how to use these concepts in treatment. Therefore, specific objectives based on the Triangle of Conflict schema have been developed (McCullough, 1993; McCullough Vaillant, 1994) to help desensitize and restructure Affect Phobias. This section presents an overview of the three broad treatment objectives that are discussed in detail in Chapters 5–10.

1. **Defense Restructuring:** Helping the patient see and give up (prevent) defensive responses.

2. **Affect Restructuring:** Helping the patient to experience affect without excessive inhibition, and to express it appropriately.

3. **Self- and Other-Restructuring:** Helping the patient improve relationships and gain positive feelings toward the self.

General Points about Restructuring

Definition of Restructuring

Restructuring—changing the structure of an Affect Phobia—occurs when positive consequences become associated with adaptive feelings and actions instead of restrictive or punishing inhibitions. From this point of view, therapy derives its power from the **corrective emotional experience**, defined by Alexander and French (1946) as "reexperiencing the old, unsettled conflict **but with a new ending**" (p. 338; emphasis added).

Desensitization Is the Tool for Restructuring

In this therapy, systematic desensitization is the main tool for removing the internal aversive consequences (i.e., the excessive inhibition) of adaptive feelings and actions. It is important to pay attention to the external aversive consequences as well. Therapy needs to be conducted in a safe, validating fashion, so that the therapist does not unwittingly increase (i.e., sensitize) the conflict (e.g., by being judgmental or critical). In the same way, therapist and patient need to pay attention to situations outside of the therapy that may reinforce maladaptive patterns.

Beyond removing aversive consequences, the change process is helped when the consequences of adaptive action are as positive as possible. This is why methods that include support, empathy, collaboration, validation, building compassion, and the like are important in this therapy.

Desensitization Occurs throughout Treatment

Each of the three treatment objectives listed above has phobic aspects that require some degree of desensitization. For example, Defense Restructuring is needed most when patients are "afraid" to look at their defenses. Patients often have shame simply over **having** defenses, and this shame needs to be reduced. In this case, exposure means that the patients must be made aware of their defenses, and anxiety regulation is used to decrease the shame. Thus the techniques of desensitization can be useful on several levels throughout treatment.

Breaking the Hold of Inhibitory Affects

The presence of anxiety or inhibitory feelings is what makes feelings conflicted or sensitized. Desensitization means loosening or breaking the hold of inhibitory affects on the adaptive affects. Compare these two statements:

PATIENT 1: Being angry [F] makes me feel guilty [A], so I just shut up [D]. [The guilt overly inhibits the expression of anger.]

PATIENT 2: Now I know I have a right to be angry [F], and I know how to express it so it helps me. [After desensitization, guilt no longer restricts anger, as long as it is modulated and presented appropriately.]

Desensitization: Expose, Prevent Maladaptive Responses, and Calm Anxieties

Remember from Section V of Chapter 1 that desensitization is a step-by-step process—moving among exposure, preventing evasive/defensive responses, and calming anxieties. This process should be repeated again and again to help patients desensitize their anxieties until their adaptive resources are more freely available.

Anxiety Regulation

Supportive or cognitive methods are used as needed to regulate anxieties, so that restructuring of the phobic situation does not become overwhelming. (For a review of anxiety regulation, see Section VI of Chapter 1.) Then, as soon as possible, exposure should be continued until the fear diminishes.

Anxiety regulation occurs within each of the objectives. Defenses are restructured because positive consequences are associated with awareness of and willingness to give up the defensive response, rather than the reinforcing comfort of ego-syntonic defenses. Affects are restructured because positive consequences are associated with the experience and expression of adaptive affect, replacing frightening or shameful inhibition. And Self- and Other-Restructuring occurs because positive consequences become associated with the experience of self and others, instead of a sense of shame, guilt, or excessive vulnerability.

Each of the Three Treatment Objectives Has Two Components

Defense Restructuring

To prevent defensive responses, patients must both recognize how defenses block feeling, and feel motivated to change them. These are the two components of Defense Restructuring:

- **Defense Recognition:** Seeing the problematic behavior.
- **Defense Relinquishing:** Wanting to stop it.

Defense Restructuring (using desensitization to regulate anxieties about defenses) is needed because patients are afraid of seeing their defenses and afraid of giving them up. Defense Restructuring functions as **response prevention** in desensitizing an Affect Phobia, because it enables patients to identify and give up (or prevent the use of) defenses that block affect.

Example: Defense Recognition

THERAPIST: You've just told me an incredibly sad story. Are you aware that you are smiling as you tell me this? [Pointing out defense]

PATIENT: I notice it now that you point it out, yes.

THERAPIST: What would happen if you didn't smile?

PATIENT: I guess it's covering something up, isn't it? It keeps me from feeling how incredibly sad I feel about the fact that I'll never see my father again.

THERAPIST: So the sadness is something you try to avoid.

PATIENT: Yeah, I don't like to go there.

THERAPIST: What's the hardest part about sitting with the sadness? What hurts the most? [Regulating the anxiety]

Example: Defense Relinquishing

THERAPIST: You learned to hide your feelings because you were shamed for showing any sign of weakness. You did the best that a child in that situation could do—put on a brave face and try to avoid the painful feelings. [Validation of the defense] But the costs to you have been enormous, the loneliness, and all these years living a quiet depression, never able to express what's truly in your heart. [Pointing out the costs of the defense]

PATIENT: You're right. It seems like such a waste! I don't want to hold back my feelings any more.

Affect Restructuring

Conflicts over affects need to be desensitized by exposure. Unearthing (experiencing) and sharing (expressing) buried feelings resolves the Affect Phobia. These are the two components of Affect Restructuring:

- **Affect Experiencing:** Feeling the avoided or phobic feeling.
- **Affect Expression:** Learning to express the feeling appropriately.

Affect Restructuring (using desensitization to regulate anxieties about feeling) is needed because patients are afraid of feeling something new, and afraid of expressing feelings to others. Affect Restructuring constitutes the exposure needed in desensitizing an Affect Phobia, because the patient has to face and bear the feared feeling.

Example: Affect Experiencing

THERAPIST: When you think of the last time you saw your father, how do you experience the sad feelings?

PATIENT: There's a lot of pressure behind my eyes.

THERAPIST: What if you relaxed your eyes a little, let go of the pressure, and just let yourself see what your body is experiencing?

PATIENT: (Pauses) There's this incredible heaviness in my chest when I remember him (*tears begin to flow*).

Example: Affect Expression

PATIENT: Sure, it's OK now to cry in here [therapy], but I'm not sure I want my girlfriend to see me when I'm sad. I could never tell her what I've just told you.

THERAPIST: What would be the worst part if you allowed her to see how moved you were?

PATIENT: She wouldn't want to be seen with a grown man weeping.

THERAPIST: Well, let's look at that. When you came here, you said she was frustrated with the fact that you didn't show very much of yourself. Now you're saying that she would be disgusted to see you express sadness. Is she really so judgmental?

PATIENT: No, I see what you're saying. I'm still expecting that I'll be judged for showing my feelings.

THERAPIST: So what would it be like to show her that side of you? Let's imagine what it would be like for you to open up with her.

Self- and Other-Restructuring

Self- and Other-Restructuring means acquiring adaptive images of self and others. It involves two specific forms of exposure to feelings, associated with images of self and other, respectively.

- **Self Restructuring:** Improving self-image and building self-care.
- **Other Restructuring:** Building more adaptive perceptions of and connections to others.

Self- and Other-Restructuring (using desensitization to regulate anxieties about attachment to self and others) is needed because patients are afraid of feeling good about themselves, and afraid of feeling close or unsure about being distant (whichever is adaptive in a particular situation).

Why Does Self- and Other-Restructuring Follow Defense and Affect Restructuring?

Self- and Other-Restructuring must at times come first in treatment, and so it may be confusing that these chapters are placed after those on Defense and Affect Restructuring. There are several reasons for this:

1. Typical STDP begins with restructuring defenses and affects.
2. The need for extensive work on self-image and image of others suggests a somewhat different form of treatment with a more impaired patient, and sometimes this work is not short-term at all.

(For more information on the origin of the three objectives, see CC, Ch. 1.)

Example: Self-Restructuring

THERAPIST: How do you think of yourself if you were to cry in her arms?

PATIENT: Like a wimp, pure and simple.

THERAPIST: Isn't it sad how harsh you are on yourself for having such a natural human response? Can you see yourself any other way?

PATIENT: Maybe, but I'll have to work on it.

Example: Other-Restructuring

THERAPIST: Did you feel like a wimp here with me when you cried?

PATIENT: Well, at first I did, but it seems a little more comfortable now. I guess you don't seem so judgmental any more.

Changing Old Behaviors Changes Character

Because these conflicted, maladaptive character patterns are at least in part learned, patients are able—through the process of restructuring—to learn more flexible and adaptive ones. By unlearning long-standing behavior patterns and learning new and more adaptive ones, patients are **changing character**.

CHAPTER 2 • EXERCISES

EXERCISE 2A: IDENTIFY POLES ON THE TRIANGLE OF CONFLICT

Directions: Identify the pole of the Triangle of Conflict that the therapist is referring to in the underlined portions of the following statements, using D (Defense), A (Anxieties/Inhibitions), or F ([Adaptive] Feeling). **Note**: When the word "feel" or "feeling" is used as a thought ("You seem to feel confused"), it does not necessarily represent F.

Example: When we talk about your feelings, you often <u>change the subject</u>. Could this be a way you avoid difficult topics?   (D)   A   F

Explanation: Changing the subject is a defense.

Exercise 2A.1.   Do you see how you <u>avoid my eyes</u> when we talk about this?   D   A   F

Exercise 2A.2.   It seems that every time you become angry, you feel <u>guilty</u>.   D   A   F

Exercise 2A.3.   Have you noticed that you <u>intellectualize</u> when I ask about feelings?   D   A   F

Exercise 2A.4.   When I ask about your mother, you seem to become very <u>nervous</u>.   D   A   F

Exercise 2A.5.   Are you feeling <u>angry</u> right now, when you think of how he betrayed you?   D   A   F

Exercise 2A.6.   Do you feel <u>uncomfortable</u> when I ask you to look at me?   D   A   F

Exercise 2A.7.   You have spoken of your <u>longing</u> for your mother.   D   A   F

Exercise 2A.8.   Could we look at the <u>grief</u> you felt over his betrayal?   D   A   F

EXERCISE 2B: IDENTIFY POLES ON THE TRIANGLE OF PERSON

Directions: Determine which pole on the Triangle of Person the underlined words in the statements below refer to. Remember that members of the family of origin are always coded as past figures (P), even though they still may be interacting in the present. This is because they were present when the problems originated, and may have contributed to the genesis of the problem.

Example:	THERAPIST: How do you feel here with <u>me</u>?	(T) C P
Explanation:	This refers to the therapist.	

Exercise 2B.1.	PATIENT: My <u>sister</u> and I are very close.	T C P
Exercise 2B.2.	PATIENT: I often feel uncomfortable in <u>here</u>.	T C P
Exercise 2B.3.	THERAPIST: Your <u>father</u> and <u>grandfather</u> meant a great deal to you.	T C P
Exercise 2B.4.	PATIENT: My <u>boss</u> lost his temper today, and I was terrified!	T C P
Exercise 2B.5.	THERAPIST: What did your <u>mother</u> praise you for doing?	T C P
Exercise 2B.6.	PATIENT: I had a long talk with my <u>wife</u> today.	T C P
Exercise 2B.7.	THERAPIST: Your <u>Aunt Margaret</u> was jealous of your mother and critical of you.	T C P
Exercise 2B.8.	THERAPIST: Did you want to avoid coming <u>to therapy</u> today?	T C P
Exercise 2B.9.	THERAPIST: Can we look at the competition between you and your <u>brother</u>?	T C P
Exercise 2B.10.	PATIENT: My <u>son</u> won't listen to anything I say.	T C P

EXERCISE 2C: IDENTIFY THE POLES OF THE TWO TRIANGLES: D-A-F-T-C-P

Directions:	Fill in the blanks after the underlined words in the statements below with D (for defenses—avoidant/maladaptive behaviors, thoughts, or feelings), A (for anxieties/inhibitory affects), F (for adaptive, activating affects for the patient, if permitted to happen), T (for therapist), C (for current persons), or P (for past persons).
Example:	THERAPIST: Can you see how you <u>drum your fingers</u> [D] and become <u>restless</u> [D] when I point out your <u>angry feelings</u> [F] with <u>me</u> [T]? Does looking at <u>angry feelings</u> [F] make you so <u>anxious</u> [A] that you have a hard time <u>asserting yourself</u> [F] <u>here</u> [T]?
Explanation:	This therapist is trying to show this patient how she is playing out certain patterns in therapy. He thus points out a common defense of drumming fingers (D) that the patient uses to avoid the anger (F—the adaptive activating affect). By showing how the patient plays her pattern out with the therapist (T), he can show her how she is continuing her maladaptive ways. Together, they can look at decreasing her anxiety (A) about her activating emotions (F), and work toward a well-guided expression of these emotions—with the therapist (T) and others in her life (C).
Exercise 2C.1.	THERAPIST: It seems you get *distant* [_] and *irritable* [_] whenever *closeness* [_] comes up between you and *your wife* [_], just like with *your mother.* [_]. You seem to have some *fear* [_] that *silences you* [_] and makes you *avoid* [_] being *close and loving* [_]. Does this pattern I describe sound right to you?
Exercise 2C.2.	THERAPIST: I notice that you *change the subject* [_] with *me* [_] whenever you become *sad* [_] over your *brother's* [_] death. These feelings may be *too painful to*

bear [_]—and may have made you *depressed* [_] and *numb* [_], rather than able to *grieve* [_]. What do you think?

EXERCISE 2D: IDENTIFY THE POLES OF THE TWO TRIANGLES: D-A-F-T-C-P

Directions: As in Exercise 2C, use the letters D-A-F-T-C-P to identify phrases on the poles of the Two Triangles in the following patient statements. This time you will not be signaled by underlining or blanks, so you need to pick out the relevant phrases yourself. Underline each word or phrase that indicates a pole of one of the Two Triangles, and insert the corresponding letter after or above it.

Exercise 2D.1. PATIENT: It's true, they really don't pay me anything like what other people get for what I do. The owner told me they can't afford to pay me any more, but I notice he just built a huge new house. I shut down when I get angry at him. I could send out my resumé, but I would feel like such a traitor to pursue another job. I just keep hoping that he'll figure out what I'm worth and give me a raise.

Exercise 2D.2. PATIENT: When my boyfriend told me that he wanted to leave me for her, I just got so depressed and so aggravated with myself. I've sacrificed everything to make him happy, and somehow I'm still not good enough. My friends tell me he's not good for me and I should leave him, but I just love him too much.

Exercise 2D.3. PATIENT: I was stone-faced at my husband's funeral, and I really haven't cried since. I look at my daughter crying uncontrollably, and it's just so embarrassing. I can't stand it!

EXERCISE 2E: WHAT DOES A DEFENSIVE FEELING LOOK LIKE?

Directions: Each exercise below has a defensive affect followed by a list of behaviors. Pick which of the behaviors could be instances of the affect used defensively by putting an × in the blank following it—as illustrated in the example below. **Note:** When an affect is used maladaptively, it is almost always defensive. Defensive feelings are often (though not always) loud, dramatic, excessive, or done for effect or show.

Example: Defensive joy

1. Acting depressed ___

2. Laughing too loudly and too often when nervous _X_

3. False smile to cover pain _X_

4. Loud displays of "How wonderful!"   <u>X</u>

Explanation: Behaviors 2, 3, and 4 are uses of joy to cover some other feeling. Behavior 1, acting depressed, can be defensive, but it is not a defensive use of joy. Depression is a response involving helplessness, passivity, and hopelessness, and may be a means of blocking or thwarting joy (or assertion, or grief).

Exercise 2E.1.   Defensive tenderness

    1. Ignoring presence of another   ___

    2. Exaggerated affection   ___

    3. Calling spouse "sweetie" when angry   ___

    4. Negativity toward others   ___

    5. Sugary sweetness   ___

Exercise 2E.2.   Defensive anger

    1. Biting humor   ___

    2. Violent reaction to minor incident   ___

    3. Finger pointing (blame)   ___

    4. Saying nonsense   ___

    5. Picking on someone   ___

    6. Tantrums   ___

Exercise 2E.3.   Defensive sadness

    1. Manic addiction to exercise or shopping   ___

    2. Crying in the middle of an argument   ___

    3. Pathological mourning that does not resolve   ___

    4. Being happy when the person one is jealous of loses out ___

Exercise 2E.4.   Defensive excitement

    1. Lack of interest   ___

    2. Frenzied planning of a wedding to an unfaithful lover ___

    3. Loud displays of "I'm thrilled!"   ___

    4. Frantic activity after a loss   ___

Exercise 2E.5.   Defensive sexual desire

    1. Frequent arguing before going to bed   ___

    2. Initiating sex when an argument seems likely   ___

    3. Sex without intimacy   ___

    4. Excessive need for a platonic closeness   ___

    5. The feeling of being ugly and unloved   ___

**Assessment
and Selection of
Treatment for the Patient**

Chapter Objectives   To describe what the initial evaluation process consists of, and how the Global Assessment of Functioning (GAF) Scale is useful in assessment and treatment.

Topics Covered

I.   Overview of the Initial Assessment

II.   How the DSM Multiaxial Assessment Guides Treatment Selection

III.   How to Rate the Global Assessment of Functioning (GAF) Scale

IV.   Indications and Contraindications for STDP

V.   Using the GAF Scale to Tailor Treatment to Patients' Needs

VI.   The Supportive–Exploratory Continuum of Interventions

I. OVERVIEW OF THE INITIAL ASSESSMENT

Tasks for the Initial Assessment

The first session or first few sessions of Short-Term Dynamic Psychotherapy (STDP) must include diagnostic assessment, psychodynamic formulation, and treatment planning. This places enormous demands on the therapist to do the following simultaneously:

- Determine the patient's overall level of functioning as rated by the Global Assessment of Functioning (GAF) Scale (described in this chapter).
- Obtain information for determining *Diagnostic and Statistical Manual of Mental Disorders*, fourth edition (DSM-IV) diagnoses (described in this chapter and Chapter 11)

- Formulate core psychodynamic conflicts to spot Affect Phobias (described in Chapter 4).
- Select the most appropriate treatment based on the assessment (described at the end of this chapter, in Chapter 4, and in the Introduction to Chapters 5–10).

In this chapter, we give an overview of the assessment process and discuss how diagnostic information—particularly the patient's level of functioning—affects **how** the patient should be treated (the process of treatment). Then, in Chapter 4, we describe how to use the initial session(s) to formulate the core psychodynamic conflict(s) and determine **what** Affect Phobia to focus on (the content of treatment).

STDP is not appropriate for every patient. As we discuss below, selection of the appropriate treatment for a patient is based more on the patient's level of functioning (GAF, Axis V) than it is upon the other DSM-IV diagnostic axes. For that reason, the bulk of this chapter focuses on how to make a rapid GAF assessment, and how to use that to guide treatment planning. Section IV of this chapter then explains how diagnostic information helps therapists know when STDP is either contraindicated or needs significant adaptation to meet a patient's needs.

Our Assessment Process

To accomplish the many goals listed above, our assessment process for outpatient psychotherapy generally begins with the first phone contact with a patient. In this 10- to 20-minute initial contact, we try to get a brief description of the kind of problems that the individual wants to address. We also try to get a rough idea of the person's level of functioning, and to determine whether there are major contraindications (e.g., substance abuse or dependence, severe medical illness, or severe life stressors) to a short-term approach. Again, these contraindications are discussed in more detail later.

PAC Forms

Then, if the person decides to enter treatment, we mail or e-mail the Psychotherapy Assessment Checklist (PAC) Forms, with instructions to fill out the forms and bring them to the first session. The PAC Forms are a comprehensive set of questions and checklist items, which can be filled out ahead of time by the patient. The forms, with instructions on how to use them, can be obtained from our Web site, www.affectphobia.org.

The forms include basic demographic data; presenting problems with severity ratings; and checklists noting major criteria for Axis I and Axis II diagnoses, problems with health/illness (Axis III), life stressors (Axis IV), and level of functioning (Axis V). The items and answers are presented in a columnar format that allows the therapist to scan a great deal of information in 3–5 minutes prior to seeing a patient. Thus, the therapist is able to obtain a great deal information about functioning and history up front—information that quickly provides indications or contraindications for STDP.

- The PAC Forms do not require scoring. They are similar to medical symptom and illness history checklists. In a clinic setting, the staff could have a prospective patient arrive 30 minutes early to fill out the checklist in the waiting room prior to the first session (as is done with medical checklists given out by physicians).
- The Axis I and Axis II criteria checklists do not provide definitive DSM-IV diagnoses, but streamline the evaluation by quickly directing a therapist to diagnostic and problem areas of greatest concern.
- More impaired patients may not complete the forms, but this can signal that more supportive measures need to be taken, including therapist assistance with completing the forms.

Interweaving of Tasks in the Initial Interview

One reason why the PAC Forms are helpful is that patients come to treatment anxious to talk about their problems, and often feel put off by beginning with assessment questioning. So, in the initial session (which we also refer to as the **initial evaluation**), we spend significantly more time hearing problems and exploring the underlying core psychodynamic conflict. If a patient fills out the PAC Forms and a therapist reviews them before the initial evaluation, the therapist has more time to focus on exploration and building the treatment alliance with the patient. However, diagnostic and functional assessment of the patient goes on in the background throughout the session.

Session Length

Ideally, the initial evaluation is conducted in a 3-hour session. Many therapists do not have this time flexibility, so the evaluation may be limited to two back-to-back sessions or spread over three separate sessions. However, the extended time is very useful, for these reasons:

- Therapists can take time to verify the information on the PAC Forms and to collect further GAF and other DSM information.
- Therapists have time to hear many examples of the presenting problems, as well as time to figure out the defenses, anxieties, and feelings that contribute to them in a number of different relationships. This gives a broader perspective, which leads to more robust formulations.

II. HOW THE DSM MULTIAXIAL ASSESSMENT GUIDES TREATMENT SELECTION

Suitability for STDP

The pioneers of brief psychotherapy generated lists of criteria to judge whether a patient could tolerate a rapid uncovering mode of therapy (see CC, Ch. 2, pp. 59–60). However, it is very difficult to hold all these criteria in mind in the speedy flow of the initial evaluation, given that therapists have to gather all the information discussed above and decide what treatment is most suitable.

Fortunately, the DSM multiaxial assessment—and in particular the GAF Scale (Axis V)—covers many factors that indicate suitability for STDP, as well as many other forms of therapy (American Psychiatric Association, 2000; Endicott, Spitzer, Fleiss, & Cohen, 1976). The five axes of the DSM diagnosis are useful in the following ways:

DSM-IV Diagnoses on Axis I and Axis II

Clinical experience has shown that patients with poor impulse control or a fragile sense of self may not be able to tolerate the rapid uncovering of a short-term treatment. For example, patients with some Axis I psychiatric diagnoses (such as schizophrenia or substance abuse/dependence), or with Cluster B personality disorders (such as borderline or narcissistic personality disorder on Axis II), are less likely to profit from short-term treatment. Thus the diagnosis can provide a quick way to rule out a patient for whom STDP may not be appropriate. Axis I and Axis II information may also indicate whether pharmacological interventions should be considered. These diagnostic indications and contraindications are discussed in detail in Chapter 11.

Finally, recall from Chapter 2 that most of the symptoms constituting DSM Axis I or II diagnoses fall on the Defense Pole (D) of the Triangle of Conflict (with some symptoms also including the Anxiety Pole [A]). Identifying and desensitizing the conflicted affect(s) can reduce or eliminate symptomatic behavior. Thus Axis I and Axis II diagnoses can be helpful in guiding treatment by identifying symptoms on the Defense and Anxiety Poles (discussed further in Chapter 11). However, diagnoses are not the guiding force in our treatment selection process, as discussed below.

Axis III

Medical problems are important to consider along with psychological problems, because patients with severe medical problems will generally need more supportive interventions, and may not benefit from the more stressful experience of having their defenses challenged.

Axis IV

Life stressors are important considerations, because patients who are undergoing severe life stressors or transitions may not have the resources available to manage a rapid, uncovering treatment.

Axis V: The GAF Scale

Axis V of DSM-IV is the Global Assessment of Functioning (GAF) Scale. Some therapists think of the GAF Scale as a burden imposed by insurance companies. In reality, it is an extremely useful tool during the initial evaluation because it organizes a tremendous amount of information in a simple format, and can help to direct the therapist to a suitable treatment for the patient.

The GAF Scale is a diagnosis-free rating of "global" or composite functioning, which takes into consideration the individual's strengths as well as vulnerabilities in three areas of functioning: psychological (symptoms), social, and occupational. The rating is a single number on a scale that runs from 1

TABLE 3.1. The Global Assessment of Functioning (GAF) Scale

Code	(Note: Use intermediate codes when appropriate, e.g., 45, 68, 72.)
100 | 91	Superior functioning in a wide range of activities, life's problems never seem to get out of hand, is sought out by others because of his or her many positive qualities. No symptoms.
90 | 81	**Absent or minimal symptoms** (e.g., mild anxiety before an exam), **good functioning in all areas, interested and involved in a wide range of activities, socially effective, generally satisfied with life, no more than everyday problems or concerns** (e.g., an occasional argument with family members).
80 | 71	**If symptoms are present, they are transient and expectable reactions to psychosocial stressors** (e.g., difficulty concentrating after family argument); **no more than slight impairment in social, occupational, or school functioning** (e.g., temporarily falling behind in schoolwork).
70 | 61	**Some mild symptoms** (e.g., depressed mood and mild insomnia) **OR some difficulty in social, occupational, or school functioning** (e.g., occasional truancy, or theft within the household), **but generally functioning pretty well, has some meaningful interpersonal relationships.**
60 | 51	**Moderate symptoms** (e.g., flat affect and circumstantial speech, occasional panic attacks) **OR moderate difficulty in social, occupational, or school functioning** (e.g., few friends, conflicts with peers or co-workers).
50 | 41	**Serious symptoms** (e.g., suicidal ideation, severe obsessional rituals, frequent shoplifting) **OR any serious impairment in social, occupational, or school functioning** (e.g., no friends, unable to keep a job).
40 | 31	**Some impairment in reality testing or communication** (e.g., speech is at times illogical, obscure, or irrelevant) **OR major impairment in several areas, such as work or school, family relations, judgment, thinking, or mood** (e.g., depressed man avoids friends, neglects family, and is unable to work; child frequently beats up younger children, is defiant at home, and is failing at school).
30 | 21	**Behavior is considerably influenced by delusions or hallucinations OR serious impairment in communication or judgment** (e.g., sometimes incoherent, acts grossly inappropriately, suicidal preoccupation) **OR inability to function in almost all areas** (e.g., stays in bed all day; no job, home, or friends).
20 | 11	**Some danger of hurting self or others** (e.g., suicide attempts without clear expectation of death; frequently violent; manic excitement) **OR occasionally fails to maintain minimal personal hygiene** (e.g., smears feces) **OR gross impairment in communication** (e.g., largely incoherent or mute).
10 | 1	Persistent danger of severely hurting self or others (e.g., recurrent violence) OR persistent inability to maintain minimal personal hygiene OR serious suicidal act with clear expectation of death.
0	Inadequate information.

to 100, with 10-point intervals that describe discrete levels of functioning (see Table 3.1). The GAF score can be a simple first step in determining whether STDP is an appropriate treatment for a particular patient, or whether another form of treatment would be more appropriate.

GAF Ratings above 50 Suggest STDP Is Appropriate

Ratings of 50 or above on the GAF encompass most of the criteria required for the rapid uncovering of STDP (i.e., sufficient ego strength and only moderate impairment in symptoms and/or functioning). Ratings below 50 signal the need for more supportive, ego-building, or defense-building interventions. This topic is discussed in detail below.

Selection of Treatment Is Based More on Axis V Than Axis I or Axis II

There are several reasons why we use GAF (Axis V) ratings, rather than Axis I and Axis II diagnoses, as the first step in the selection of treatment:

- This model is based on the idea that a relatively small number of Affect Phobias (conflicted feelings) give rise to a broad range of defenses and symptoms. Thus Affect Phobias represent the psychological underpinnings of many Axis I and Axis II diagnoses, together with whatever biological contributions are present (to be discussed below). Although diagnoses are important considerations in treatment, diagnostic criteria are seen as surface manifestations or symptoms of underlying Affect Phobias. STDP is designed to focus on these Affect Phobias as a means of resolving diagnostic symptomatology and other problems.
- Diagnoses can occur across a wide range of levels of functioning and capacities to respond to treatment. Some patients may be incapacitated by major depressive disorder, while others may have coping mechanisms that allow them to continue to function even while experiencing significant emotional pain. In a similar way, some patients with Axis I and/or Axis II diagnoses have the resilience to benefit from STDP, while others may not.
- Although DSM-IV diagnoses tend to be presented as discrete entities, and disorder-specific treatment is a popular concept, actually it is rare for a patient to have a **single** Axis I or Axis II diagnosis, or to have Axis II criteria that fall entirely within a single disorder or even a single diagnostic cluster. It is more common for patients to present with a complex and unique mixture of diagnoses and traits.

A Biopsychosocial Model: Nature and Nurture Combined

In the discussion of diagnoses, it is important to take into consideration the issue of biological contributions. This treatment model is entirely compatible with a holistic biopsychosocial framework, which views problems as resulting from a combination of biological, environmental, interpersonal, and psychological factors.

Multiple Interventions Advocated

One individual may have a family history of depression, learned helplessness due to societal discrimination, and intrapsychic conflict about anger/assertion as a function of parental injunctions. And just as problems may have several contributing factors, a number of interventions may prove helpful, individually or in combination. For depression, medication, coping skills, **and** psychodynamic exploration can all be useful.

Biology and Learning Intertwined

In this model, Axis I symptoms with biological underpinnings can often be viewed simultaneously as defensive patterns. DSM disorders are not only biologically predisposed, but also reflect what is learned and conditioned through life experience; for example, genetic makeup and learned helplessness both contribute to a mood disorder such as depression. During development, any individual who is repeatedly ignored, neglected, abused, or shamed would tend to suppress such natural responses as speaking up, asking for help, being curious about things, and so on. This blocking of adaptive responses often results in feeling depressed, "down," or "blue." Of course, some people are genetically predisposed to develop major depression, but the environment can also trigger that vulnerability.

All behavior is ultimately rooted in biology, but patients' problems reflect the interaction of the genetic makeup with learned behavior. Nobel Prize winner Eric Kandel (1998) has written,

> Just as combinations of genes contribute to behavior, including social behavior, so can behavior and social factors exert actions on the brain by feeding back upon it to modify the expression of genes and thus the function of nerve cells. Learning, including learning that results in dysfunctional behavior, produces alterations in gene expression. Thus all of "nurture" is ultimately expressed as "nature." (p. 460)

As recent brain imaging studies have shown (e.g., Baxter, 1995), psychotherapeutic change, a form of nurture or new learning, leads to new neuronal connections or structural changes in the brain. In the end, it is not nature "versus" nurture, but a combination of both.

Summary

In summary, in determining how to proceed with treatment, we have found the following principles useful:

- The GAF is the most helpful part of the DSM multiaxial assessment in guiding the **initial** broad form of treatment selection—that is, exploratory (Defense and Affect Restructuring) versus supportive (Self- and Other-Restructuring) interventions (see Section VI).
- Next, the core conflict formulation (covered in Chapter 4) teaches how to determine the core Affect Phobias. These become the focus of the treatment interventions (covered in Chapters 5–10).
- Finally, Axis I and Axis II diagnoses, with all their biopsychosocial complexities, can provide further information about components of the Affect Phobia(s) and how to work with them during treatment (as described in Chapter 11).

Because of the importance of the GAF Scale to the first step in this treatment process, the next section explains how to arrive at a GAF rating. The remainder of the chapter explains how the GAF—combined with other DSM information—can be very helpful in providing a rough guideline for

(1) whether rapid uncovering short-term work might be done; and (2) if so, how such work ought to be done.

III. HOW TO RATE THE GLOBAL ASSESSMENT OF FUNCTIONING (GAF) SCALE

When to Do a GAF Rating

The GAF rating can be made following the initial evaluation, along with preliminary DSM-IV Axis I/Axis II diagnoses and other information derived from the session. This can be done either in an unstructured interview style, or by scanning the Psychotherapy Assessment Checklist Forms (PAC-Forms) described above, which the patient fills out prior to the first session in order to provide an overview of diagnostic and functioning information.

Two GAF Ratings Given: Current and Past Year

Generally, a therapist makes two GAF ratings: one for a patient's current level of functioning, and one for the past year. For example, if a patient is functioning very well today, but was hospitalized for a suicide attempt or substance misuse in the past few months, the current GAF rating would not be stable enough to guide treatment decisions. Therefore, one would also consider the patient's GAF rating for the previous year to decide how best to treat the patient.

To arrive at a GAF rating, it helps to think about three separate areas: **psychological functioning** (i.e., symptoms), **social functioning**, and **occupational functioning**. Here are some questions that can help you assess these areas.

Questions for Determining the GAF Rating

Psychological Functioning

Consider the severity of the patient's symptoms (incapacitating vs. absent or minimal):

- Are there problems with addictions or impulse control? (Below 50)
- Is absence of symptoms due to medication or other supports?
- Have there been prior hospitalizations or suicide attempts?

Social Functioning

Consider the patient's degree of connection to others and satisfaction with it. Also consider factors that indicate trust in others—a crucial capacity for patients in a short-term exploratory process.

- Is there at least one close, give-and-take interpersonal relationship? (Above 50)
- Is there evidence of being able to interact flexibly with the therapist?
- Is the patient able to give and receive praise and criticism?

Occupational Functioning

Consider the patient's level of satisfaction at work or school:

- Is there interest and enthusiasm, or boredom and lack of interest?
- Have there been repeated firings or conflicts, serious difficulty obtaining or maintaining employment, or completing tasks?

Other Helpful Questions: Best and Worst Times

In addition to the questions above, here are a few questions that can help in quickly determining a GAF score, and that also elicit a great deal of important historical information (overall life functioning, strengths and vulnerabilities, suicide attempts, hospitalizations, object relatedness, etc.). These questions provide a broad overview of the patient's best and worst experiences, and will contribute to a more sound GAF rating.

1. "What were the worst times in your life?"
2. "In those moments, who helped?"

Did the patient go through crisis alone, or was he or she able to reach out and ask for help, and/or receive the help or solace that was offered?

3. "What were the best times in your life? When were you most proud?"
4. "With whom did you share these times?"

Could the patient feel proud or receive praise comfortably? or did the patient reject praise and affirmation, leaving him or her isolated?

Finding the 10-Point Interval

After the historical information has been gathered, the patient should be placed in the appropriate 10-point interval on the GAF Scale (see Table 3.1). To do this, find separate 10-point intervals for psychological, social, and occupational functioning. To select the interval for each area, it can help to read the descriptions of the intervals above and below the one you have selected, and compare the patient's functioning with the descriptions offered.

Once the 10-point intervals have each been identified for psychological, social, and occupational functioning, the **lowest** of these three intervals is the one in which the patient's overall GAF rating falls. For example, one patient has a satisfying job (occupational functioning rated 71–80), but has chronic conflicts with significant others (social functioning rated at 51–60), and has major depressive disorder with vegetative signs (psychological symptom functioning rated at 41–50). In this case, the GAF score would fall in the 41–50 range, the lowest of the subscale ratings.

An important exception to the rule that the GAF score falls in the lowest of the three subscale ratings is that serious impairment (41–50) in **several** ar-

TABLE 3.2. Interventions on the Exploratory–Supportive Continuum

Exploratory/expressive	Supportive
Uncovering, confrontation, interpretation	Validation, praise, advice, reassurance
Breaking down defenses, experiencing intense affect	Building defenses, teaching about feeling
Bringing painful things into consciousness	Building social supports and coping skills
THERAPIST: Your difficulty with men seems to stem from sexual feelings toward your father. Could we explore that further?	THERAPIST: Your difficulty with men seems to cause you much pain. Can we talk about what is uncomfortable for you, and find some ways to help you cope with these situations?

eas moves the overall score down to 31–40, and inability to function in **almost all** areas moves the overall score to 21–30.

Locating the Patient within the 10-Point Interval

Once you have found the 10-point interval that most accurately describes the patient being rated, you must find where within that 10-point interval the patient falls. The interval descriptions on the GAF Scale (Table 3.1) were designed to fit someone whose functioning falls in the middle of the scale.

For example, on the GAF, the description for the 51–60 range best fits a 54–56 rating. Think of higher ratings within the interval as being in the top third (57–60) and representing functioning that is somewhat better than described, but not as good as functioning in the interval above (61–70). The bottom third of the interval (51–53) represents functioning that is somewhat worse than described for that interval, but not as impaired as functioning in the interval below (41–50).

Of course, it is impossible to give an exact numerical rating. Distinctions among, say, 51, 52, or 53 are likely to be subjective. Your goal should be to try to give a rating that would agree with other raters within 5–10 points.

To place a patient within a 10-point interval, it can help (as noted above) to examine the intervals above and below the interval selected. For example, if a patient has mild impairment in all three areas of functioning (in the 60s), then examine the 70s and the 50s to see which interval more closely resembles the functioning of this patient. If the category description seems to fit your patient very well, then give a score in the middle of the scale—in this case, 65. If functioning shares characteristics with the higher category, then consider scores in the high 60s. If functioning is closer to the lower category, then consider scores in the low 60s.

What If a Patient Is "All over the Scale"?

A trainee just learning to rate the GAF Scale often complains, "I can't give a GAF rating. My patient is all over the scale—symptoms are in the 40s, social functioning is in the 50s, and job functioning is in the 70s."

A wide variation in ratings is not unusual. **The way to rate patients with wide variations in scores is to remember that the GAF rating is the lowest of the three scores.** In the case described here, the symptoms would determine the GAF rating (e.g., depression with suicidal ideation is in the 41–50 range). Then the rater would have to determine where within the 40s the patient falls. The fact that the patient is able to work—and has some, if conflicted, relationships—shows that patients has the strength to cope, even with severe symptoms. For this reason, the rating would probably be in the high 40s (say 46–49).

Sometimes a patient has strong interpersonal connections (above 70), moderate symptoms (61–70), and a moderate to serious impairment in work functioning (51–60). This patient would receive a GAF in the 51–60 range due to the job performance. However, the ratings in the social and symptom categories still provide valuable information for STDP. It is a positive prognostic sign when there are strong interpersonal connections, and when symptoms are not severe. This shows that the patient has areas of strength to help deal with the job problems, and may be able to better handle an in-depth therapy than patients who have all three ratings in the 51–60 range.

IV. INDICATIONS AND CONTRAINDICATIONS FOR SHORT-TERM DYNAMIC PSYCHOTHERAPY

GAF Rating Guides STDP

The treatment interventions described in this manual were originally developed for patients with Cluster C personality disorders, mood disorders, and anxiety disorders, who demonstrate a moderate or better GAF rating (above 50), but not a severe or incapacitating (50 or below) level of functioning (Winston et al., 1991).

Indications for STDP

A rating of 50 on the GAF Scale is used as a rough cutoff for providing A rapid, focused short-term treatment such as STDP to patients. Patients who respond best to Defense and Affect Restructuring and can tolerate desensitization of Affect Phobias have, at a minimum, the following characteristics:

• Moderate level of overall functioning.

- A few friends, but conflicts in relationships.
- Ability to hold a job, but occupational conflicts and dissatisfaction.
- Moderate difficulty with symptoms, but not incapacitated.

This profile describes typical patients for whom STDP was initially designed: moderately impaired individuals with Cluster C personality disorders.

As we discuss below, the closer the GAF score is to 50 or below, the more supportive interventions and/or Self- and Other-Restructuring will be called for. The higher the GAF score, the more rapidly the therapist can offer "deep" interpretations and begin to desensitize conflicted emotions with Defense and Affect Restructuring.

It is important to note that even when rapid uncovering is contraindicated, the Affect Phobia schema can be extremely useful in guiding a more supportive treatment in ways that will foster a patient's growth.

Contraindications for STDP: Treatment Modifications for Patients with GAF Scores below 50 and Other Factors

We do not recommend that therapists proceed with uncovering of affect (Defense and Affect Restructuring) with patients whose GAF ratings fall below 50, and who have the following characteristics:

- No friends.
- Severe difficulties in day-to-day functioning.
- Inability to contain affect well enough to control addictions or aggressive impulses.

Such individuals usually should not have their deepest rage and pain uncovered, because they may not be able to bear it. Active interventions that rapidly uncover feelings could be too overwhelming and could increase the already significant impairment or lead to acting out of destructive impulses. In such cases, restructuring the sense of self and others is indicated, not affect or defense work.

PATIENT: I have been in so much pain in the 3 weeks since coming here that I can hardly stand it. I'm having frightening dreams, and I'm so distracted at work that I'm not getting my tasks done.

THERAPIST: Then we need to slow down what we're doing, so that it doesn't interfere too seriously with your daily living. Therapy can be painful and difficult at times, but it should not have to cause you this degree of stress. Tell me what were the most difficult parts of the past weeks, and let's see if we can work together to help you feel stabilized.

In addition to a GAF score below 50, several other factors are contraindications for STDP:

- Poor impulse control.
- Low motivation.
- Severe stressors.
- Lack of psychological-mindedness.

Here is a brief discussion of these four important areas to consider in your patients.

Disturbances of Impulse Control

STDP is contraindicated for patients with disturbances of impulse control until the behaviors have been well under control for 1–3 years. Individuals with substance use disorders, acting out, eating disorders, aggressive outbursts, or the like will have GAF ratings below 50. Listen carefully for indicators of such problems, because patients often minimize or deny problems related to these areas. Moreover, rapid uncovering of strong feelings can actually lead to an increase in substance misuse and other impulsive behaviors.

PATIENT: I was so upset when I left here last week that I really needed a drink. I haven't been like this in 2 years.

THERAPIST: I'm so glad you could tell me that . . . it's signaling that maybe we need to slow down, because starting to drink again is the last thing you need. Can you tell me what it was that has been so uncomfortable for you?

Low Motivation

When patient motivation is low or absent, either treatment should not be attempted, or the **only** focus of therapy should be building the patient's motivation for treatment. Here are some ways to assess degree of motivation:

- Did the individual seek treatment, or was it mandated by others or the law?
- Is there recognition that there is a problem?
- Is there interest in changing the problem?

Example 1: A 13-year-old student only comes to therapy because he is offered the choice between therapy or expulsion following his second incident involving cheating. (Low motivation)

Example 2: A lawyer enters therapy to work on his problems with intimacy in an effort to reconcile with his wife, from whom he is currently estranged and whom he very much wants back. (High motivation)

Severe Life Stressors

High levels of stress in a patient's life (such as illness or legal battles) can make it difficult to engage in a rapid uncovering process of short-term treatment.

PATIENT: I want to get to the root of the problems related to my mother's abandoning me.

THERAPIST: Let's remember that tomorrow you have to be in divorce court. Why don't we focus on how prepared you feel for that? We can look at these more painful and deeper issues when the court case is over.

Lack of Psychological-Mindedness

When psychological-mindedness is absent, and the patient has no desire to acquire it, then consider such alternatives as behavioral, cognitive, or interpersonal therapies.

Example: A university professor enters therapy due to difficulty maintaining intimate relationships. When he is asked his goals for therapy, the following exchange ensues:

PATIENT: Don't waste my time asking me questions about my mother. I just want to know how I can keep a girlfriend for longer than a month.

THERAPIST: It seems like you don't see much of a connection between your relationship with your mother and your girlfriends.

PATIENT: No, I don't, and I'm sick of you therapists trying to tell me there is one.

V. USING THE GAF SCALE TO TAILOR TREATMENT TO PATIENTS' NEEDS

As noted in the preceding section, the first signal that STDP may be appropriate is a GAF rating over 50. This section looks at how the GAF Scale can be used to guide treatment decisions in a more finely tuned way.

Five GAF Intervals Guide Use of Treatment Objectives

The GAF Scale can be helpful in determining which of the STDP treatment objectives to use. Higher GAF ratings are indicators for Defense Restructuring and Affect Restructuring, and lower GAF ratings call for Self- and Other-Restructuring (see Section IV of Chapter 2). We have found that five rough intervals of GAF ratings can give therapists some quick clues about what type of treatment might be indicated for patients within each interval. Of course, these are not rigid categories, just guidelines to assist in treatment decisions.

GAF 81–100: High-Functioning Individuals

The highest GAF category reflects good to superior functioning, with symptoms that are absent or minimal. Such individuals have many strengths to draw upon. They have few if any symptoms, and experience joy, satisfaction, and competence in work and relationships. They have a wide range of interests, and are generative with and respected by others as leaders or role models. This high level of functioning can represent a standard to work toward in treatment. Such people rarely seek therapy, but when they do, they can be treated similarly to those in the 71–80 range.

GAF 71–80: Moderately Well- Functioning Individuals

The second GAF category reflects transient or expectable symptoms, and fewer positive traits than those described above for high-functioning persons. Often patients in this range or above have some awareness of their defenses, so the therapist can start with or move quickly to Affect Restructuring (Chapters 7 and 8), often with rapid change.

PATIENT: I hate being evasive [D] every time I am with a man [C]. I want to stop it.

THERAPIST: So let's look at the feelings [F] that come up in those situations.

Although some individuals rated above 70 may seek treatment for psychological problems, most outpatients will fall in the next two categories, with GAF ratings between 41–50 and 51–70.

GAF 51–70: Outpatients with Mild or Moderate Impairment

The next GAF interval is the category of typical STDP patients: It involves mild to moderate but long-standing character pathology, and moderate impairment in social and occupational functioning. Such an individual is able to work and does have relationships. However, there are conflicts in these areas or symptoms that are problematic but do not impair functioning. With such patients, the therapist generally needs to begin with Defense Restructuring—identifying defenses and assessing motivation to give them up (see Chapters 5 and 6)—and then to evaluate how the patient responds before proceeding to Affect Restructuring.

PATIENT: I have trouble with men [D—vague] and I don't know why.

THERAPIST: Let's look at how you react [exploring conflict] when you're with them. Can you give me a specific example?

In addition, patients at the 51–70 GAF level often have problems with sense of self. In such cases, we find that including Self- and Other-Restructuring can greatly assist the patient's ability to proceed with Defense Restructuring, and later, Affect Restructuring. Medication may also be provided if functioning is compromised or symptoms are burdensome.

PATIENT: When you point out all the ways I avoid my feelings, I feel so stupid!

THERAPIST: Then, before proceeding, let's help you become more compassionate toward yourself. Don't you think most people do things to avoid feeling? [Normalizing to reduce shame]

GAF 41–50: Outpatients with Severe Impairment in Functioning

Patients in the next category have numerous impairing symptoms, but generally are able to maintain outpatient status. They may have difficulty functioning, difficulty keeping a job, have no close friends, and struggle with substance misuse and/or other severe impulsivity.

Such patients already have difficulty maintaining stability. Confronting their defenses or their deepest and rawest emotions in outpatient treatment could be destabilizing (see Section IV, above), so they are not candidates for a rapid uncovering short-term therapy. However, focusing on Self- and Other-Restructuring (Chapters 9 and 10) can often help patients in this GAF range to develop a more adaptive sense of self and others; this has the potential to develop their capacity to tolerate confronting defenses against deep feeling. In such cases, therapy requires a longer time, because so much needs to be built (e.g., self-structure, better connections) before conflicted feelings can be uncovered. Specifically, the therapist can focus on (1) empathically helping such patients see and give up self-destructive or masochistic behaviors, and (2) helping the patients build better images of self and others.

PATIENT: I don't think I can have a relationship with a man. I never want to [D] let someone close [F] enough to find out what a loser I am [D].

THERAPIST: Why don't we look at how you feel about yourself, and how that is hurting you?

In addition, for these patients with GAF ratings below 50, therapists generally should focus on supportive interventions and building coping skills rather than on uncovering and removing defenses, as in standard STDP. Medication should also be strongly considered in this severe range of functioning, as many of the major Axis I disorders (e.g., bipolar I disorder, schizophrenia, severe attention-deficit/hyperactivity disorder) will be more responsive to pharmacological intervention than to psychotherapy.

GAF 1–40: Patients with Severe or Incapacitating Impairment

Patients in the last category often require inpatient treatment or other supervised environments: hospitalization (generally below 40), structured living (31–40), or custodial care (1–10 or 11–20). Patients at these levels need not only support, but also observation, medication, and training in daily living and social skills.

Treatment Objectives Are Interwoven, Not Sequential

Although we have offered suggestions for when to focus on the different objectives, Defense Restructuring, Affect Restructuring, and Self- and Other-Restructuring **do not** need to be dealt with in isolation, or in a fixed linear sequence. They represent parallel strands to be woven together in proportion to each patient's needs and as called for throughout the treatment process.

Self- and Other-Restructuring Mixed with Affect Restructuring

It is important to keep in mind that Self- and Other-Restructuring is not restricted to more impaired patients. As noted above, even higher-functioning patients can need some Self- and Other-Restructuring to be intermingled with Affect Restructuring.

PATIENT: It's so hard to talk about these sexual feelings. [Affect Experiencing of sexual feelings had been going on for 10–15 minutes.]

THERAPIST: What's the hardest part for you? [Anxiety regulation]

PATIENT: I keep wondering if you think I'm perverted or strange.

THERAPIST: Let's take a few minutes to talk about this before proceeding. You need to feel safe with me when you discuss such personal things. What do you think I might be feeling about you? [Self- and Other-Restructuring]

Often there will be some combination of the objectives:

THERAPIST: Do you notice that when you reach the deepest feelings [F] about your mother, you tend to pull back [D]? I wonder if you can stay focused on the feeling a little longer. [Defense Restructuring, response prevention, and moving toward Affect Restructuring]

But sometimes the focus of the objectives will be based on what the patient presents:

PATIENT: Whenever you encourage me to get angry [F], I am terrified it means I'm a violent person [A].

THERAPIST: Let's see what makes you feel so terrified. [Anxiety regulation] Treatment should not make you feel worse about yourself. [The therapist is beginning Self-Restructuring.] Later we can try some anger work again to see if you can tolerate it better. [Affect Restructuring is put off for the moment until the patient's sense of self is better able to bear the feelings.] How is it that an inner feeling makes you a bad person? Is it how a person **feels** that makes them a violent person, or is it what they **do**? We're not talking about acting on any of these feelings; we're talking about just letting yourself have them.

Objectives Can Be Used in Short-Term or Long-Term Treatment

In conclusion, these objectives help to guide short-term treatment when a patient is not seriously impaired, but they are also helpful in longer-term treatment when patient impairment necessitates it. The therapist is free to focus on whatever objective seems the most helpful to the patient at the time. Again, there are guidelines, but there is no hard and fast rule.

A Dream: Intensive STDP in Inpatient Settings

For patients with GAF ratings below 40, rapid uncovering work may be possible only in a structured and supportive environment such as an inpatient setting, with a highly trained staff. It is our dream to be able to do in-depth exploratory therapy in such settings. In environments that provide ample supports, inpatients may have the potential to restructure character disorders through intensive work on Defense, Affect, and Self- and Other-Restructuring in relatively short amounts of time. Of course, the intensive uncovering would need to be paired with strong outpatient aftercare to help these patients maintain the gains and continue the emotional growth. Indeed, this approach is being pursued in some hospitals around the country at the grassroots level, but it needs research and study to be implemented wisely and well. (For disorder-specific applications for treatment, see Chapter 11 of this book and CC, Chs. 10 and 11.)

VI. THE SUPPORTIVE–EXPLORATORY CONTINUUM OF INTERVENTIONS

The GAF Scale: A Flexible Guideline for How to Intervene

According to Luborsky's (1984) **supportive–exploratory continuum**, as a general rule, the higher the patient's level of functioning on the GAF Scale, the more one can employ expressive or exploratory interventions. The lower the patient's GAF score, the more one must employ supportive interventions. As we have emphasized above, these general principles are not meant to be laws of nature, but flexible guidelines. Therapists should rely on clinical judgment and intuition to treat each patient, assisted by data such as the GAF rating.

The Supportive– Exploratory Continuum

People often make a false dichotomy between supportive and exploratory (or expressive) interventions. We want to underscore that these two forms of interventions represent two ends of a continuum, as described by Luborsky (1984). The issue is not to choose one or the other, but **a relative proportion** of supportive and exploratory interventions. There is generally no sharp line between the two, and often the best interventions artfully combine both elements.

Defense and Affect Restructuring Are More Exploratory

For better-functioning individuals (scoring above 50 on the GAF Scale), the more exploratory interventions can be used to challenge defenses and rapidly uncover conflicted affects. This fits with the treatment objectives of Defense and Affect Restructuring. However, it is important to remember that in our treatment model, supportive techniques are always used to assist the uncovering process. As the Affect Phobias are being desensitized, supportive interventions are included to strengthen the alliance and to help regulate the anxiety resulting from the exposure.

Self- and Other-Restructuring Is More Supportive

For more impaired individuals (with scores below 50 on the GAF Scale), more supportive interventions are used to help keep anxiety within bearable limits. Self- and Other-Restructuring can also be used to build self-esteem and better relationships (see Chapters 9 and 10). However, occasional exploratory interventions—such as those used in Defense Restructuring (Chapters 5 and 6)—can help such patients recognize self-attacking, self-destructive, or masochistic behaviors. If such interventions are done very gently and compassionately, they can often be very helpful for more impaired patients.

Table 3.2 describes various types of interventions that fall toward each end of the supportive–exploratory continuum.

Examples of the Supportive–Exploratory Continuum for Each GAF Interval

The following therapist statements at each end of the continuum may be used separately or in combination with each other. Often treatment works well with a blending of exploratory and supportive comments.

GAF above 50: Defense Restructuring and Affect Restructuring Are Indicated

At GAF levels above 50, therapist interventions are intended primarily to confront defenses and uncover affects.

More Exploratory Interventions	More Supportive Interventions
"Do you see how you change the subject when we discuss your mother's death?"	"It is probably very painful to face these feelings, but you have shown me that you have the strength to do so. Do you think you could continue?"
"Each time we look at anger, you become tearful and withdrawn. I wonder if you could let the anger surface."	"People often learn in childhood to withdraw, and it leads to a lot of problems. No wonder you're having difficulty now. But I wonder if you can let the anger surface now?"
"When you look at me, you tend to look away very quickly. Can we look at the feelings here between us?"	"It's natural for all kinds of feelings to come up—but sometimes it's difficult, isn't it? Therapy can move a lot faster if we can look at all of them."
"When we talk about sexual feelings, you tend to change the subject. Could you try to stay on this focus a little longer?"	"It seems like it's very upsetting for you to talk about sexual feelings. It's very hard to speak openly about such private matters, but this is a safe place to do so."

GAF below 50: Self- and Other-Restructuring Is Indicated

At GAF levels below 50, therapist interventions are intended to build defenses and bolster patients' sense of self and others. Defense Restructuring is used only to point out self-attacking behaviors; Affect Restructuring is used only to focus on self-care or self-compassion.

More Exploratory Interventions	More Supportive Interventions
"Often you become weepy and withdrawn when someone confronts you. I wonder what you might do instead?"	"Withdrawing is probably something you learned to do to protect yourself as a child."
"You are awfully hard on yourself. Why do you think you give yourself such a hard time?"	"I know it can be difficult when I point out things here, but I do not want you to feel criticized. There are good reasons why you do this. We need to understand it."
"When you have become anxious in groups of people, what have you done that helps calm yourself down?"	"Sometimes it can help to talk about the anxiety, so you can learn how to cope with it."
"How are you feeling about coming to therapy today? Do you feel comfortable here with me?"	"It takes time to be comfortable with someone and we'll proceed slowly until you feel safe with me."

Summary: General GAF Guidelines for Treatment

The list below summarizes the general guidelines for the types of treatment interventions that are typically considered (but not dictated) on this supportive–exploratory continuum at various ranges of functioning. In general, higher GAF scores and more exploratory methods imply shorter-term treatments; lower GAF scores and supportive methods imply longer-term treatments.

- GAF above 70: Emphasis on Affect Restructuring (predominance of exploratory/expressive interventions).
- GAF from 50 to 70: Defense Restructuring followed by Affect Restructuring (balance of exploratory interventions) with Self- and Other-Restructuring and support as needed. Medication as needed.
- GAF below 50: Self- and Other-Restructuring, medication (predominance of cognitive and supportive interventions).
- GAF below 40: Increased support, such as residential or custodial care.

This chapter has focused on using the patient's level of functioning (as indicated by the GAF rating) to guide the selection of treatment objectives, as well as to guide **how** a therapist intervenes—that is, choosing among the three objectives, and finding the appropriate balance of supportive and exploratory interventions. (See CC, Ch. 2, for more discussion on assessment and treatment selection.) However, more evaluation and assessment are needed before the therapist proceeds with treatment. Next, in Chapter 4, we present a method for determining what core conflict or Affect Phobia to focus on. The combination of these two elements then guides the use of the specific interventions that are covered in Chapters 5–10. Chapter 11 describes how to use diagnostic information for further understanding of the Affect Phobias.

CHAPTER 3 • EXERCISES

EXERCISE 3A: MATCH THE PATIENT WITH A GAF INTERVAL

Directions: Referring to the GAF Scale in Table 3.1, assess each of the following patients and choose (1) the 10-point GAF interval in which the patient currently functions, and (2) the highest GAF interval in which the patient functioned in the previous year.

Example: A 38-year-old divorced former office manager drinks heavily on weekends, and has been socially isolated for years. He has no close friends and is estranged from family members. He had been on probation at work for conflicts with colleagues, before being fired 3 months ago. Since being fired he has been depressed, has had trouble getting out of bed, and has considered suicide, but says that he would not act on the idea. He has been fired from several jobs due to missing days.

Answer: **Specific functioning: Psychological:** _41–50_ . **Social:** _41–50_ . Occupational: _41–50_ .

   Current GAF rating: _31–40_ . GAF rating for the past year: _41–50_ .

Explanation: His depression with suicidal ideation—but no clear plan—puts him in the 41–50 category for psychological symptoms. In addition, his daily functioning is seriously impaired, and he drinks heavily on weekends. He is socially isolated, with neither friends nor family connections. His job functioning is seriously impaired because of the firing and the inability to stay employed. In addition to psychological symptoms, both social and occupational functioning are seriously impaired, and would also receive GAF ratings of 41–50.

When all three of the specific category ratings fall in the 41–50 category (indicating major or serious impairment in all areas), his GAF score would be lowered to the 31–40 range (see the description of this range in Table 3.1).

His GAF rating for the previous year is higher (41–50), based on serious impairment in two, but not three, areas (heavy drinking and social isolation). Last year he was still employed, though with conflicts (51–60 range), so he did not as yet have serious impairment in all three areas.

Exercise 3A.1.   **The Crying Daughter**

A 27-year-old environmental advocate sought therapy as a result of her mother's sudden death in a car accident 4 months ago. She typically has a very satisfying life: She loves her job, and has a strong marriage and an enjoyable social network. However, since her mother's death, she has found herself going to the bathroom at work, crying, and feeling guilty about all the things she wished she'd said to her mother. Her sleep is more restless than usual due to her feelings of guilt, but she is able to complete her work. Her husband of 2 years is very supportive, and she's been able to confide in him and in her closest friend.

Specific functioning: Psychological: ____. Social: ____. Occupational: ____.

Current GAF rating: ____. GAF rating for the past year: ____.

Exercise 3A.2.   **The Student with Suicidal Thoughts**

A 16-year-old high school student, whose mood had been generally good, has begun to feel seriously depressed. He says he cannot get thoughts of suicide out of his mind. He constantly mulls over plans for suicide, but has taken no action. He has skipped school several times in the past 2 months. In the current semester, he has dropped from his usual grade level of A's and B's to C's and D's. He has a few friends, but has never been a "joiner" or played team sports. He feels alienated from most of his classmates. There is intermittent conflict with his parents, but no drug use.

Specific functioning: Psychological: ____. Social: ____. Occupational: ____.

Current GAF rating: ____. GAF rating for the past year: ____.

Exercise 3A.3.   **The Anxious Head Nurse**

A 40-year-old gay man is a competent and well-respected head nurse of a burn unit. He has been sought as a consultant on setting up such units in other hospitals in the city. He has been in a committed and loving relationship for 12 years. He reports that he confides in his partner, and that when they have fights they are able to resolve the conflicts well. He has a wide circle of friends. He has been sober and attending Alcoholics Anonymous (AA) for 2 years, and has generally been in excellent spirits. But he currently does not have a sponsor in AA, and does not feel secure about his sobriety. He has come to therapy because in the past few months he has become increasingly worried that he'll return to drinking; this has led to intermittent panic attacks and chronic low-grade anxiety.

Specific functioning: Psychological: ____. Social: ____. Occupational: ____.

Current GAF rating: ____. GAF rating for the past year: ____.

Exercise 3A.4.   **The Irritable Stockbroker**

A 34-year-old stockbroker has been employed by the same firm for 10 years. Intermittent clashes with his supervisor throughout his job history have resulted in his being passed over for an important promotion this last year. For many years, whenever there are job stresses, it has taken him hours to fall asleep. The lack of sleep then leaves him irritable and make his workday more difficult. He has a girlfriend and a group of "buddies" he goes to sports events with. However, he says he would not confide in them about this work problem, as he has an image to keep up. His girlfriend has asked him to seek therapy due to his irritability.

Specific functioning: Psychological: ____. Social: ____. Occupational: ____.

Current GAF rating: ____. GAF rating for the past year: ____.

EXERCISE 3B: RATE THE PATIENT AND CHOOSE A PREDOMINANT INTERVENTION STYLE

Directions: For each of the following patients, rate the patient's social, psychological, and occupational functioning, and then give an overall current and past rating on the 1–100 GAF Scale. Since there is always some degree of subjectivity in a GAF rating, consider ratings that fall within 5 points of our ratings to be good agreement. Next, choose whether you would lean toward supportive or exploratory interventions in treatment.

Example: **The A Student Who Flunked an Exam**

A 20-year-old Japanese American female in her sophomore year of college was referred to treatment due to a teacher's concern that this normally straight-A student had failed an exam and was quite upset about it. In the initial evaluation, the student revealed that she had a close friend who was having thoughts of suicide and had been calling at all hours for support. Because the calls had occurred during the week of finals, she had been distracted from her studies.

The night before coming to see the counselor, the student had set firm limits with her friend and made appropriate calls to the friend's family in order to assure that her friend received help. On the initial visit, the student, although appropriately concerned about her friend, did not appear overly distressed over the incidents of the past week. In fact, as a result of taking a firm stand, she appeared to experience great relief. She chided herself gently for being the kind of person whom other students seek out to talk about their problems, and for not having set limits with her friend sooner.

A partial history revealed a student with many strengths and a generally healthy coping style, except that she tended to work quite hard and occasionally became stressed about exams or papers. In her first 2 years in college, she had already made many good friends, appeared to be thriving as a student, and was elected to the student governing board. Her other grades were all A's. She was able to do extra work to make up for the test she had failed. At a follow-up appointment 2 weeks later, the student appeared happy and content. She was then terminated from counseling.

Specific functioning: Psychological: _75_. Social: _91_. Occupational: _75_.

Current GAF rating: _75_. GAF rating for the past year: _75_.

Would you use relatively more supportive or exploratory interventions?   S (E)

Explanation: **Psychological functioning: 75.** Although the student's symptoms at the time of flunking the exam may have dipped to the 61–70 range (possibly lower), at the time of the intake she had returned to her baseline, which was marked by only "transient and expectable" stresses regarding her schoolwork. In a difficult situation, she was eventually able to set good limits and experience relief from doing so.

Social functioning: 91. She had close friends after 2 years in college and tended to be sought out by others.

Occupational functioning: 75. This student got straight A's normally. By the time of the intake she had returned to baseline, and, other than failing the one test, her overall grades were not affected by the distraction. This would be rated as in the 71–80 range—temporarily falling behind in schoolwork—because she was able to do extra work and make up for it. If the failed test had had a more negative impact on her grades, she could also have been rated for a mild problem (61–70 range).

Current GAF rating: 75. GAF rating for the past year: 75. She was functioning at very high levels both academically and socially (probably in the 91–100 range, because she was a leader and was sought out by others). However, her occasional stress and overwork would place her symptoms in the middle of the 71–80 range ("transient and expectable" stresses regarding her schoolwork). The GAF score for the past year would be the lowest of the three category ratings (75), even though her social and occupational scores would be much higher.

Would you use relatively more exploratory or supportive interventions? If treatment were necessary, exploratory interventions would be indicated, because her level of functioning was well above 50. However, the patient returned to her normal high level of functioning between the initial evaluation and the second session, and was no longer distressed. She felt that she understood what had happened, and that she could handle such a situation better the next time. Therefore, treatment was not continued, with the understanding that she could return if she experienced further distress.

Exercise 3B.1

The Divorced Secretary

A divorced 39-year-old female with two children (ages 16 and 6) from different marriages has sought therapy after ending a 2-year relationship with a successful businessman, whom she found to be unfaithful to her. The patient is depressed and describes herself as extremely angry at herself for trusting this man. Twice married to passive, alcoholic men, she believed that this latest boyfriend represented a "different kind of man." In fact, in many ways this relationship did seem more stable and loving than her previous relationships, with fewer conflicts and greater communication. However, discovering that he was unfaithful to her and dishonest in his representation of his commitment to her has been "proof" to her that she does not deserve to have someone in her life who is reliable and successful.

The patient has supported herself and her children by working long hours and overtime, with almost no financial help from either husband. In the past 4 years she has put herself through a community college, found work, and for the first time is able to sustain herself and her family comfortably with only one full-time income. She prides herself on her reliability with money, her sense of organization, her work ethic, and the fact that she has recently become a homeowner for the first time. Although she has had great difficulty functioning for the past month due to the depression she is experiencing over the loss of this relationship, she has not missed a day of work in 2 years.

As a mother she can be overly strict and inflexible with her children, at times lashing out at them when under stress, but overall she is a very committed and loving parent. She has no contact with any of her relatives, including her mother and father, who both live within an hour of her. She has developed a small but close group of friends with whom she socializes. Still, she feels very isolated and longs for the sense of family and belonging that she has never had.

Since being rejected by her latest boyfriend, she has experienced intense rage— which she quickly turns on herself, berating herself for trusting someone this much. She questions her own values and choices in the face of a world that she experiences as corrupt and untrustworthy. She has not acted out physically and has no suicidal ideation.

Specific functioning: Psychological: ___. Social: ___. Occupational: ___.

Current GAF rating: ___. GAF rating for the past year: ___.

**Would you use relatively more supportive or exploratory   S   E
    interventions?**

Exercise 3B.2.   **The Estranged Architect**

The patient is a 56-year-old unemployed architect who has been referred by her day hospital for therapy because of severe depression that has impaired her functioning. She has been nonresponsive to a series of antidepressant medications. Although she once functioned adequately as an architect, she became increasingly unable to complete her work over the past 5 years, and was let go from her firm. She has been living at a friend's house since the bank foreclosed on her house last year. The social worker in the day hospital wants her to complete some paperwork so that she can continue to receive health benefits, but the patient "can't find the papers." In the past few weeks, she has become more slovenly in appearance. She does not appear to be taking regular baths and lately eats only with much encouragement from her friend. She is estranged from her daughter and two grandchildren, and refuses to call them for help. The social worker has tried phoning the daughter, but reports that she refuses to answer his calls. The patient's relationship with her friend appears positive, but she has no other meaningful social contacts.

Specific functioning: Psychological: ___. Social: ___. Occupational: ___.

Current GAF rating: ___. GAF rating for the past year: ___.

**Would you use relatively more supportive or exploratory   S   E
    interventions?**

Exercise 3B.3.   **The Depressed Engineer**

This 36-year-old engineering student has come to therapy with depression following the breakup of a 1-year relationship. He has a history of drug abuse (marijuana and cocaine) with a few years' abstinence. His ex-girlfriend broke off the relationship suddenly, saying that she was tired of the fact that he did not have the time or money to do a lot of the things that she wanted to do. Four months after the breakup, he obsesses about things he might have done to make the relationship successful, despite evidence that he had always worked much harder than she to make the relationship work.

He believes that his ex-girlfriend is right in not wanting to continue with him. He comes from a family of very high achievers and is the only one in his family without a successful professional career. The fact that he has managed to turn his life around in the past four years—stopping drugs, and succeeding as a student in a very competitive program while working a full-time job—does nothing to dissuade him from feeling that he is a failure. Currently he feels overwhelmed with the pressures of school and work. There has been no change in his work performance, but he is "falling slightly behind" in school. His energy level is poor, and his feelings of sadness are quite intense; he often feels as though he will break out in tears. Well liked by both professors and peers, he still feels like a loner who must put on a cheerful face to the world, so that people will not be "brought down" by his pervasive sadness.

Although he claims not to have had any recent impulses to use drugs, he has begun to attend weekly Narcotics Anonymous meetings, realizing that the pressures he is under could make him vulnerable to relapse.

Specific functioning: Psychological: ___. Social: ___. Occupational: ___.

Current GAF rating: ___. GAF rating for the past year: ___.

**Would you use relatively more supportive or exploratory   S   E
     interventions?**

How to Formulate a Core Psychodynamic Conflict: Spotting Affect Phobias

Chapter Objectives   To show how to formulate an Affect Phobia or core psychodynamic conflict efficiently, in order to (1) focus treatment and (2) guide the patient toward resolving phobias about feelings.

Therapist Stance   Collaborator in the discovery of Affect Phobia patterns.

Anxiety Regulation   Awareness of the pain and anxiety associated with the Affect Phobia.

Topics Covered
- I. An Overview of the Formulation Process
- II. Identifying Defenses: How Adaptive Feelings are Avoided
- III. Identifying the Adaptive Activating Feelings: What Feelings Are Feared and Avoided
- IV. Identifying Anxieties/Inhibitions: The Reason Why Adaptive Feelings Are Avoided
- V. Summarizing the Formulation in Terms of Affect Phobia
- VI. Examples of How to Formulate Core Conflicts
- VII. Identifying Pitfalls in Making Formulations
- VIII. Repetition to Revise and Refine the Formulation

I. AN OVERVIEW OF THE FORMULATION PROCESS

As described at the beginning of Chapter 3, the initial evaluation process for Short-Term Dynamic Psychotherapy (STDP) includes four tasks, generally carried out over the first 3 hours of therapy. Chapter 3 has covered the determination of the patient's Global Assessment of Functioning (GAF) score and diagnosis. This chapter explains how to formulate the patient's core psychodynamic conflicts, and continues the discussion of treatment se-lection begun in Chapter 3. (For a more detailed discussion of the initial evaluation, also refer to CC, pp. 358–359.)

Defining Core Conflict Formulation

The purpose of the core conflict formulation is to generate a hypothesis about the predominant Affect Phobia patterns underlying the patient's most salient problems. Formulating these core conflict patterns consists of identifying defenses, anxieties, and adaptive feelings on the Triangle of Conflict (the D, A, and F Poles), and connecting those behavior patterns to specific people on the Triangle of Person (the T, C, and P Poles). Put an-other way, a formulation explains the pattern of the main Affect Phobias, why they happen, and with whom. For example, denial (D) is an effective way to avoid grief (F), if it is too painful (A) to bear thinking about the loss of one's mother (P).

Core conflict formulation is primarily the observation and identification of what the problem is. Its purpose is to generate a hypothesis about the un-derlying Affect Phobia pattern—formulated by identifying the behaviors on the poles of the Triangle of Conflict.

It is possible for a patient to present with several problems (e.g., difficulties at work, with a spouse/partner, and with children) that all stem from a sin-gle core conflict (e.g., over anger/assertion). More typically, a patient will have two or three core conflicts that underlie a range of presenting prob-lems. The core conflicts most frequently seen in clinical practice concern only four of the eight categories of adaptive affects: assertion/anger, grief, closeness, and positive feelings toward the self.

Beginning Formulation

The therapist begins the core conflict formulation during the initial evalua-tion, by asking the patient what problems he or she wants help with. It helps to elicit two or three main problems. If the Psychotherapy Assess-ment Checklist (PAC) Forms are used (see Chapter 3), patients are asked to describe three main problems and provide ratings of severity on a 1–10 scale.

Asking for Specific Examples

Once the patient has identified a few problems, the therapist asks the pa-tient to describe a **specific example** of the problem he or she wants help with. For example, if the patient wants help with a speaking phobia, the therapist must ask for a specific incident, not generalities:

THERAPIST: Could you describe the last time you froze and were unable to speak?

PATIENT: Last week sometime. I just blanked out.

THERAPIST: Could you describe the specific incident?

PATIENT: I think it was last Friday morning in my office. My client [C] walked in unannounced and I couldn't think of anything to say [D].

THERAPIST: At that moment, what were you feeling toward your client?

Only through specific examples, including specific persons, can the patient effectively reach into experience and access affect. It is not enough to hear the patient say, for instance, "I have trouble with men." The therapist needs to elicit: "When Dan touched me last night, I couldn't respond."

Using the Triangle of Conflict

As you listen to patients describe specific examples of their problems, use the Triangle of Conflict to guide your questions and organize your thinking. The affect being avoided is often unconscious (outside of a patient's awareness), so it can be easier to begin by identifying the defenses that can be seen in the more clearly visible symptoms and maladaptive problems presented by the patient. Also bear in mind that while there are many, many different defenses, there are only a few activating affects, and even fewer inhibitory affects (see Section III of Chapter 1).

Formulating a core psychodynamic conflict is challenging, but it does not have to be a daunting process. Ask yourself these simple questions about patient behaviors to help identify each pole of the Triangle of Conflict:

Questions for Identifying the Poles

1. **How** is an adaptive feeling avoided ? (D)
2. **What** is the activating feeling that is being avoided? (F)
3. **Why** is that feeling being avoided? What is the excessive inhibitory affect? (A)

Figure 4.1 shows the Triangle of Conflict, together with several questions at each pole—each from a different perspective. Sometimes questioning a patient from different angles can help a therapist better understand the underlying Affect Phobia patterns.

Formulating an Affect Phobia Narrative

The preliminary answers to the three questions above can then be formulated into a narrative of the patient's conflict. The formulation is presented to the patient as a suggestion that the problems or defenses (D) lie in fear (A) of a specific feeling (F). Put another way, anxieties (A) linked to the feeling (F) arouse the defenses (D), causing the patient to avoid the conflict. The therapist then shares this preliminary formulation with the patient to check its accuracy.

Therapist Stance: Collaborating with the Patient

The therapist and patient become collaborators from the outset in discovering the maladaptive patterns underlying the patient's presenting problems. The therapist tentatively constructs hypotheses about the conflict patterns, yet does not consider them valid until corroboration by the patient.

THERAPIST: You've said that you gave your mother [P] the silent treatment [D] because you knew it would just get worse [A] if you told her you were mad [F].

IDENTIFY DEFENSES

The Phobic Avoidance Reaction

What is the maladaptive response?

How is the response "self-protective?"

[What **anxiety** would emerge if the patient **did not defend**, but tried to experience the **adaptive affect**?]

How is adaptive feeling avoided?

IDENTIFY ANXIETIES (Inhibitory Affects)

The Cause of the Phobia

What's the reason for the maladaptive response?

How is the response self-attacking?

Why is the adaptive feeling avoided?

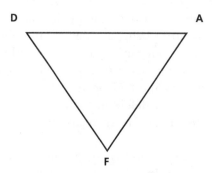

IDENTIFY THE ADAPTIVE FEELING

The Phobic (Feared) Feeling

What Feelings are being avoided?

What would be an adaptive response?

What feeling would motivate the person to act adaptively?

What response would be nurturant, self-caring, or self-soothing?

SUM UP THE FORMULATION

Put together all three poles of the Triangle of Conflict:

What *feeling* is feared, **how** is it avoided, and **why**?

FIGURE 4.1. Four steps of core conflict formulation.

PATIENT: Well, not exactly. It wouldn't get worse [A- possibly suggested anxiety]. I just felt like she was so fragile I would destroy her [A-guilt].

THERAPIST: In that case, it sounds like you weren't so scared [A] about her attacking you, but guilty [A] about hurting her. [Determining the type of inhibition]

PATIENT: Yeah, that's right.

Regulating the Patient's Anxiety

The process of formulating core conflicts (identifying the main Affect Phobias) will raise patient anxieties and emotional pain. From this initial evaluation to termination, the therapist must always use the patient's pain and anxiety level as the barometer to guide the pace of therapy. The therapist needs to pay careful attention to the patient response to each intervention, to make sure that the patient's discomfort level does not become so high that it will sensitize (rather than desensitize) the conflict, or otherwise jeopardize treatment. As discussed in Chapter 3, anxiety can be regulated through appropriate supportive interventions. For example, during the initial evaluation, it can be particularly effective for the therapist to express awareness of the patient's pain stemming from the Affect Phobia.

THERAPIST: You said you feared coming here all week. What could happen here that would be so bad? Can we look at the worst part?

PATIENT: I felt like I would come in here and just look ridiculous—all needy and disgusting.

THERAPIST: What a terrible way to feel! It must have taken a lot of courage to come. Let's look at what's the worst part of that ridiculous feeling, so it won't be so difficult coming here next week. [Anxiety regulation]

Summary of Steps in the Formulation Process

To summarize, there are four main steps in formulating a core conflict, or the main Affect Phobia. The sequence of the steps listed below is meant to be a helpful guide, not a fixed linear progression. Depending on the flow of a discussion with the patient, these topics can arise in varying sequences. As the patient describes a specific example of the presenting problem, the therapist does the following:

- **Identifying defenses:** The therapist identifies **how** the patient might be defending and points out the maladaptive behavior to the patient, while monitoring and regulating the patient's anxiety (D).
- **Identifying the adaptive feelings:** The therapist and patient speculate on **what** an adaptive feeling response might be, while the therapist monitors and regulates the patient's anxiety (F).
- **Identifying anxieties/inhibitions:** The therapist and patient explore the conflicts centering around the adaptive feeling, to discover **why** one or more of the associated excessive inhibitory affects are used to block feeling (while monitoring and regulating anxiety.) The inhibitory feeling (A) is the cause of the Affect Phobia.
- **Summing up the formulation:** The therapist empathically sums up the Affect Phobia pattern and presents it to the patient—focusing on conflicted affect as the central theme to be worked toward, but making sure that the patient can see the defensive avoidance of the affect. **It is very important for the therapist to assess the patient's response to the interpretation of the pattern, regulating anxiety as necessary.**

Formulation Process Is Repeated for Other Conflicts

When the therapist and patient have been through the steps in formulation, the process is repeated, looking at other presenting problems and looking for recurrences of problems across relationships. It is very important to link conflicts (D-A-F on the Triangle of Conflict) with actual people in the patient's life (T-C-P on the Triangle of Person).

Core Conflicts plus GAF Level Guide Treatment

Once the formulation process is complete, the mutually agreed-upon Affect Phobias become a guide for treatment intervention, along with the information about the patient's level of functioning (GAF) and his or her capacity to proceed with specific treatment objectives.

In the remainder of this chapter, we discuss the steps in the formulation process in greater detail.

II. IDENTIFYING DEFENSES: HOW ADAPTIVE FEELINGS ARE AVOIDED

Remember, a defense can be **any behavior, thought, or feeling** that blocks the experience or expression of adaptive affect. There are as many ways to defend as there are snowflakes or fingerprints, so during the fast pace of a therapy session, it is not necessary—or possible—to classify the patient's specific defense mechanisms (e.g., projection, acting out, denial, reaction formation, etc.). It is only necessary to pick out the avoidant or defensive behaviors, thoughts, or feelings that cause the patient's problems.

Looking for Defenses in Specific Examples

Listen carefully as the patient describes the specific problem. The **clue** to **recognizing defenses** is to look for any behavior that seems to be one of the following:

- Maladaptive, destructive, dysfunctional, or hurtful.
- Avoidant (the patient seems to be dodging something).
- Odd, quirky—not a typical reaction. (You think, "Why did the patient do that?")
- Even a little bit "off"—something doesn't seem right.

Examples of Defensive Behavior

Some examples of frequently encountered defensive behaviors include passivity, withdrawing, not speaking up, acting out, rapid speaking, smiling when talking about something sad, avoiding eye contact, forgetting appointments, changing the subject abruptly, somatic preoccupations (headaches, abdominal discomfort), self-attack, and intellectualization/rationalization. It can also help to remember that most of the symptoms and criteria of Axis I/Axis II disorders are thought of as defensive behaviors in this model (see Section I of Chapter 2). As soon as you sense that a behavior may be defensive (dysfunctional, maladaptive), imagine writing it down at D on the Triangle of Conflict.

Questions for Identifying Defenses and Suggesting Them to Patients

Here are some helpful questions for identifying suspected defensive behaviors and pointing them out to patients. The more ways you have to consider these issues, the better.

Questions to Consider	**How a Therapist Might Inquire**
Do the problematic or maladaptive behaviors appear to be avoiding or disguising another, more adaptive response?	"What might be going on when you call your wife 'Sweetie' in that sugary tone that always makes her so furious?"
	"Do you notice how you smile as you are telling me that sad story?"
What feels "off" or "not quite right" about the patient's story, which might signal that defensiveness is occurring?	"When your girlfriend stood you up the other night, do you notice how you didn't react? You said that it didn't matter to you. Is that really true?"
What feeling is the patient expressing that is exaggerated, muted, or inappropriate?	"So your boyfriend was really nice for your birthday, taking you to a restaurant and buying you flowers. Isn't it interesting that all you could think about was that his beard annoyed you?"
What behaviors are helpless, "victimized," futile, or do not lead to resolution?	"If you never say anything when your coworker keeps making those cracks, can you see how you stay his victim?"

Sometimes it will be necessary to help the patient bear the anxiety, guilt, shame, or pain that the defense analysis elicits:

Regulating Anxieties about Defenses

THERAPIST: You just lowered your head when I pointed out your [defensive behavior]. Is that hard for you to hear?

PATIENT: Yes. It's so hard to face what I have been doing to myself.

THERAPIST: What's the hardest part right now? Let's not proceed until you feel more comfortable with this process. [Anxiety regulation]

As the defense analysis proceeds, the patient's anxieties are regulated whenever the formulation is difficult to bear. Then the patient and therapist work together to modify the formulation, or help the patient cope with facing the defenses.

III. IDENTIFYING THE ADAPTIVE ACTIVATING FEELINGS: WHAT FEELINGS ARE FEARED AND AVOIDED?

Adaptive Feeling: The Missing Capability

Form a hypothesis about the underlying adaptive activating affect that is blocked by the defenses. The ability to experience the adaptive feeling can be thought of as a **missing capability** that the patient needs to acquire (Gustafson, 1986). Sometimes the warded-off feeling is obvious, as in cases where people can't cry when a loved one has died. Often, however, the warded-off feeling is hard to determine, because the patient may not be fully aware of the underlying feelings. Adaptive activating feelings are often outside of awareness and may need some "detective work" on the part of the patient and therapist. **This is the challenge of dynamic psychotherapy: to make the unconscious conscious.**

Eight Main Families of Activating Feelings

Identifying underlying feelings in clinical work is made much easier by the fact that there are only eight main categories of activating affects to choose from, and four categories are the most common.

Four Most Common Activating Affects

- Assertion/anger.
- Sorrow/grief.
- Closeness/tenderness.
- Positive feelings toward the self.

Four Additional Activating Affects

- Interest/excitement.
- Enjoyment/joy.
- Sexual desire.
- Activating fear (i.e., fear that moves one to run away).

The way to discover the underlying adaptive feeling can be fairly simple: Ask yourself, "What is the patient **not** feeling (or doing) that could help at this moment or resolve the problem at hand?" Examples include not crying when sad, not speaking up when angry, not reaching out when feeling loving, and not soothing oneself when agitated. Here is another way to put the question: "What does the patient need to learn to do that he or she is not doing, and what is the underlying feeling that would motivate that action?"

Questions for Identifying Adaptive Feelings and Suggesting Them to Patients

Questions to Consider	How a Therapist Might Inquire
What are the self-soothing, nurturing, or protective responses that are not occurring?	"When you lie next to your wife and obsess about the taxes, what feelings might you be avoiding?"
	"You want that raise so badly, but I wonder if you've let the boss know?"
	"You are not well, yet you are working far too hard. What would you suggest that someone else do in your situation?"
What might the person do that would make life better?	"How would it feel, next time you're lying in bed with him, to share what's been bothering you?"
What self-compassion or self-care is needed?	"If other people had been through all that you have, do you think they should be so hard on themselves?"

IV. IDENTIFYING ANXIETIES/INHIBITIONS: THE REASON WHY ADAPTIVE FEELINGS ARE AVOIDED

Exploring the Avoidance

As noted earlier, there is no hard-and-fast rule that you should explore the Anxiety Pole after the Feeling Pole. Some patients are able to access their anxieties more easily than their adaptive feelings, so proceed whichever way is easiest for a particular patient.

Remember that psychodynamic conflict arises because of excessive inhibition, which is represented at A on the Triangle of Conflict. This high level of inhibition causes the patient to use defenses to avoid the conflicted adaptive feeling. Exploring the reasons for the avoidance elicits the anxieties so they can be identified and resolved.

Four Main Families of Inhibitory Affects

Like the task of identifying adaptive feelings, the job of identifying anxieties/inhibitions is easy because there are so few relevant affect families to consider:

- Anxiety (fear that paralyzes).
- Shame/guilt/humiliation.

- Emotional pain/anguish.
- Contempt/disgust.

Identifying Anxieties while Regulating Them

Recall our discussion of anxiety regulation (Section VI of Chapter 1): A standard question used in STDP to elicit anxieties is "What's the hardest [scariest, worst, or most painful] thing about _____?" In the following example, the patient identifies but then avoids an adaptive response. The therapist explores the avoidance to identify the anxieties behind it and help the patient begin to cope:

PATIENT: It was 5 P.M. and I needed to leave to get dinner for my kids, but I just couldn't [D] tell my coworker that [F—anger/assertion].

THERAPIST: Why not? [Exploring the avoidance]

PATIENT: Oh, I just wouldn't feel right about it [A].

THERAPIST: What would be the most difficult thing about telling her that? [Anxiety regulation to assist in exploring the underlying adaptive feeling]

PATIENT: I don't know, I'd just feel bad [A—pain] . . . selfish [A—shame] . . . I tried to tell her [F], but she just started telling me about what a mess her life is, and I just felt selfish [A] for wanting to leave [D—self-attack in response to her aversion to the coworker and desire to meet other responsibilities].

Here is what this problem looks like on the Triangle of Conflict:

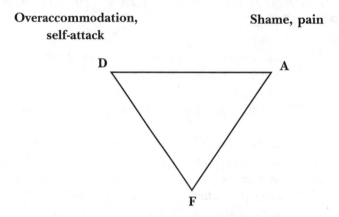

Overaccommodation, self-attack   **Shame, pain**

D   A

F

Assertion of need to leave

This cognitive technique of asking about "the worst thing" is very effective at eliciting inhibitory affects, while also regulating the anxiety so it can be brought within adaptive limits. (We discuss anxiety regulation further in Chapters 6 and 7.) In this example, it can be followed up in this way:

THERAPIST: What's so selfish about wanting to leave work on time to feed your kids?

Not only is this question likely to elicit further information about the conflict; by exposing the patient's distorted thinking to the light of day, it will help her "dispute the logic" of her self-attack.

Following the Trail of Anxieties

It may take a series of questions to follow the trail of anxieties closer to its source. Over and over, you will need to ask, "What's the worst thing about it?" Here's another example:

THERAPIST: What would be the hardest part about letting yourself feel sad [F] over your brother's death?

PATIENT: I just wouldn't want everyone to see me looking sad or down [A]. I usually try to keep a stiff upper lip [D].

THERAPIST: What would be the worst thing about looking sad?

PATIENT: I guess I worry [A] that they'd get mad at me. I remember my mother [P] getting mad at me if I got sad [F] after my dad [P] died.

On the Triangle of Conflict, this patient's problem would look like this:

"Stiff upper lip"   **Anxiety or shame over mother's criticism**

D _____ A
   \   /
    \   /
     \   /
      \   /
       \   /
        \   /
         \   /
          \   /
           \   /
            \ /
             F

Grief over brother's death

Excessive versus Too Little Inhibition

The examples above have illustrated excessive inhibition, but in other cases there may not be enough inhibition. The questions that follow probe both ends of this continuum involving too much versus too little inhibition.

Questions for Identifying Anxieties/Inhibitions and Suggesting Them to Patients

Questions to Consider	How a Therapist Might Inquire
Is there too much fear? (anxiety, panic, phobias)?	"When you ask your daughter to sleep in your room when your husband is away on a business trip, what is happening that makes you unable to be alone?"
Is there too much shame/guilt (self-hate)?	"A lot of people have had their minds go blank when giving a talk, but saying that you'll never try it again seems far too shaming or harsh on you. What do you think?"
Is there too much pain (depression, anguish)?	"What was it about your mother lying there in that hospital bed that makes you unable to talk about it?"
Is there not enough fear? (e.g., thrill seeking, impulse control problems, failure to protect self)?	"You are taking dangerous risks by having unprotected sex. Why would you not be more protective of yourself?"
Is there not enough shame/guilt? (e.g., some antisocial or sadistic behavior)?	"What is so enjoyable about watching your employees squirm when you're in a bad mood?"
Is there not enough sensitivity to pain (e.g., masochism, acceptance of abuse)?	"You let people treat you so badly, and you don't seem to feel it."

V. SUMMARIZING THE FORMULATION IN TERMS OF AFFECT PHOBIA

Working Hypotheses
The initial evaluation period (the first 2–3 hours of therapy) can be considered a "trial therapy," in which the therapist scans the main issues and underlying feelings and arrives at a preliminary formulation. The preliminary formulation is only a working hypothesis (or even a hunch) about the ways in which the patient is avoiding underlying affects. **The formulation does not have to be perfect or "right."** By speculating—and collaborating—therapist and patient come to an understanding of how defenses (D) and anxieties (A) block adaptive feelings (F). These working hypotheses are shared with the patient in the initial evaluation and throughout treatment, with the

understanding that the formulation will be sharpened and deepened as the therapy progresses.

Putting the Affect Phobia in Narrative Terms

Here is an example of a formulation. A patient constantly keeps himself busy or in contact with others (the defense—D) because he is unable to calm or care for himself when alone (adaptive feeling—F), probably due to shame or guilt (anxieties—A) about the self caused by his harsh, critical parents.

A therapist should propose a formulation to the patient gently, tentatively and compassionately—as well as asking for the patient's corroboration—as follows:

THERAPIST: Can you see now what you have described to me? Let me say it back to you, and you can tell me if you agree or if you would want to revise it. It seems that you always keep yourself busy or stay around other people [D] because you have had such a difficult time calming yourself when you are alone [F—self-care]. This seems to be because you have learned to be so harsh and critical of yourself [A-shame] because your parents [P] were so critical of you. If this is the case, how sad that you learned these patterns so early and have carried them all these years! [This empathizes with and validates the defensive pattern, to make it easier for the patient to bear facing it.] Am I describing this pattern correctly, or would you say it differently? [Soliciting patient's reaction]

The therapist must pay close attention to the patient's response, both to regulate the anxiety that may be present and to confirm that the formulation "rings true" for the patient. If the patient's response does not resonate with the formulation, this needs to be noted.

THERAPIST: This is what I think might be happening. What do you think?

PATIENT: I don't think it's quite the way you described.

THERAPIST: Let me hear how you see it. It's not valid until it rings true to you.

The therapist can revise a hypothesis as the patient provides more information. It is not important for the therapist to be "right" all the time. The important point is to collaborate with the patient and use the Two Triangles to find one or more agreed-upon Affect Phobias (core conflicts) that underlie each of the presenting problems. (For more on developing working hypotheses, see CC, pp. 101–103.)

Determining a Rough "Map" of the Territory

The therapist then shares this map with the patient, with the understanding that the formulation about Affect Phobias will be sharpened and deepened as the therapy progresses. Then the therapist must carefully note the patient's response, regulate the anxiety that is present, and proceed at a pace that the patient can bear. The following section offers examples of core conflict formulations and how they are arrived at.

VI. EXAMPLES OF HOW TO FORMULATE CORE CONFLICTS

Below, the steps of core conflict formulation are applied to case examples to illustrate how to generate a psychodynamic formulation of an Affect Phobia. While listening to the patients' description of their problems, keep in mind the key questions to help formulate a hypothesis:

1. **How** is the patient defending or avoiding? (D)
2. **What** adaptive activating feeling is being avoided? (F)
3. **Why** is that feeling being avoided? (A)

In the dialogues that follow, the patients' key phrases are underlined and labeled.

Example 1: The Bereaved Brother

Opening Question   THERAPIST: Can you tell me the main problem you would like help with?

PATIENT: I don't know what's happening to me. I have no energy. I can't work. I'm a mess [A—shame].

Specifics   THERAPIST: Can you give me a specific example of when you feel like this?

PATIENT: In the last few months I haven't been myself. I was always the strong one in the family. (*Chuckles*) [D] All my life I have taken care of other people. I worked with disabled kids when I was younger. And I took care of my older brother [P], who was ill for a long time. My brother [P] died more than a year ago. I wanted to cry [F] but couldn't bring myself to [D], not even at the funeral. I felt like I had to be strong [D]. Also, there was no time [D]. My father and I went to clean out my brother's apartment. There I am going through my brother's closet, and it's like a dream, like it wasn't happening [D—dissociation]. (*Laughs half-heartedly*) [D] I used to be so proud of how strong I was. But look at me now. I'm a mess [A—shame]. (*Laughs*) [D] I just feel numb [D] and like there's no purpose to anything any more [D]. I'm afraid I'm going to lose my job if I don't snap out of it, yet I'm too embarrassed [A—shame] to talk to my boss about the problems I'm having.

Preliminary Formulation for the Bereaved Brother

Figure 4.2 shows how this material looks charted on the Triangle of Conflict. Some therapists like to do this on paper, while others are comfortable

THE DEFENSIVE BEHAVIORS

"I couldn't bring myself to cry."

"I had to be strong." (*laughs*)

"There was no time."

"It's like a dream, like it wasn't happening."

"I feel numb. There's no purpose."

THE INHIBITING ANXIETIES

"I'm a mess." (A—shame/pain)

"I'm too embarrassed." (A—shame)

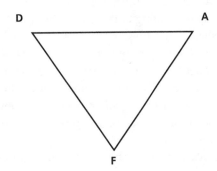

THE AVOIDED ADAPTIVE ACTIVATING FEELING

"I wanted to cry." (F—grief)

FIGURE 4.2. Preliminary formulation for the Bereaved Brother.

doing it in their heads. There are some patients who benefit from going over the Triangle of Conflict explicitly in a therapy session.

Defensive Behaviors (D)

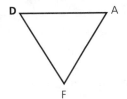

What are the defensive behaviors? The Bereaved Brother minimizes his own feelings by laughter, numbness, dissociation, rationalization, self-attack, and taking care of others' needs. This is a very common clinical presentation—a patient who has become depressed following the inability to grieve for the death of a loved one. To point out this defense, the therapist might say:

THERAPIST: Your numbness may have felt like it helped you get through the funeral and all the planning that accompanied your brother's death. Yet the numbness is no longer helpful to you. In fact, it may be the primary cause of your depression.

In beginning to explore this patient's defenses, the therapist might start by gently pointing out the defensive chuckle.

THERAPIST: I notice that you chuckle when you're telling me these very painful memories of your brother. What do you think the laugh might be doing?

Activating Feelings (F)

What is the adaptive form of the activating feeling that this patient is avoiding? He is avoiding grief/sorrow over the death of his brother. The initial

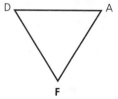

hypothesis about the patient is that the flat affect and numbness of the depression are blocking him from the shame of being weak by grieving. If he could bear his shame and pain and grieve for his loss, the depression would no longer be needed as a barrier between him and his embarrassing feelings.

Inhibitory Affects (A)

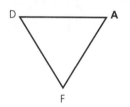

Why are these feelings being avoided? This patient feels shame over needing help (including coming to a therapist), shame over expressing emotion, and shame that he has become depressed. Bringing his defenses to his attention has the potential to further increase his shame about feeling vulnerable. Therefore, this process of addressing his defenses and managing his shame needs to be done thoughtfully. The therapist must constantly check his anxiety (including shame) as a barometer to determine how fast to proceed in trying to access the grief over the brother's death.

THERAPIST: What's the hardest part about allowing yourself to feel your sadness over your brother's death?

Summary of the Core Conflict

The Bereaved Brother has been unable (D) to grieve (F) for his brother's (P) death. Our hypothesis is that his shame (A) about his feelings of loss (F) causes him to numb himself (D), rationalize (D), and get depressed (D).

The therapist might present this formulation to the patient in the following way:

THERAPIST: You've spent so much of your life being strong and stoic and taking care of others [D]. But now, when you really need to let yourself grieve [F] for your brother's [P] death, you stop yourself [D] because of worries [A] about how you might look to others. Does that sound right?

Example 2: The Man Who Has Everything

Opening Question

THERAPIST: Can you give me a specific example of the problem you would like help with?

Specific

PATIENT: On the outside, everything looks great for me. I have a house, a dog, a great wife, and a baby on the way—and I was just given a raise at work. But I can't bear to be alone [D]. My wife just went away for the weekend, and I couldn't stay alone in my house [D], even with my dog. So I went over to my brother's house and went out with friends I don't even like that much [D]. Usually I work to keep myself busy and not let my thoughts wander [D], but I just finished up a big case and had nothing to work on over the weekend.

Note that this man only demonstrates defensive behavior. He is unable to say what his conflict is about, other than being alone. Figure 4.3 shows the limited information to be gleaned from the exchange above.

WHAT IS THE DEFENSIVE BEHAVIOR?

"I can't bear to be alone"

"I couldn't stay alone in my house"

"I went out with friends I don't even like"

"I work to keep myself busy and not let my thoughts wander"

WHY IS THAT FEELING BEING AVOIDED?

Anxiety?

Shame/guilt? pain? contempt/disgust?

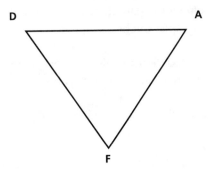

WHAT IS THE ADAPTIVE FORM OF THE ACTIVATING FEELING THAT IS BEING AVOIDED?

Positive feelings for self?

Self-care (capacity to self-soothe when alone)?

FIGURE 4.3. Preliminary formulation for the Man Who Had Everything.

Defensive Behaviors (D)

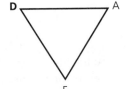

What are the patient's defensive behaviors?

- Constant stimulation by friends or work.
- Avoiding being alone.

These are the maladaptive responses that help the patient avoid the feeling and have been "self-protective"—though at some cost. In pointing this out to the patient, the therapist might say:

THERAPIST: So you see that you go to great lengths not to be alone. On the one hand, you get to avoid how painful it is to be by yourself, but on the other hand, it sounds exhausting and depleting to have to be on the run all the time.

Activating Feelings (F)

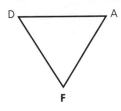

What is the adaptive form of the activating feeling that is being avoided? The underlying feelings here seem to be largely unconscious. We can only hypothesize what this man might need to acquire. If someone is not able to tolerate being alone, it suggests some lack of capacity to soothe oneself, and/or to bear what feelings come up in solitude. So we might guess the following in this case:

- Positive feelings about the self (i.e., being comfortable with himself when alone)
- Self-care, self-compassion, self-interest.

These feelings would constitute the adaptive response (or "missing capability") that is "being avoided" (i.e., self-soothing).

In helping the patient discover, accept, and express the underlying feeling, the therapist might ask:

THERAPIST: How could you feel better when you are alone? What gets in the way of enjoying time alone?

Inhibitory Feelings (A)

Why are the feelings being avoided?

D △ A
F

- Anxiety?
- Shame? Guilt?
- Emotional pain?
- Contempt/disgust?

There are not sufficient data to know what inhibitory feeling is blocking more adaptive feeling, but there are only a few possibilities. We could guess that he feels anxiety about aloneness due to a poor sense of self or inadequacy (shame or guilt), but we are only speculating and would have to ask more questions. To encourage the patient to explore inhibitory feelings, the therapist might ask:

THERAPIST: Why is it so difficult to be alone? What's the worst thing about it?

Summary of the Core Conflict

The Man Who Has Everything requires constant stimulation or contact with work or others (D) because he is unable to calm or care for himself (F) when alone, perhaps due to shame, guilt, or possibly contempt or disgust (A) about the self. The therapist might say:

THERAPIST: We've seen how hard it is for you to be alone [D] because you have a hard time calming yourself down or caring for yourself [F]. I wonder if there are some negative feelings [A] you have toward yourself?

VII. IDENTIFYING PITFALLS IN FORMULATING CORE CONFLICTS

Pitfalls

Pitfalls in formulating core conflicts occur in the following areas:

- Emotional accuracy of the formulation.
- Efficacy of the formulation.

- Painfulness of the process.
- Lack of readiness for insight.

Emotional Accuracy of the Formulation

Because the formulation process goes so quickly, there is a danger of "jumping to conclusions" and misunderstanding the patient, leading to empathic failures. To increase the effectiveness of the formulation and to minimize empathic failures in the patient–therapist relationship, a therapist should offer formulations **tentatively**, and invite the patient's feedback. Both the therapist and the patient must feel strongly that the formulation fits the information. The patient might say:

- "You're right, that describes me exactly."
- "You seem to understand what makes me tick."
- (When the formulation does not feel right to the patient:) "It's not quite like that. I don't see it that way. Here's how I would describe it . . . "

Efficacy of the Formulation

It can never be known for certain whether a formulation accurately matches the patient's life experience (i.e., is historically "accurate"). Therefore, a formulation's worth can only be evaluated by its efficacy—that is, its **power to guide treatment toward change** and its ability to move the patient beyond the maladaptive conditioning of the past. This means that **the formulation can be considered "right" if it helps desensitize an Affect Phobia and resolves long-standing problems.**

Painfulness of the Formulation Process

Having the therapist point out defensive patterns can be very difficult for the patient and can thwart therapy progress. If anxiety, shame, or pain becomes too strong for the patient to bear, the therapist needs to focus on anxiety regulation until the inhibition is reduced to a manageable level.

PATIENT: I've just been so upset since our last meeting. I look back over my life, and I can see a string of mistake after mistake.

THERAPIST: What's the worst part about looking back? [Often this is a self-attack, or fear of separation from someone the patient is dependent on.] What would help you now? We shouldn't go any further until we can find a way to resolve this so it's not so painful [or frightening, shameful, etc.].

Some patients are so overwhelmed by feeling that they need to slow down the treatment process, either covertly or overtly—sometimes for quite a long time. In many cases, though, the positive regard of the therapist will be enough to help the patient to proceed:

THERAPIST: I really appreciate how hard you're working at this, and how willing you are to hang in there through painful stuff.

Patients should not be pushed too hard to experience feelings that are too difficult for them to bear. But even when therapists are conservative in this regard, some patients drive themselves too hard or try to be too agreeable, so that they "bite off more than they can emotionally digest." When this happens, a therapist needs first to use supportive statements to bring such a patient's anxiety down, and then to help the patient understand what was so difficult to bear. Here are two examples:

THERAPIST: I think you are pushing yourself too hard. I appreciate how hard you want to work on this, but I think we'll get there sooner by being a little gentler. Can you tell me what the hardest part is about all of this? [Anxiety regulation]

THERAPIST: We do not have to face these things until you are ready. But can you tell me what your fears are about facing them?

Using this anxiety-regulating approach helps patients take incremental steps toward tolerating feeling and adaptive behavior.

Patient's Readiness for Insight and Change

Despite such careful and stepwise work, some patients may not be ready for insight or change. Such patients may not have the necessary ego strength, or a sufficiently positive sense of self, that will permit growth and change. Others may be bound to destructive relationships that do not allow change. In such cases, restructuring of the sense of self and others will be needed in order to proceed in treatment. Many capacities and skills will need to be built before the patient will be able to give up lifelong defenses that may have supported the patient's identity and maintained his or her relationships (see Chapters 9 and 10 for Self- and Other-Restructuring).

Sometimes in-depth exploration can uncover a traumatic memory or feelings of such intensity that the patient becomes overwhelmed. If this happens, it can often be effectively handled by the use of supportive interventions to soothe the anxieties until the patient feels more steady and grounded.

PATIENT: You're moving too fast for me. I've never been really close to anyone, and you're asking me all these questions about how I feel about you and all. It feels like you're ripping all my clothes off and seeing me naked!

THERAPIST: That is not at all what I want to do. Let's back off a little. We don't have to focus on you and me so much until you feel more comfortable.

This level of discomfort with the formulation process is relatively rare in patients with GAF scores above 50. The collaborative empathic understanding of their problems in terms of defenses, anxieties, and adaptive feelings gives them hope and builds the therapeutic alliance for treatment.

VIII. REPETITION TO REVISE AND REFINE THE FORMULATION

The therapist should not assume that the Affect Phobia or core conflict formulation determined in the initial evaluation is cast in stone. It is common for the formulation to shift during treatment and to become more refined—or to be revised as more material is uncovered and comes into the patient's awareness. The therapist needs to examine the core conflict or Affect Phobia patterns repeatedly, across many situations and in many relationships, until a clear and consistent pattern or set of patterns emerges.

CHAPTER 4 • EXERCISES

EXERCISE 4A: HOW PEOPLE DEFEND

Directions   Think of some examples of defensive behaviors that might be used to avoid adaptive feelings. Please remember that there are many ways that people defend against such feelings. You need only think of a few. The purpose of this exercise is to encourage you to begin speculating about the kinds of defensive behaviors that people might employ to avoid conflicted feelings.

Example 1:   If someone is afraid to cry, what might that person do instead?

Answer: _Act as if nothing mattered, laugh, or change the subject._

Example 2:   If someone is ashamed to speak up, what response might that person make?

Answer: _Stay numb and silent, or leave the scene._

Try to think of what defenses might be employed in the following examples:

Exercise 4A.1.   If a patient is too frightened to get angry, what might that patient do?

_____

Exercise 4A.2.   If someone is too embarrassed to show enthusiasm, what might that person do?

_____

Exercise 4A.3.   If someone is afraid to be close, what might that person do?

_____

Exercise 4A.4.   If someone feels too guilty about feeling self-compassion, how might that person react?

_____

EXERCISE 4B: IDENTIFY D-A-F-T-C-P

Directions: This exercise is similar to the exercises in Chapter 2 on the Two Triangles. We include this for more practice because the Two Triangles form the basis of a core conflict formulation. In the following therapist statements, identify the components of the core conflict formulation, underline them, and write D, A, F and T, C, P above the line as appropriate.

Example   THERAPIST: There appears to be a pattern, in how you can't concentrate be-
                    ^D above "can't concentrate"
                    cause you feel nervous about bringing up what's really concerning you with
                    ^F above "nervous" ^F above "bringing up what's really concerning you"
                    your supervisor, as well as in here with me. What do you think?
                    ^C above "supervisor" ^T above "in here with me"

Exercise 4B.1.   THERAPIST: It seems as though whenever you're in a situation where authority figures can evaluate you, you get anxious and withdraw rather than feel self-confident. Do you see it that way?

Exercise 4B.2.   THERAPIST: Can you see how you may be using anger to avoid closeness and to push away your wife?

Exercise 4B.3.   THERAPIST: So your tendency to lighten up seems to result from feeling ashamed of showing your sad feelings. And this happens not only with me—but with anyone. Does that sound right to you?

Exercise 4B.4.   THERAPIST: Instead of allowing your tender feelings to emerge, it seems like you need to make yourself aloof and distant from people close to you so you won't be hurt.

Exercise 4B.5.   THERAPIST: It seems like you deny feeling proud about yourself because of the discomfort you feel about this emotion. We have seen it with your parents and your wife, and maybe in here with me as well. What do you think?

EXERCISE 4C: FORMULATE CORE CONFLICTS OR AFFECT PHOBIAS

Directions: In this exercise, read each narrative and then describe, in your own words, the defensive behaviors, inhibitory affects, and underlying adaptive feelings. The following example demonstrates how this is to be done:

Example: **The Compliant Friend**

PATIENT: I was so angry with my friend Susie I didn't know what to do. I had already promised her that I would drive downtown with her, but I really didn't want to go. She's been very good to me in the past, so I couldn't tell her I didn't want to be with her . . . it's easier to just swallow it and not make waves. Susie's been like a mother to me. I don't want to risk losing her friendship. So here I am getting the short end of the stick once again. (*Begins to tear up*) What's wrong with me?

Answer: **Defensive behaviors:** _Defensive anger, passivity,_ _rationalization, self-attack, defensive weepiness._

Inhibitory feelings: _Fear of losing friendship. Shame—she_ _may not believe she is worthy of voicing her needs; she_ _can't risk being honest with friends._

Adaptive activating feelings: _Assertion, care for self_

Exercise 4C.1.   **The Worried Roommate**

PATIENT: I can't seem to enjoy myself without worrying about every little thing. I end up losing sleep at night going over and over things in my mind. Silly things that shouldn't mean anything. My roommate is from a hot climate. She keeps the heat turned up at night, and it drives me crazy. Not that it is really too hot; actually I kind of like it. It's just that the idea of spending all that money for heat makes me feel horribly guilty. And I'm doing OK for money; it's only a few extra dollars a month. It's just the idea of it. It's crazy. I am here in college and I should be having the time of my life, but I cannot stop thinking about silly things like this.

Defensive behaviors: _____

_____

Inhibitory feelings: _____

_____

Adaptive activating feelings: _____

_____

Exercise 4C.2.   **The Distressed Virgin**

PATIENT: I'm extremely picky. I always find something wrong with the person I'm dating, even if it's not a big deal. And they're little things: like one guy was a little short, and another went to a college that I didn't respect, and another had a funny way of talking. All these guys had a lot going for them, but I only focused on the things that annoyed me. Of course, if I do get involved with someone I'm attracted to, the physical attraction goes away as soon as he shows interest. I'm 26 and a virgin, not by choice. What's wrong with me?

Defensive behaviors: _____

_____

Inhibitory feelings: _____

_____

Adaptive activating feelings: _____

_____

Exercise 4C.3.

Top of the Class

PATIENT: I am at the top of my class and always have been. Until recently I was able to write my papers with relative ease. Now I can't seem to type the first word without feeling this immense dread and anxiety over writing. At first I thought this was writer's block, but I think it's something bigger. I can't even get close to my computer without my chest tightening and my stomach feeling queasy. My parents will be so mad if I can't turn in my work for the semester.

Defensive behaviors: _____

_____

Inhibitory feelings: _____

_____

Adaptive activating feelings: _____

_____

Exercise 4C.4.

The Blown Top

PATIENT: Sometimes I get so angry at my wife or children that I just can't talk to them, for fear I will blow my top. I usually just go to the office and work there. I come home late and leave early rather than risk an explosion. I used to think that this was a good solution until my wife and kids told me they felt I was distant.

Defensive behaviors: _____

_____

Inhibitory feelings: _____

_____

Adaptive activating feelings: _____

_____

Exercise 4C.5.

The Wallflower

PATIENT: I find that I have trouble in social settings. I get worried and tense, because I'm afraid I'll say the wrong thing and offend someone. I usually just sit by myself and act like a wallflower. Sometimes I'll have a couple of drinks to relax.

Defensive behaviors: _____

_____

Inhibitory feelings: _____

_____

Adaptive activating feelings: _____

_____

Exercise 4C.6.

The Overtime Worker

PATIENT: I have trouble asking for things. I think on some level, I'm afraid that the other person will say no. For example, I really need a raise, but I'm afraid to ask for it. I've been doing a lot of overtime in hopes my boss might notice and give me a raise.

Defensive behaviors: _____

_____

Inhibitory feelings: _____

_____

Adaptive activating feelings: _____

_____

Exercise 4C.7.

The Overspender

PATIENT: I've been living with my parents' help for several years now. I have no sense of responsibility. My family is very wealthy and pays all my credit card bills. I'll go on a $2,000 shopping spree whenever I feel like it. I can't stop, and it's not just shopping. When I start drinking or eating, I can't stop either. The only way I can stop is when my parents put their foot down.

Defensive behaviors: _____

_____

Inhibitory feelings: _____

_____

Adaptive activating feelings: _____

_____

Exercise 4C.8.

Her Mother's "Crutch"

PATIENT: I think I just went numb when my father died. I made myself useful for my mother, doing things for her, like cooking and taking care of my little sisters. She called me her "crutch." It was a lot of responsibility, but it made me feel good about myself. I learned very early that it was bad to cry or show weakness in front of people. To be honest, I never thought about him that much until last winter, when I started to get depressed. I was always the cheerful, resourceful one who everyone relied upon, not this pathetic crybaby that I've become now.

Defensive behaviors: _____

_____

Inhibitory feelings: _____

_____

Adaptive activating feelings: _____

_____

PART II | DEFENSE AND AFFECT RESTRUCTURING

Introduction to Part II

Overview of the STDP Treatment Objectives

Part I has covered the basics of theory, evaluation, and formulation of Short-Term Dynamic Psychotherapy (STDP). Parts II and III cover the STDP treatment objectives, showing how therapists can use the assessment and formulation information gathered above to resolve their patients' underlying Affect Phobias.

Restructuring of a patient's maladaptive patterns is achieved through systematic desensitization, using exposure, response prevention, and anxiety regulation. To achieve this goal, the treatment process has been broken down into three main objectives: Defense Restructuring, Affect Restructuring, and Self- and Other-Restructuring. Earlier we have presented various aspects of the objectives, and some readers may find it helpful to review that material at this transitional point (Section IV of Chapter 2 and Section V of Chapter 3). As discussed there, each of the main objectives is divided into two components:

Defense Restructuring

- Chapter 5: Defense Recognition—seeing one's maladaptive patterns.
- Chapter 6: Defense Relinquishing—wanting to give up the destructive patterns.

Defense Restructuring can be thought of as a form of **response prevention.**

Affect Restructuring

- Chapter 7: Affect Experiencing—feeling affects in the body, but also containing them.
- Chapter 8: Affect Expression—expressing feelings appropriately in face-to-face interactions.

Affect Restructuring is **exposure** to inner feelings and interpersonal expression. Defense and Affect Restructuring are covered in Part II.

Self- and Other-Restructuring

- Chapter 9: Self-Restructuring—improving one's care and compassion for the self.
- Chapter 10: Other-Restructuring—improving one's relationships with others.

Although **anxiety regulation** is used throughout this therapy, Self- and Other-Restructuring uses anxiety regulation the most. Because of its somewhat specialized nature, we cover Self- and Other-Restructuring separately in Part III.

Weaving Together Affect Phobias and Treatment Objectives

Following the formulation process, the therapist should begin treatment to resolve the main Affect Phobias. This means selecting:

1. The initial affect to focus on (when there is more than one Affect Phobia—as is often the case).

2. The most suitable treatment objective, given the patient's level of functioning.

Guidelines for sequencing of objectives have ben provided in Section V of Chapter 3, and are overviewed below.

How Does a Therapist Choose Which Affect Phobia to Start With?

When there is more than one core Affect Phobia, therapists commonly look to the most pressing problem, clinical intuition, or even trial and error to select the initial focus. There are no hard-and-fast rules, but here are some general guidelines that may be helpful in selecting the initial focus when the situation is not clear:

- Problems with self-feelings (lack of self-esteem, self-confidence, and/or self-compassion) should precede work on grief and anger, because the sense of self may not be strong enough to tolerate exploratory work.
- Problems with closeness often suggest that there will be problems with the alliance, which will need to be worked through before proceeding with uncovering other conflicts. Deep exploratory work needs a strong alliance.
- When there are losses that have not been mourned, then a focus on grief may need to precede work on anger, because unresolved mourning will have de-energized or depressed the patient (Davanloo, 1980). Desensitizing the phobia about grief will help energize the patient for work on anger and other affects. On the other hand, some patients need to feel angry first before being able to shed tears of grief over loss.

First Select the Affect Phobia, Then the Objective

Once an Affect Phobia has been chosen, the therapist needs to begin to desensitize that affect (or build the skills to eventually do so), using the objective (Defense, Affect, or Self- and Other-Restructuring) that is most appropriate to the patient's level of functioning. To review, whatever the Affect Phobia focus, the therapist must choose which way to start:

1. Pointing out defenses against that affect with Defense Restructuring.

2. Moving to exposure of the feeling with Affect Restructuring.

3. Doing remedial work to improve the patient's ability to tolerate or share the feelings, using Self- and Other-Restructuring.

Specific indications for selecting these objectives are as follows.

Focus on Defense Restructuring When . . .

The therapist can begin with a focus on Defense Restructuring when all of these criteria are met:

- The patient's Global Assessment of Functioning (GAF) score is 50 or above.
- The patient's sense of self is strong enough to bear looking at defenses.
- His or her impulse control is good.

Focus on Affect Restructuring When . . .

The therapist can start with a focus on Affect Restructuring when one or both of these criteria are met:

- The GAF score is around 70–80 (often such a person can proceed very quickly to Affect Experiencing).
- Defenses are seen clearly and no longer wanted.

Focus on Self- and Other-Restructuring When . . .

The therapist should begin with a focus on Self- and Other-Restructuring if one or more of these criteria are met:

- The patient's GAF score is below 50.
- His or her impulse control is poor.
- Defenses remain entrenched despite much Defense Restructuring work.
- Lack of self-compassion makes direct work on Defense or Affect Restructuring too painful.
- Self-esteem or relationships with others are seriously impaired.
- Motivation for change is low or absent.

Objectives Are Not Sequential

With the exception of using Self- and Other-Restructuring first with severely impaired patients, the three objectives do not have to be employed in any fixed sequence, as noted in Section V of Chapter 3. Here is a review of the general guidelines from Chapter 3, indicating how the objectives might be interwoven:

Blending of Objectives

For many patients with GAF scores above 50, it is typical to start with Defense Restructuring and move into Affect Restructuring, with occasional Self- and Other-Restructuring as needed. Some patients who are less aware of their patterns and/or have less motivation for change (particularly those with GAF scores between 50 and 60) will need more extensive work on learning to recognize and relinquish their defenses (Defense Restructuring) before beginning to desensitize affects (Affect Restructuring). Patients will **not** be able to proceed with systematic desensitization of Affect Phobias if they are not ready to relinquish their defenses at least partially.

Other patients at a higher level of functioning (often with GAF scores of 70–80, but some with GAF scores above 60) may be able to start immediately with Affect Restructuring. Even so, therapists often encounter resistance in high-functioning patients and need to move back to Defense Restructuring; they may then discover a problem with the patient's sense of self that needs to be addressed.

It is common for a therapist to move back and forth among the three objectives, according to a patient's needs and ego strength or self-structure at the moment. In fact, we find that once STDP gets started, the three objectives often become woven together in varying proportions throughout most sessions.

Self- and Other-Restructuring Comes First When Self Is Impaired (GAF < 50)

As noted above, exceptions to this more fluid way of working are patients with significant impairment (e.g., GAF scores below 50), who may first need a **sole focus** on Self- and Other-Restructuring before they are able to tolerate the exploration of defense and affect work. Without this initial focus, attempts to restructure Affect Phobias can often become blocked—for example, because of excessive shame or excessive distrust of others.

Self- and Other-Restructuring Implies Longer Treatment

Thus **an adaptive sense of self and others can be thought of as a prerequisite for intensive Defense and Affect Restructuring.** When these capacities are lacking, the therapist must take the time to build them, before or during work on other core conflicts. **This generally means a longer time in treatment.** Nevertheless, a clear affect focus (on self-care, self-compassion, etc.), combined with specific steps to follow for desensitization, can make even longer-term treatments more effective and efficient.

Conclusion

Though the process of weaving these strands together may seem daunting, it comes to feel quite natural with practice. To start you toward that mastery, we turn to the individual objectives.

CHAPTER 5 — Defense Restructuring, Section 1: Defense Recognition

Chapter Objective	To show how to help patients recognize the defenses blocking phobic affects.
Therapist Stance	Active and empathic collaborator in the discovery process.
Anxiety Regulation	Teaching compassion for self and validating defenses.
Topics Covered	I. Overview of Defense Recognition
	II. Pointing Out Defenses against Phobic Affects
	III. Validating Defenses
	IV. Pointing Out Strengths That Exist Alongside Defenses
	V. Managing Difficult Defenses
	VI. Repeating Interventions Until Defenses Are Recognized
Indications for a Focus on Defense Recognition	• The patient's Global Assessment Functioning (GAF) score is over 50 (particularly 50–70).
	• The patient's sense of self is strong enough to tolerate facing maladaptive patterns.
	• Affect Restructuring becomes blocked during treatment.

I. OVERVIEW OF DEFENSE RECOGNITION

Overview

Chapter 4 has shown how to develop a core conflict formulation for Affect Phobias by identifying defenses, anxieties, and feelings. Defense Recognition, discussed in this chapter, places more emphasis on the following:

• The defenses themselves—their many and varied forms.

- Helping patients see their defenses and understand the role defenses play in avoiding the conflicts of Affect Phobias.
- Interventions to change the way a patient thinks and feels about the defenses—the first step in preventing defensive responses.

How Defense Restructuring Differs from Core Conflict Formulation

Although Defense Recognition has many areas of overlap with core conflict formulation, they are somewhat different processes and have different purposes. Core conflict formulation is primarily the observation and identification of **what the problem is.** Its purpose is to generate a hypothesis about the underlying Affect Phobia pattern, which is formulated by identifying the behaviors on the Defense, Anxiety, and Feeling Poles (D, A, and F) of the Triangle of Conflict. Defense Recognition works with this same information, but instead of just identifying a pattern, this objective is a more active process concerned with **how to change the pattern.** This chapter details the ways to begin altering the maladaptive defensive pattern by restructuring the patient's perceptions of and feelings about the Defense Pole behaviors on the Triangle of Conflict.

Key Interventions for Defense Recognition

Some key interventions for how to point out defenses include the following:

- A compassionate therapist stance.
- Regulation of anxieties about facing defenses.
- Validation of the defensive patterns.
- Pointing out strengths to put the defenses in perspective.

Insight Is Only the First Step

Although it has been said that "awareness is all" or "insight is all," in this model insight into the defensive patterns is only the first phase of Defense Restructuring. In the second phase, Defense Relinquishing (Chapter 6), therapists help patients build motivation so that maladaptive responses can be given up. Remember that defenses represent the unconscious responses patients use to avoid conflicted affect. Defense Restructuring is the **response prevention** component of the systematic desensitization of Affect Phobia. Defense Recognition is the important first part of this process: heightening the patient's awareness of (or insight into) unconscious processes. Later, during Affect Restructuring (Chapters 7 and 8), therapists help patients experience and express adaptive affect.

But patients can't change a maladaptive behavior if they cannot recognize when they are doing it. Even after the conflict formulation process, many patients do not notice when they lapse into defensive behavior. Continual "consciousness raising" to encourage insight is how we teach patients to recognize defensive patterns.

Changing Defenses from Ego-Syntonic to Ego-Dystonic

Not only can defenses remain unconscious, they are often **ego-syntonic**; that is, patients often feel that the defenses are a natural, protective part of their being (e.g., "It's true I haven't cried about it, but I'm just a cheerful person"). A change in awareness of the defenses often involves altering the patient's perception of the defenses from positive to negative—that is, from ego-syntonic (something that feels like a valid part of the self) to **ego-dystonic** (something that feels alien and unpleasant). When a defense is ego-dystonic, a patient may say, "I see what I do, and I don't like it!" Note that **when defenses are strongly ego-syntonic, therapy will often take longer.**

When to Focus on Defense Recognition

Defense Recognition generally can be the starting point of Short-Term Dynamic Psychotherapy (STDP) when a patient has a GAF rating of 50 or above. At this level of functioning, the person generally has the discipline and ego strength to bear uncovering of painful feelings, together with the following:

- Only moderate impairment in functioning, and moderate symptoms.
- Some relationships and the capacity to work.
- No active substance use disorder or other disturbance of impulse control.

When Not to Focus on Defense Recognition

It may not be necessary to focus on Defense Recognition when the patient has the insight and the strengths to work with affects. Therapists can unnecessarily lengthen treatment by underestimating the capacities of higher-functioning patients. It can shorten treatment to try Affect Experiencing to see whether a patient can manage the feeling with the help of some anxiety regulation. If the patient becomes resistant, it can be helpful to return to Defense Restructuring.

However, when the patient has a GAF score of 40–50 (serious symptoms, no close relationships, and/or no job), Defense Recognition should **not** be used to uncover conflicts, because the patient may not have the stability to tolerate the unearthing of painful feelings. Instead, remedial work needs to be done to build self-esteem, relatedness, and coping skills.

When to Focus on Self- and Other-Restructuring

Impaired Functioning or Poor Self-Esteem: In cases of severe impairment in functioning, the therapist should help the patient recognize only maladaptive or self-attacking defenses that block compassion for self. In addition, when a patient's sense of self is not strong enough to tolerate looking at defenses against anger or grief (even with a compassionate therapist who is trying to validate the defenses, point out strengths, etc.), then more remedial work on restructuring the self is indicated. In cases of serious impairment in functioning or poor sense of self, restructuring of the self becomes the top priority, as discussed in detail in Chapter 9.

Poor Alliance or Strong Projection: When patients become resistant, oppositional, or angry at the therapist during the defense recognition process, it is a sign that there is either a problem with self-esteem, a problem in the patient–therapist alliance, or both.

PATIENT: I hate being scrutinized. I feel like you just want to focus on what I do wrong. You make me feel really stupid [D—projection].

THERAPIST: That's certainly not what I'm here to do! [Supportive comment] Maybe we should change our focus and work on your feeling safe and feeling trust here with me before we go any further. [Move to Self- and Other-Restructuring].

PATIENT: Yeah, I think that would help.

When a patient's ability to trust or be open with the therapist—or others—is impaired, then work on restructuring the relationships to others is indicated (Chapter 10).

Entrenched Defenses: Finally, when the defenses remain steadfastly entrenched and ego-syntonic or the patient is unable or unwilling to go through these change processes, then Self- and Other-Restructuring must be done first.

Self- and Other-Restructuring Implies Longer-Term Treatment

As noted earlier, in cases where remedial Self- and Other-Restructuring work is needed, therapy unavoidably becomes a longer process. Nevertheless, the therapist should endeavor to work as efficiently as possible—even in the longer-term treatments. With proper support and encouragement, many patients can collaborate with the therapist and use the Triangle of Conflict schema to begin to recognize defensive patterns, the related inhibitions, and conflicted feelings.

Steps in Defense Recognition

When Defense Recognition work is indicated, therapists can follow the following basic steps:

1. Identify the defense (D) by watching for a specific example of maladaptive behavior in the problem being discussed with a specific person (the therapist, a current person, or a past person—T, C, and P on the Triangle of Person).

2. Gently point out the defensive behavior to the patient.

3. Begin speculating with the patient **what** is defended against (F—adaptive feelings) and **why** (A—anxieties/inhibitions).

4. Assist the patient in this difficult process by providing support:

   a. Using an empathic and collaborative stance.

   b. Validating the defense.

   c. Recognizing the patient's strengths.

Both Triangles Guide Defense Recognition

Then the Triangle of Person schema can be used to show the patient how defenses started in past relationships, and how they continue to be used in current relationships. Defenses (D) can be pointed out alone or with anxieties (A) and feelings (F), and must be linked to how they occur with specific people (T-C-P). But, in the beginning, it is easier for the patient to absorb if only one or two of these links are made at a time.

Therapist Stance: Empathic Collaboration

Sensitivity to Patient Shame

Pointing out defenses means bringing the patient's weakest, most vulnerable, or most shameful parts into awareness. Because this can process can feel painful and even humiliating, the therapist needs to maintain an empathic stance and great sensitivity to the patient's discomfort. Anxiety regulation should be carefully attended to throughout the process, especially in regard to how the patient feels viewed by the therapist.

THERAPIST: How do you think I feel toward you after hearing what you have been through and how you have had to use these defenses to protect yourself?

Acting as "Companion in Discovery"

Defense Recognition works best if the patient sees the therapist as a trusted ally or "companion in discovery" who helps point out difficult-to-see, problematic responses. The patient must be encouraged to have a strong collaborative role in the process.

Empathic Collaboration

THERAPIST: Here is how I have heard what you've told me. It sounds so painful [A] to have been ignored by your parents [P] when you said, "I love you." It's no wonder you find it scary [A] to love [F] someone. That seemed to lead you to run [D] from closeness [F] to protect yourself from being hurt again. Am I describing it accurately? What do you think? Do you see it this way, or would you describe it differently?

Pointing out defenses should be done tentatively enough to enlist the patient's involvement in confirming or disconfirming the assertion. No interpretation can be considered valid without the patient's acknowledgment. Even when the therapist feels certain of the correctness of an interpretation, **no interpretation is useful until it is said to the patient in a way that represents the patient's personal experience.**

PATIENT: Yes, that's the way I see it. You said it exactly the way it was.

Or:

PATIENT: No, it's not like what you said.

THERAPIST: OK, then let me hear how you see it.

Putting Tools in the Patient's Hands

Putting the therapeutic tools in the patient's hands as soon as possible is a major goal of STDP. Therapists should encourage patients to work actively toward identifying defenses in sessions, between sessions, and even after therapy is completed.

Anxiety Regulation: Teaching Compassion for Self

Replacing Shame With Self-Compassion

As noted above, the main difficulty in Defense Recognition is the patient's shame in having defenses pointed out. Often patients feel stupid, ignorant, and/or humiliated when they see their maladaptive behaviors. Therefore, the main role of anxiety regulation in Defense Recognition is to decrease a patient's shame and guide the patient toward a more compassionate self-appraisal.

Working with Self-Attack

Defenses are used to protect a hurt part of the self, which can be seen as an emotional "injury." Patients should not "add insult to injury" by blaming or punishing themselves for using defenses that were protecting those hurts or vulnerabilities. Self-compassion needs to replace the self-attack and self-criticism that often arise from acknowledging defensive behaviors. It is common for patients to recognize defenses but to feel terribly embarrassed about them. Therefore, when patients use self-attack (and thus avoid self-compassion and acceptance of the self), therapists might respond in one of the following ways illustrated below:

Ways to Respond to Self-Attack

PATIENT 1: I can't believe I've been so stupid as to act this way all my life.

THERAPIST 1: It's so sad to hear how hard you are on yourself! How can you call yourself stupid, when you've never realized what you've been doing before?

PATIENT 2: I feel naked and ashamed—like you've seen the worst parts of me.

THERAPIST 2: You seem to imagine that I'm thinking badly of you. Why would you think I would do that? Can you see how harshly you are judging yourself?

PATIENT 3: I bet I'm the only who is dumb enough to behave this way.

THERAPIST 3: Why would you single yourself out in such a critical way? Don't you think there are many people who struggle with the very same issues?

PATIENT 4: I feel like you're criticizing me when you scrutinize how I act.

THERAPIST 4: I am certainly not here to criticize you. I am here to help you recognize some behaviors that may be hurting you. Do I feel like an ally—or do I feel like I am attacking? [If the patient continues to feel attacked, this is a signal to move to Self- and Other-Restructuring as covered in Chapters 9 and 10.]

PATIENT 5: When she said that to me, I realized that I stayed passive, but I just couldn't stop myself. I'm such a jerk! If I know that I'm doing it, why can't I just stop?

THERAPIST 5: That is really great that you could see it right at the time that you were doing it. [Reinforcement of partial success] But you're so hard on yourself! You know it took years to set up this pattern, and it's going to take more than a week to change it.

Creating a Safe Place

To make the patient comfortable, the therapist has to create a safe, nurturing, or "holding" environment.

THERAPIST: It makes perfect sense that you would be uncomfortable having angry feelings and would become a "people pleaser" to avoid conflict. After all, your mother was so destructive with her anger. How could you do otherwise? But you've paid such a huge price for not letting yourself have those feelings. After all, anger used responsibly is how people defend themselves and set limits. That's something that's been so hard for you.

As noted above, when a patient persists with self-attack, despite interventions of this kind, the therapist may need to concentrate on Self-Restructuring (Chapter 9) or Other-Restructuring (Chapter 10) rather than Defense Recognition.

II. POINTING OUT DEFENSES AGAINST PHOBIC AFFECTS

Catching Defensiveness

Remember from Chapter 4 that the quickest and easiest way for a therapist to pick up on defensive behavior is to note behaviors that are **maladaptive, avoidant, odd, quirky, or a bit "off."** This will signal the possibility that defensiveness may be occurring. Then the therapist can use several methods to point out this behavior to the patient and begin speculating about what purpose it serves.

Clarifying Defenses

The therapist can use **clarifications** to reflect back defensive behavior:

THERAPIST 1: I notice that you smiled [D] when talking about a sad [F] subject. What do you think the smile is doing?

THERAPIST 2: You just rolled your eyes [D]. Why do you suppose that is?

THERAPIST 3: You seem very withdrawn [D] with me [T] today. Is that the case?

THERAPIST 4: You looked away [D] when I mentioned your sister [P]!

Confronting Defenses

The therapist can use **confrontations** to bring repressed defenses and warded-off feelings into awareness. Note that this is "confrontation" in the technical sense of bringing something unconscious to the patient's attention. Confrontation is done in a gentle, supportive way, and there is no "bright line" between this technique and clarification.

THERAPIST 1: When situations like this come up, you talk a lot about what you **think** [D], but you seem to avoid talking about how you **feel** [F].

THERAPIST 2: I notice that you hung your head [D] just now when I mentioned your aunt's leaving [P]. Is there some sorrow [F] you're avoiding?

THERAPIST 3: You changed the subject just as I asked about your feelings here with me [T]. Are you uncomfortable [A] about what you feel [F]?

THERAPIST 4: Whenever we talk about your father [P], it seems like it's very hard for you to look [D] at me [T]. Do you have any sense of what feelings might be involved? [Probing for F]

Interpreting Defensive Patterns

The therapist can use **interpretations**—explanatory statements that link the defenses, anxieties, and feelings with significant others. As noted above, this informative process is similar to presenting a core conflict formulation to the patient. However, in the process of Defense Recognition, many patterns of defensiveness are noted—not only the most salient ones.

THERAPIST 1: Now we can see that you often chuckle [D] when you're really angry [F] at your mother [P], but you have been afraid [A] to show it. Does that make sense to you?

THERAPIST 2: Sexuality is an important part of any intimate relationship [anxiety regulation of shame]. But could it be that part of the reason why you get so focused on the sexual aspect of the relationship [D] might be because the closeness [F] with your wife [C] can be so frightening [A]?

THERAPIST 3: I wonder if spending all that time at work [D] might be a way of avoiding the virtually unbearable [A] feelings of grief [F] that are an inevitable part of the breakup with your lover [C].

THERAPIST 4: Did you notice that when we talked about the mean things your stepmother [P] used to say to you, you started feeling more depressed [D]? Instead of speaking firmly [using anger appropriately—F] to her [P], you have felt guilty [A] about those angry feelings [F] and turned them on yourself. Then you wind up attacking yourself [D] and getting depressed [D]. Am I understanding that correctly, or would you say it another way?

Overlap with Conflict Formulation

As noted above, Defense Recognition is an integral part of the formulating process, and some of the examples above may seem similar in format to core conflict formulations. However, pointing out defenses does not always have to concern "core" conflicts. Any defensive pattern can be noted in the process of treatment—whether it is a core conflict pattern or a less central pattern. Defense Recognition is a separate process because patients often need an intensive, repetitive focus on defenses until they can recognize their defenses on their own and begin to see them as ego-dystonic.

Working with Defensive versus Adaptive Affects

As noted in Chapter 2 and again in Chapter 4, any affect can function as a defense. It is fundamentally important for the therapist to figure out whether a feeling is adaptive or defensive. This can be very challenging, particularly since affects can be a blend of both. Here is an example of a therapist working with a blend of defensive and adaptive affect.

Diverting Defensive Crying (D) into Genuine Grief (F)

A woman enters therapy looking as though she has been crying; her face is quite red and contorted.

PATIENT: I've been crying all week, and the kids are getting worried about me. I can't stop. It just keeps getting worse.

The indicator that this form of crying is defensive is that it "keeps getting worse"; there appears to be no relief. It is not uncommon for defensive forms of sadness (e.g., feeling helpless or "victimized" or depressed) to block the expression and relief of genuine grief. This can be caused by the unbearable pain of a loss, negative feelings about the self, or the like. The following exchange is an example of how to work with this conflict.

Empathically Exploring the Defense

THERAPIST: Is there any image that brings on such painful crying [D]?

PATIENT: I keep seeing this image of my mother dying. She looked so pitiful there, and I couldn't do anything.

THERAPIST: You wanted so much to be able to hear her, to help her.

PATIENT: But I couldn't. I went by there all the time during the last weeks. But now I wish I had never left.

THERAPIST: So is it that you feel you've failed her? [Exploring the meaning of the defensive crying] Would your mom have felt that way?

PATIENT: No, I get what you mean. It's me being hard on myself again. Why do I do that? [Patient recognizes own defense.]

THERAPIST: Let's look at that. It seems like your tears [D] carry a lot of anger and blame at yourself [D] and just make you feel worse [D]. You're awfully hard on yourself [D]. It also seems like it helps you avoid [D] feeling how sad [F] it is that you will never see your mother again.

PATIENT: Oh, it's much easier to blame myself [D] than to feel [F] that.

THERAPIST: Then there must be more pain [A] than you can bear. Can you let me help you face it, so you don't have to blame yourself [D] any longer?

Summary of Example

By exploring the maladaptive affect—in this case, self-attacking crying—the therapist was able to guide this patient to greater self-acceptance and better coping with the painfulness of the loss, so that she could grieve in a way that would provide some relief.

A prime indicator of whether affect is adaptive or defensive has to do with the physiological characteristics of the feeling (i.e., how the feeling moves or otherwise affects the patient's body). Table 5.1 has some guidelines for identifying defensive feelings by the ways the body responds. Table 5.2 compares the behavioral manifestations of defensive and adaptive forms of specific affects. (For more detail on the adaptive and maladaptive/defensive forms of affects, see CC, pp. 198–199 and 216–217, as well as Ch. 7, "Specific Affects in Clinical Work.")

III. VALIDATING DEFENSES

Validating defenses is one of the most effective techniques for helping patients face painful defenses. When patients can see the valid reasons for their defenses, their self-destructive behavior becomes understandable to them. As a result, the shame that comes with looking at one's defenses is significantly reduced. Patients no longer have to make excuses for their defensiveness, and they begin to see their defensive responses in a more compassionate light.

PATIENT: Of course I had to intellectualize everything! We weren't allowed to feel!

With this understanding, patients' anxiety (and guilt and shame) can become regulated. The goal of Defense Recognition is to work with patients until they can look upon their defenses without flinching, and know that they were doing the best they could at the time.

TABLE 5.1. Physiological Characteristics of Defensive and Adaptive Affects

	Maladaptive or defensive affect	Adaptive affect
Physiological: Direction of energy flow	Either inward or outward, but hurtful to self and/or others. Self-attacking, tense, constricted, and withdrawn, **or** a bottled-up feeling with wish to explode or act out.	Flowing out from the area of the torso to the extremities. Surging, resonating, responsive to the moment.
Action tendencies: Stimulation or inhibition	Results in excessively thwarting or self-attacking inhibition of action, **or** impulsive or explosive acting out. Both lead to greater conflicts or problems with self and others.	Surge or flow generates an action tendency, and expression leads to a sense of relief or satisfaction.
Anxiety release: Inhibition increase or decrease?	Inhibition is maintained if inner-directed, and inhibition is only temporarily reduced if acted out.	Inhibition is decreased, and person is calmer after expression.
Lasting effect: Relief after expression?	Momentary, but not lasting, and only if acted out. If not, frustration collects and builds into perverse or self-punitive form.	Yes, with lasting satisfaction.

TABLE 5.2. Defensive and Adaptive Expression of Activating Affects

	Maladaptive or defensive affect	Adaptive affect
Grief	Tears, leading to feeling worse.	Tears over loss, with positive and negative memories. Leads to feeling relieved.
Anger	Frustration, leading to greater hopelessness.	A rush of energy to the limbs, and feeling of greater energy to set limits or make a change.
Closeness/tenderness	Idealized, perfectionistic image of the other based on self-need and longing. Longing- and need-based.	Gentle, unexaggerated, tender connection based on acceptance of the whole person (strengths and weaknesses).
Self-esteem/positive feelings about self	Exaggerated or grandiose feelings about the self, covering insecurity. Contempt toward others to bolster self-image.	Quiet, comfortable feelings of pride or self-compassion based on acceptance of all aspects of the self and acceptance of similar qualities in others.
Joy	Inauthentic, dissociated, false peacefulness. Exaggerated calmness. Fake smile of serenity on face.	Genuine relaxation and enjoyment. Deeply savoring the pleasurable or spiritual experience.
Excitement	Manic arousal. Urgency about the experience.	Vital enthusiasm or curiosity. Life energy. Deep interest and involvement. Spirit.
Sexual desire	Demeaning or hurtful to self or others, compulsive, addictive quality.	Passion flowing freely—deeply satisfying to self and partner.

THERAPIST 1: When you were growing up, you were desperately longing for attention and weren't getting it. No wonder you got attention by getting into trouble. A child craves any kind of attention, and isn't negative attention better than being ignored?

THERAPIST 2: Wasn't this the only way you had to protect yourself? What else could you have done under the circumstances?

THERAPIST 3: In your family, it wasn't safe for you even to offer an opinion. So no wonder you've been reticent all your life!

The therapist should continue validating defenses this way until the patient begins to show some self-compassion, as in the following example:

PATIENT: Now I can see that it wasn't my fault! I couldn't have reacted any other way!

IV. POINTING OUT STRENGTHS THAT EXIST ALONGSIDE DEFENSES

It is helpful to point out patients' strengths and adaptive coping abilities **at the same time** as you work on their weaknesses and destructive capacities. Recognizing defenses can be deeply embarrassing; pointing out positive capacities helps put the maladaptive behavior in a proper perspective.

THERAPIST: You're so good at thinking and reasoning [strengths]—it's helped get you through [validation]! But I wonder if sometimes all those thoughts can crowd out [D] your feelings [F].

The combination of such supportive statements with confrontation of defenses helps move the Defense Restructuring process along rapidly. This provides a broader and more constructive view for the patient than simply focusing on what is negative. Patients are often very relieved and grateful that the therapist can see their positive or constructive capacities, and not only their vulnerabilities and weaknesses.

THERAPIST: You've told me that you have trouble being close to people [D], and that is important to look at. But you have also spoken with great tenderness [strength] of your friend Sue and your daughter [C].

PATIENT: I keep forgetting that—because I've driven so many people away.

THERAPIST: Right. We have seen many examples of how you push people away [D]. But let's also remember that you have been able to be tender and confide in some people—sometimes [strength].

If a patient has very few evident strengths, the therapist can point out the strength and courage it took to come to therapy.

V. MANAGING DIFFICULT DEFENSES

Patients respond in various ways to having their defenses pointed out, and these responses vary in the degree of resistance they indicate. The following loose categories represent a rough hierarchy of patient responses—from agreement to more difficult levels of defensiveness—when the therapist points out a defensive behavior.

THERAPIST: Do you notice you chuckle when you tell this sad story? I wonder if that is a way of avoiding your sadness?

Range of Patient Responses

PATIENT 1: You're right! I never thought about my laugh that way. [Agreement]

PATIENT 2: Yes, I see it, and I want to stop doing that. [Defense seen as ego-dystonic]

PATIENT 3: I have no idea what you're talking about. [Failure to see]

PATIENT 4: I'm not sad. I'm chuckling because she's so pathetic. [Disagreement]

PATIENT 5: You're the expert. I'm sure you're right. [Overcompliance]

PATIENT 6: I just smile because I'm a cheerful person. [Ego-syntonic defense]

PATIENT 7: I'm such a stupid jerk. I hate myself for laughing. [Self-attack]

The following discussion describes methods for managing these various types of responses.

Patients Who Agree or Who Readily See Their Defenses as Ego-Dystonic

In addition to the responses above, other typical agreeing and ego-dystonic responses include the following:

THERAPIST: Do you notice you chuckle [D] when you tell this sad story [F]?

PATIENT 1: Did I really? I didn't notice. This must mean I'm avoiding something [D].

PATIENT 2: I see. It makes no sense, does it? I wonder why I'm doing that?

PATIENT 3: Do you think I might be avoiding getting sad?

PATIENT 4: [Some patients will add to the therapist's observation.] You know, now that you mention it, I do the same thing with my mother [P]— when she talks about missing my dad [P]. I can't even look at her [D], and I feel like I need to get out of there [D].

When patients see their defenses this readily, they can complete Defense Recognition rapidly and move on to Defense Relinquishing (Chapter 6). When the defenses are ego-dystonic (not only recognized but actively disliked), they can generally move on to Affect Experiencing (Chapter 7).

The following sections cover responses that suggest the need for more Defense Recognition work. Some of the techniques used in the examples can help move patients "up the hierarchy" toward seeing their defenses and readiness to proceed with the subsequent objectives.

Patients Who Can't See Their Defenses

When patients find it difficult to see their defenses, the therapist should try to create situations where they might attain greater insight into them.

Interrupting Defensive Behavior

For defensive behaviors that happen during a session (such as smiling when sad or angry, avoiding eye contact, speaking rapidly, etc.), it can be helpful simply to ask the patient to avoid doing the defensive behavior and observe what feelings arise. This "experiment" will sometimes allow the patient to experience the underlying Affect Phobia directly. Sometimes it helps to ask the patient to repeat the same experience with and without the defensive behavior, and to note the difference.

Pointing Out Defenses against Sadness

THERAPIST: Could it be that when you chuckle [D] you don't want to feel sad?

PATIENT: I don't know.

THERAPIST: Well, let's imagine if you didn't chuckle when you told me that sad story, what would you feel then? Want to try it?

PATIENT: (*Tells story again and then pauses*) Oh! I see what you mean. I feel sad just as soon as I stop myself from smiling.

Pointing Out Defenses against Closeness

THERAPIST: I wonder why you would avoid my eyes [D]?

PATIENT: I can't imagine.

THERAPIST: Could it be that you don't want to feel something?

PATIENT: Oh, all this psychobabble annoys me.

THERAPIST: Well, lets imagine if you didn't avoid my eyes, what might you feel?

PATIENT: I would feel ashamed. I don't want to see your eyes judging me.

Changing Perspectives

Another technique to help a patient gain insight into his or her defenses is to have the patient "change perspective"—that is, put him- or herself in someone else's shoes.

THERAPIST: When John took credit for your idea, how did it make you feel?

PATIENT: I thought, "There he goes again."

THERAPIST: That's what you **thought**, but I'm wondering what you **felt**.

PATIENT: I didn't really feel anything. I just continued cleaning out the files.

THERAPIST: I wonder if cleaning out files [D] was a way of keeping yourself from feeling?

PATIENT: I have no idea.

THERAPIST: If a friend told you that they'd been in a meeting and a coworker had taken credit for their idea, what do you think your friend might feel? [Changing perspectives]

PATIENT: They'd probably feel angry.

THERAPIST: Probably so. And if they told you that they didn't feel angry, what would you think?

PATIENT: I'd think they were pretty stupid. [Recognizing defense, but also self-attacking]

THERAPIST: Well, I don't know about stupid, but wouldn't it make you curious about what was so unsafe about feeling angry for them? [Building intermediate defenses—intellectualization rather than immature self-attack] There must be some good reason. [Validation]

The technique of changing perspective is covered in more detail in Chapters 9 and 10.

Patients Who Disagree

Pointing Out the Defense

When a patient disagrees, it is not necessary to confront him or her head-on. Instead, the therapist encourages the patient to watch for the behavior that is being called defensive and explore what purpose it might serve.

THERAPIST: I wonder what that chuckle [D] might be doing?

PATIENT: I just chuckle because I see the irony in situations.

THERAPIST: Could it be that you don't want to feel sad [F]?

PATIENT: No, I don't think so. I think you're making too much out of a trivial thing.

THERAPIST: Well, let's watch for that chuckle, and see if it happens in sad situations.

PATIENT: (*Tells story again and laughs*) Maybe there's something to it, because I just chuckled again.

As with patients who can't see their defenses, it can be helpful to experiment with stopping defensive behavior.

THERAPIST: I wonder why you would avoid my eyes [D]?

PATIENT: I'm not avoiding your eyes. I look at you a lot.

THERAPIST: You do usually look at me a lot, so it was particularly striking that when we started to talk about your father's funeral, it seemed as though you almost couldn't look at me.

PATIENT: I think I just like to look away when I'm thinking.

THERAPIST: Well, if you didn't avoid my eyes, what would you feel then? Want to try?

PATIENT: Oh! It feels uncomfortable to look at you too long.

THERAPIST: What's the most uncomfortable thing about it? [Anxiety regulation]

Overly Compliant Patients

Overcompliance in a patient must be addressed, but it is not necessarily a strong deterrent to treatment. In fact, overly compliant patients are often more willing to examine defenses and try some interventions, which can be helpful in getting the treatment process moving. When they note changes (such as feeling more comfortable with anger and speaking up for themselves), then they often become motivated to continue for themselves. However, when superficial compliance or lack of autonomous functioning interferes with progress in therapy, it must be addressed. In general with such patients, the establishment of autonomous functioning should be one of the main goals in treatment.

**Working with
Compliance:
Example 1**

THERAPIST: Could it be that you look away in order not to feel sad?

PATIENT: You must be right (*still avoiding eye contact*).

THERAPIST: Are you saying that to go along with me, or does it really make sense to you?

PATIENT: I really don't know.

THERAPIST: Would you try looking into my eyes and see if any feeling comes up? Are you willing to give that a try?

Example 2

THERAPIST: I wonder if some of that anger that you felt toward your wife is actually a way to keep her at a safe distance.

PATIENT: That's what she says, so you're probably right.

THERAPIST: Well, I'm wondering what **you** think.

PATIENT: She always says I'm trying to push her away, but the things she does really get to me.

THERAPIST: Maybe you need some distance to feel safe [Shift into anxiety regulation and validation]. Could that be possible?

Example 3

THERAPIST: We've talked about how you tend to get passive and just go along with other people at times when you might be feeling angry . . . I wonder if the same thing might be going on in the situation at work you told me about?

PATIENT: You're the expert.

THERAPIST: Only **you** are the expert about you. What do you think?

PATIENT: I'm sure you're right.

THERAPIST: You know, I'm having a hard time figuring out if what I'm saying feels right to you, or if you're just going along with whatever I say.

PATIENT: No, no. You've been at this a long time; what would I know?

THERAPIST: Well, I can always be wrong. It's got to ring true to you. But it seems to me you're going along with me when your heart's not in it.

PATIENT: Yeah, I guess maybe that's true.

THERAPIST: So let's watch for when you agree too much [D] and help you say what you really feel [F].

Oversocialization

Agreeableness and politeness (as in the examples above) are not necessarily defensive if they are appropriate to the situation—for example, if they enhance the probability that a request will be granted. But excessive politeness (oversocialization) can be inauthentic; it may serve as a defense against assertion, or protect against a feeling of not being good enough. Therefore, it is important to explore excessive politeness, correctness, or mannerliness for possible defensiveness.

Ego-Syntonic Responses: When Patients See Behavior, but Don't See the Defense

Some patients can see their behavior but don't recognize it as defensive. As mentioned at the start of this chapter, this means that their defenses are ego-syntonic, or intrinsic to their sense of self. Typical ego-syntonic responses include

THERAPIST: Do you notice you chuckle [D] when you tell this sad story [F]?

PATIENT 1: Yeah, this is the way I am.

PATIENT 2: So what? Isn't everybody like this?

PATIENT 3: Of course I chuckle. I like being lighthearted.

PATIENT 4: I wouldn't know who I was if I wasn't like this.

How to Make Defenses Ego-Dystonic

Such patients have not realized that their defensive behaviors help them avoid important aspects of themselves. The key—which we cover in Chapter 6—is to help patients see the costs of their defenses. Gently make the defenses unpleasant (ego-dystonic) by helping them to see that their behaviors may function in ways they haven't realized.

THERAPIST: I wonder what that chuckle might be doing?

PATIENT: I don't think it's doing anything. It's just what I do.

THERAPIST: Could it be that you don't want to feel sad?

PATIENT: It could be, but I think I'm just a happy person.

THERAPIST: Well, let's keep watching this behavior. You've told me that you sometimes feel lonely and sad, and I don't think it's a coincidence that a chuckle comes out when we talk about these things.

However, when defenses are strongly ego-syntonic ("That's the way I am. That's the only way I know myself") **don't push too rapidly for change**. Taking away such defenses too rapidly can be destructive to the patient's sense of self. Before you take away defenses that sustain the self, you need to build a more adaptive sense of self that can tolerate giving up whatever defense is being used (Self-Restructuring; see Chapter 9).

Patients Who Respond with Self-Attack

As discussed above (Section I), self-attack needs to be met with anxiety regulation.

THERAPIST: Can you see how you pull away from me in the same way that you pull away from your girlfriend?

PATIENT: You're right. I don't see how she can stand being with a jerk like me!

THERAPIST: Wow, are you hard on yourself! How sad that you attack yourself so harshly when some self-acceptance might be more helpful to you. [Shame regulation]

When patients respond to Defense Recognition work with consistent self-attack, it is a signal that the therapist needs to shift more to Self-Restructuring (Chapter 9) to build the patient's sense of self-compassion.

VI. REPEATING INTERVENTIONS UNTIL DEFENSES ARE RECOGNIZED

Continue Pointing Out Defenses Over and Over Again

When a patient has used a defense tens of thousands of times, pointing out the defense once or twice is generally not sufficient for change. The therapist needs to continue pointing out the defensive behavior patterns, gently and compassionately, time after time, session after session, until the patient is able to identify them without assistance. Each time the pattern is identified, the therapist should encourage the patient to put it into his or her own words.

THERAPIST: As we've seen, when you start to feel joy [F] with your daughter [C], you begin focusing on her faults [D]. Is this how you would describe it?

The goal is for patients to recognize their defenses on their own. Listen for patients' description of catching themselves being defensive, and give support when appropriate.

PATIENT: I saw it so clearly this week—when my daughter hugged me, how I tightened up. It's amazing that I really do it, and never realized it.

THERAPIST: That's great that you're able to catch that as it happens, and it will really help you change your pattern.

If Defenses Are Ego-Dystonic, Move On!

When a patient responds with insight into the defensive behavior, and the defenses are clearly ego-dystonic (disliked by the patient), then the therapist can move to the next objectives—Defense Relinquishing (helping the patient give up defenses; Chapter 6) and Affect Experiencing (Chapter 7)—in order to desensitize the patient's core Affect Phobia(s).

Interweaving of Objectives

However, it is important to remember (as noted in Chapter 3) that the treatment objectives are often not dealt with in sequential fashion. In reality, the therapist often moves back and forth among Defense Restructuring, Affect Restructuring, and Self- and Other-Restructuring as needed. Sometimes the defenses have only been partially restructured, and affect work becomes blocked. Then the therapist needs to return to Defense Restructuring or Self- and Other-Restructuring to lessen blocks to feeling before resuming Affect Experiencing.

Summary of Defense Recognition Steps   The basic steps in Defense Recognition are summarized in Table 5.3.

TABLE 5.3. Steps in Defense Recognition

* Identify the defense in a discussion of a specific problem.

     Look for specific maladaptive behavior (D) with a specific person (T-C-P).

     Distinguish maladaptive defensive affects from adaptive affects.

* Gently point out defensive behavior to patient.

* Speculate about **what** is defended against (F—adaptive feelings) and **why** (A—anxieties/inhibitions).

* Provide support to patient.

     Use an empathic and collaborative stance.

     Validate the defense.

     Recognize the patient's strengths.

CHAPTER 5 • EXERCISES

EXERCISE 5A: POINT OUT DEFENSES

Directions: Read the example and then think what you as a therapist might say to point out the defenses in the following patient statements. These responses can also include any supportive comments that you think might help the patient better tolerate what is being said. The tone is more collaborative and respectful if the responses are framed in a tentative, questioning manner.

This exercise (5A) and the next one (5B) may seem difficult at first, as they challenge you to come up with fairly complex responses. However, they are good practice for preparing what you might say when a patient is sitting in front of you. If you find a particular item frustrating, we suggest that you look ahead at the answer (see the Appendix) and then try the next item to see whether you can respond with greater ease. The answers given represent just a few of many possible responses.

Example 1:   PATIENT: I don't care what anyone says; it was my father who hurt me and my mother who protected me. <u>I don't have any negative feelings</u> [D] toward her.

Answer: **What the therapist might say to point out the defense:** I realize that sometimes it can seem impossible to have negative feelings toward someone that you love. [Supportive comment] But can it be that there are *no* negative feelings in a relationship you have had your whole life? Could being angry with her be so hard to bear [A] that you might <u>not want to face it</u> [D]? What do you think?

Example 2:   PATIENT: I see what you mean about how I shut out [D] my wife and my kids by working so much [D]. I used to think I did it so they could have a better life. But now I can see how I avoid [D] them. <u>Maybe I should just give my wife a</u>

divorce [D] if she wants it. She's wonderful, and she could find someone who would love her better than I can.

Answer:

What the therapist might say to point out the defense: It's good that you can see how you have shut out your wife by working so much. [Supportive comment] But even though you regret that you have left her and the kids alone a lot, you now suggest <u>leaving her by a divorce</u> [D]. I wonder if it seems easier to leave her than work through your <u>fears</u> [A] of <u>closeness</u> [F]—and also <u>feelings of inadequacy</u> [D] that block a <u>healthy sense of self-worth</u> [F]? Does that sound like a possibility, or do you see it another way?

It is painful to face such defenses and supportive comments can help put the defenses in perspective, as well as help the patient accept himself as a worthwhile person despite his defenses (i.e., thereby reducing his shame). The therapist might then continue:

Also, saying that she would be better off without you seems to be <u>awfully harsh punishment you give yourself</u> [D], isn't it? Often when people first see these things, they feel particularly bad. [Supportive comment] But do you think your wife would really be so much better off? Aren't there things you give her that you may not be acknowledging? [Supportive comments and consciousness raising]

Remember, these answers are just possible responses. There are many valid ways to respond.

Exercise 5A.1.

PATIENT: [She has described a close, caring relationship with her husband.] Whenever I start to get in bed with my husband, I tense up [D].

What the therapist might say to point out the defense: _____

_____

Exercise 5A.2.

PATIENT: When I speak up, nobody listens [D]. I keep thinking I'm annoying people [D].

What the therapist might say to point out the defense: _____

_____

Exercise 5A.3.

PATIENT: I just grin and bear things [D]. I mean, it's no big deal [D]. This sort of stuff happens to everyone [D].

What the therapist might say to point out the defense: _____

_____

Exercise 5A.4.

PATIENT: (_Patient nods head and agrees_ [D] _with everything the therapist says._)

What the therapist might say to point out the defense: _____

_____

EXERCISE 5B: LINK DEFENSES, FEELINGS, AND ANXIETIES

Directions: For each patient behavior, answer the following questions:

- How would you point out the defensive behavior in an empathic and supportive way?
- How would you link it to the underlying feeling?
- How would you explore the anxieties, inhibitions, or conflicts?

This exercise asks a lot of you, but, again, it is a good way to practice what you might say when a patient is sitting in front of you. If you find a particular item frustrating, again, we suggest just looking ahead at the answer (see the Appendix) and then trying the next item to see whether you can respond with greater ease. We have suggested possible underlying feelings.

Example: Patient speaks very rapidly [D] when in social situations where she is getting to know people [F—closeness].

Answer: **What the therapist might say to point out the defense:** I notice that you sometimes speak very quickly, and I wonder if that might be helping you to avoid some feeling.

What the therapist might say to link defense to feeling: It seems to me that this rapid speech [D] happens at times when you are talking about people trying to get to know you better [F—closeness].

What the therapist might say to explore anxieties: What do you fear would happen [A] if you slowed down and let people get to know you [F]?

Exercise 5B.1.   Patient speaks rarely or not at all [D]. [F—assertion, or all feelings]

What the therapist might say to point out the defense: _____

_____

What the therapist might say to link the defense to feeling: _____

_____

What the therapist might say to explore anxieties: _____

_____

Exercise 5B.2.   Patient says, "It's hopeless [D]. I'll never get what I want [D]." [F—hope. What is wished for: interest/excitement and a sense of self-worth, entitlement.]

What the therapist might say to point out the defense: _____

_____

What the therapist might say to link the defense to feeling: _____

_____

What the therapist might say to explore anxieties: _____

_____

Exercise 5B.3.   Patient begins to cry in a helpless, "victimized" way [D] when therapist focuses on anger [F].

What the therapist might say to point out the defense: _____

_____

What the therapist might say to link the defense to feeling: _____

_____

What the therapist might say to explore anxieties: _____

_____

Exercise 5B.4.   Patient avoids eye contact [D] and speaks while looking past (D) the therapist. [F—closeness]

What the therapist might say to point out the defense: _____

_____

What the therapist might say to link the defense to feeling: _____

_____

What the therapist might say to explore anxieties: _____

_____

Exercise 5B.5.   Patient changes subject (D) away from difficult topic focusing on her self-esteem [F—positive self-feelings].

What the therapist might say to point out the defense: _____

_____

What the therapist might say to link the defense to feeling: _____

_____

What the therapist might say to explore anxieties: _____

_____

Exercise 5B.6.   Patient lightens up [D] when talking about her father's death [F—grief].

What the therapist might say to point out the defense: _____

_____

What the therapist might say to link the defense to feeling: _____

_____

What the therapist might say to explore anxieties: _____

_____

EXERCISE 5C: VALIDATE DEFENSES

Directions: Give a response that would validate the following patient defenses.

Example 1:   THERAPIST: I wonder what that chuckle [D] might be doing?

PATIENT: I notice I chuckle [D] because I try to lighten up what hurts.

Answer: **What the therapist might say to validate the defense:** That makes a lot of sense, considering the pain [A] you've been in for so many years.

Example 2:   THERAPIST: I wonder why you would avoid my eyes [D]?

PATIENT: I avoid your eyes [D] because I'm so afraid [A] I'll see criticism or judgment.

Answer: **What the therapist might say to validate the defense:** I wouldn't want to look in someone's eyes either, if that's what I thought I was going to see.

Exercise 5C.1.   PATIENT: It's really hard [A] for me to cry [F]. I feel numb [D]. I haven't done it for 30 years.

What the therapist might say to validate the defense: _____

_____

Exercise 5C.2.   PATIENT: It's true what you say about how I get sarcastic [D] with my wife [C] instead of telling her that I'm angry [F], but she just wouldn't speak to me for days if I were actually to tell her directly what I am angry about [A].

What the therapist might say to validate the defense: _____

_____

Exercise 5C.3.   PATIENT: I know I shut my feelings off [D] after my sister [P] died. But who wants to stay stuck [A—possibly fear or pain] in that grief [F] forever?

What the therapist might say to validate the defense: _____

_____

Exercise 5C.4.

PATIENT: I try to avoid talking [D] about closeness [F] or things like that because I feel so uncomfortable [A]. Maybe my wife [C] is right—I have a problem with intimacy [F].

What the therapist might say to validate the defense: _____

_____

Exercise 5C.5.

PATIENT: Whenever I see people laughing hard [F—enjoyment], I just feel,
"How completely immature" [D—devaluation]. My parents [P] were very
strict and forbidding about any kind of spontaneous reactions, and my board-
ing school teachers were even worse! [P—teachers would fall in the early-life
caretakers' category because of their formative influence on the patient].

What the therapist might say to validate the defense: _____

_____

EXERCISE 5D: POINT OUT STRENGTHS

Direction: How would you point out strengths in the following patient statements?

Example: THERAPIST: I wonder what that chuckle might be doing?

PATIENT: I notice I chuckle because I try to lighten up what hurts. I have been
in so much pain for so long.

What the therapist might say to point out strengths: That takes a
lot of strength—to lighten up—considering the pain
you've been in.

Exercise 5D.1.

PATIENT: I avoid any social situations [D] because I'm so afraid I'll be made fun
of [A].

What the therapist might say to point out strengths: _____

_____

Exercise 5D.2.

PATIENT: I've had a horrible life. I've been hospitalized seven times for suicidal
feelings [D]. I can't seem to get it together [D]. Some mornings I think I almost can't face going to work [D]. If my boss knew what a mess I am [D],
he'd fire me.

What the therapist might say to point out strengths: _____

_____

Exercise 5D.3.

PATIENT: I know I spend a lot of my time taking care of my aunt. But I am terrible at organization [D]. I just hate myself [D—self-attack] when I get in such a disarray!

What the therapist might say to point out strengths: _____

_____

CHAPTER 6	# Defense Restructuring, Section 2: Defense Relinquishing

Chapter Objective	To demonstrate how to work with entrenched defenses and motivate a patient to give them up.
Therapist Stance	Active, involved, and wrestling with defenses.
Anxiety Regulation	Keeping anxiety, guilt, shame, and pain in a bearable range while helping patient give up defenses.
Topics Covered	I. Overview of Defense Relinquishing II. Identifying Consequences of Defensive Behavior: Costs and Benefits III. Distinguishing the Origin from the Maintenance of Defenses: Then versus Now IV. Grieving Losses Due to Defenses V. Building Self-Compassion When There Is No Grief VI. Identifying the Secondary Gain of Defenses: Hidden Meanings and Rewards VII. Repeating Interventions to Enhance Motivation to Give Up Defenses
Indications for a Focus on Defense Relinquishing	• The patient's Global Assessment of Functioning (GAF) score is above 50. • The patient has the ego strength to make character changes, • The patient has some awareness of his or her defenses, but motivation to change is low. • Affect Experiencing becomes blocked during treatment.

I. OVERVIEW OF DEFENSE RELINQUISHING

Giving Up Defenses

In Defense Recognition (Chapter 5), patients learn to recognize their defenses and to understand how their maladaptive behaviors block more adaptive expression. Yet, despite gaining such insight, many patients will not be able to give up their defensive patterns because fear of change can seem overwhelming.

> PATIENT: Yes, I can see what I do, and I know it's not great to do it. [Defense Recognition] But I'm not sure I want to change it. [Lack of motivation to give up defenses]

What Does Giving Up Defenses Mean?

Relinquishing defenses means replacing a maladaptive defensive response with an adaptive affective response and/or a more mature defense. In systematic desensitization (discussed in Chapter 2), the ability to give up defensive responses represents response prevention, and is essential for Affect Experiencing (exposure to feeling; Chapter 7). When patients choose to give up their maladaptive defenses they stop responding in automatic and avoidant ways, and instead are potentially able to respond in constructive ways, guided by adaptive affect.

> PATIENT: I've learned to stop myself [response prevention] from obsessing in silence [D] when I get angry [F—Affect Experiencing]. Now I make sure I talk to my wife [Affect Expression] about what's bothering me.

In this chapter, therapists will learn the many ways patients cling to their long-standing maladaptive behaviors. Therapists will also learn how to increase patients' motivation, when necessary, to give them up.

Grief about Defenses Is the Signal to Move On

Sorrow or grief about the damage caused by the defenses is a signal that the patient sees the defenses as destructive and wants to give them up. When the patient begins to grieve the losses due to the defensive behavior, it can be a signal that defenses are no longer desired and that there is sufficient motivation to move to Affect Experiencing.

> PATIENT: (*With tears in eyes and voice breaking*) Oh! All the years that I have been making myself miserable! What a tragedy! I don't want to do that any more!

It is important to remember that some higher-functioning patients (e.g., GAF scores > 70) may enter therapy already seeing their defenses and wanting to give them up. When patients want to give up defenses, the therapist can proceed immediately to exposure (Affect Experiencing).

When Grief Is Not Present

When grief is not forthcoming after extensive work on Defense Relinquishing, often much more work is needed to help a patient feel greater self-compassion. Lack of concern about self-destructive behaviors indicates a lack of self-compassion and the need to build a new view of self and others (Chapters 9 and 10), so that the patient can begin to feel and bear the sorrow of what they have lost by using maladaptive defenses. This is an essential precursor to giving up such defenses.

PATIENT: It's true that I've avoided [Defense Recognition] speaking up for myself [F—anger/assertion]. But I don't care about myself. I only care that I might take something away from someone else, and that would be horrible! [A—Shame].

When to Focus on Giving Up Defenses

Patients must first be able to recognize defenses (Defense Recognition; Chapter 5) before they can be expected to give them up. Patients cannot be expected to stop intellectualizing, minimizing, or repressing if they have no idea that they are doing so. Only when the defensive behaviors become recognizable to the patient can the therapist begin to encourage the patient to give them up. As noted above, the patient should be functioning with only moderate impairment (GAF score above 50) and have sufficient ego strength to bear to make character changes.

Therapy Process Is Circular, Not Linear

Defenses may also need to be given up when conflicted feelings arise later in treatment. It's important to bear in mind that during Affect Experiencing, new or deeper aspects of the feelings—or new feelings altogether—can emerge. If the emergence of feeling is accompanied by significant resistance or inhibition that makes the experiencing too painful or difficult, it may be necessary to return to more work with Defense Relinquishing (as well as anxiety regulation) to help Affect Experiencing proceed more smoothly. As we have said before, working through the treatment objectives is not always a linear process. Defense Relinquishing is most needed whenever patients are highly resistant and their defenses are entrenched. Such resistance can be evident at the very beginning of treatment, or may emerge later when the patient is exposed to conflicted feeling. Whenever this happens, intensive work on Defense Relinquishing can get a blocked treatment moving again.

When Not to Focus on Giving Up Defenses

The active uncovering of Short-Term Psychodynamic Therapy (STDP) is typically contraindicated with impairment in sense of self (e.g., narcissistic or borderline personality disorder). Narcissistic defenses must be dealt with very gently, if at all, because they protect a vulnerable and easily injured sense of self. Pointing out defenses can elicit enormous shame and induce a "narcissistic injury." Thus defense analysis threatens the treatment and should only be attempted when the sense of self is resilient enough to bear close scrutiny. Problems with sense of self call for Self- and Other-Restructuring (see Chapters 9 and 10). More vigorous defense and affect work may become appropriate once the patient's sense of self has been stabilized through extensive Self-Restructuring or other ego-strengthening treatments, such as Dialectical Behavior Therapy (Linehan, 1993).

Methods for Defense Relinquishing

As discussed in Chapter 5, the therapist must help patients see their defenses as ego-dystonic (undesirable or harmful) rather than ego-syntonic ("This is the way I am and the way I should be"). However, some patients can have the intellectual insight that defenses are hurtful, but still keep using them. In such cases, therapists need to help increase the patients' motivation and willingness to give up the defenses, by doing the following:

- Pointing out the benefits (primary or secondary gain) of the defenses to the patients.
- Helping patients understand the origin of the defenses and their responsibility for change (origin vs. maintenance of defenses).
- Motivating patients by helping them understand and **feel** the costs of the defenses.
- Encouraging patients to grieve for the costs and losses of the defenses, and, when necessary, building the self-compassion to do so.
- Using an active therapist stance that wrestles with the patients' resistance.
- Regulating anxiety to help decrease avoidance and build supports while defenses are being given up.

These methods for helping patients with Defense Relinquishing are presented in many examples throughout the remainder of this chapter.

Therapist Stance: Active, Involved, and Wrestling with Defenses

Therapist as Catalyst

In Defense Relinquishing, the therapist needs to be an active catalyst of change. For many therapists, this is a difficult therapeutic stance to adopt, but it is essential for helping patients give up entrenched defenses. Many patients will not be able to change lifelong maladaptive patterns without energy and involvement from their therapists. Therefore, the STDP therapist must be active both intellectually (to formulate the problem and build insight) and emotionally (with appropriate encouragement and involvement). This is a dramatic departure from the traditional analytic stance of abstinence or neutrality. In contrast, the STDP therapist must care that the patient's suffering be reduced or eliminated—but the caring must be conveyed in a professional manner with good boundaries.

How to Wrestle with Defenses

In Defense Relinquishing, the involved therapist "wrestles with the patient's defenses" by doing the following:

- Actively and energetically pointing out the defenses.
- Emphasizing the negative effects of the defenses and pointing out the rewards.
- Crawling in the "foxhole" where the patient is hiding, and working to understand why the patient is engaging in defensive behaviors.
- Being vigilant for the sadness of the situation.

- Demonstrating concern (in a professional manner).
- Dramatizing what is at stake and highlighting the patient's indifference.

Sometimes it is the very "lending of concern" that will ignite the patient to change.

THERAPIST: How sad to see you hurting yourself [D] again and again! It seems tragic to repeatedly do things that make you suffer. [Emphasizing the negative consequences] I just listen to your telling me about this, and it's so poignant and sad. [Modeling concern and sharing affect] But how much more painful it must be for you, because you have to live with it every day! [Emphasizing the costs of the defenses]

Note Patient's Responses to Therapist's Concern

When the therapist shows such personal involvement, the patient's response should be noted carefully. There can be a range of such responses. Some patients will be moved to tears because the therapist's concern is something they are so unused to; other patients may defensively devalue or dismiss the therapist's concern because it is too painful to let themselves feel it. Both types of responses can be useful to explore the dynamics in the patient–therapist relationship. However, it is important to emphasize to the patient that the therapist has no power to make the patient change. Unlike surgery, **therapy requires a patient's full participation.** It has to be the patient's choice to change.

THERAPIST 1: I can show you my concern, but I have no power to make you change. Only you have the power to change your life.

THERAPIST 2: Do you notice that I am feeling more concerned than you are right now? And I am just hearing this story as an observer. You are living it every day!

Anxiety Regulation: Keeping Anxiety, Guilt, Shame, and Pain in a Bearable Range While Pushing for Defenses to Be Given Up

Anxiety regulation is greatly needed when a patient is letting go of defensive behaviors. It is understandable and expectable that patients react negatively to giving up behaviors that have been a lifelong source of protection. Therefore, the therapist must help manage the fears and losses that are unavoidable when a patient is making changes in long-standing character patterns.

How to Manage Patient Fears

Recall from Chapters 1 and 4 that the cornerstone of anxiety regulation is asking the patient, "What's the hardest [scariest, worst, or most painful] thing about _____?" Here are some examples of how a therapist might help to regulate a patient's anxieties to assist in the giving up of defensive patterns:

THERAPIST 1: It can be terrifying to change behavior that has let you hide out and feel "safe" for most of your life. What is the most frightening part of it?

THERAPIST 2: Can we talk about what is the most difficult [or frightening, or guilt-inducing] part of giving these defenses up? Can we look at what would be the most overwhelming [or painful, or shameful] thing if you no longer did this?

THERAPIST 3: How would it help you to change this behavior? Can we think about it? Let's try to imagine what benefit you might get from changing this pattern. [Positive consequences of change]?

Giving Up Defenses Too Fast

It is important to remember that there can be dangers in giving up defenses too fast. Challenging long-held beliefs may threaten a patient's sense of identity and stability. Although change can be painful, it should not be torturous. Rather than flooding the patient with too much anxiety, graded exposure is recommended to allow the patient to adjust to change in a step-by-step manner.

THERAPIST: Can we work more slowly, so you do not get overwhelmed? You do not have to force yourself through change more rapidly than you can bear.

II. IDENTIFYING CONSEQUENCES OF DEFENSIVE BEHAVIOR: COSTS AND BENEFITS

Changing Defenses from Ego-Syntonic to Ego-Dystonic

To give up defenses, patients must see these behaviors as something they do not wish to maintain (ego-dystonic), rather than something that is integral to the sense of self (ego-syntonic). As we have discussed in Chapter 5, the shifting of defenses from ego-syntonic ("This is the way I am") to ego-dystonic ("I don't want to act like this") starts during Defense Recognition and becomes a major goal in Defense Relinquishing. To enable this shift in perspective, patients must learn how defensive behaviors are both hurting and helping them—the costs and benefits. When it is clear (1) that the defenses have been damaging, and (2) that there are other, more helpful ways of responding, patients will be more motivated to give the defenses up.

Identify Costs of Defenses

Costs of defenses can be anything an individual has lost in life—for example, closeness to others, job satisfaction, joy in living. Costs also include the painful symptoms (e.g., depression, anxiety, somatic symptoms) and suffering that have been endured. As in the treatment of alcoholism, a key motivator in giving up destructive defenses lies in finding costs that the patient sees and agrees are undesirable (see, e.g., Miller & Rollnick, 1991).

Entrenched defenses will be almost impossible to change unless something preferable occurs in their place. If the defenses help the patient to avoid adult responsibility, then the defenses will not be given up until adulthood and autonomy are seen not only as less terrifying but also as desirable. If defenses maintain a childlike, dependent stance of being taken care of, then change will be blocked until the patient learns how to care for and nurture the self, and how to receive appropriate care from others.

Point Out Costs and Benefits

PATIENT: I can see how I learned to hate and fear [A] any angry feeling [F]. My sister's temper was so out of control that it scared me [A], and I did the opposite and became the super-good girl [D].

THERAPIST: But as we've discussed, instead of expressing anger [F], you protected yourself [past benefit] by withdrawing [D]. It may seem that avoiding [D] anger [F] preserves your relationships [benefit], but as you've said, your relationships wind up suffering. [This is a cost that the patient has previously agreed with.]

PATIENT: Yeah, it doesn't work as well any more [cost] to keep my mouth shut [D].

THERAPIST: I also think that avoiding anger is one of the main causes of the clinical depression you've suffered from [cost].

PATIENT: That's really true. I'm sick of being so accommodating to everyone all the time. [High motivation to give up defenses] But it's hard to do anything else.

THERAPIST: So we've got to help you learn how to use anger [F] in the form of assertion, to make your relationship better. [Learning how to replace the defense—a future benefit]

PATIENT: Yeah, it's become so much clearer how much better things are for me [benefits] when I don't have to stuff down [D] my feelings [F]. But it's scary [A].

The Rewards of Defenses

The benefits that the defenses provide can be seen as the "rewards" or "gains" the patient receives for using them. These rewards not only keep patients using their defenses; they make patients hate to give them up. There are two main categories of benefit or reward from defenses: **primary gain** and **secondary gain**.

Primary Gain

As we have noted in our discussion of the Triangle of Conflict (Chapter 2), defenses (D) help patients to avoid the discomfort of excessive inhibitory affect (A), which has been linked to adaptive affects (F) through early-life experience. The avoidance of inhibitory feeling (anxiety, guilt, shame, or pain) is known as the **primary gain** of the defense. When defenses are maintained by primary gain alone, treatment often can proceed relatively rapidly through the process of systematic desensitization, because it is relatively easy to help a person work through these inhibitory feelings with cognitive and anxiety-regulating techniques.

Secondary Gain

Furthermore, defensive avoidance of feeling often can provide **secondary gain,** an additional—and often more powerful—relief or reward.

PATIENT: I have learned that I stay passive [D] because of fear of rejection [A] [primary gain], but it also gets people to do things for me [secondary gain].

Secondary gain is often the linchpin that holds the defensive behavior in place, because it's hard to see (unconscious) and very powerful. The greater the patient's resistance, the more the therapist needs to be on the lookout for the secondary gain or hidden rewards of the defenses. **One of the greatest obstacles to giving up defenses is the often delicious and subtle reward of secondary gain.** Although the terms **secondary gain** or **hidden rewards** might suggest a pejorative connotation of willfulness, these are common and natural human responses that are often totally outside of patients' awareness and thus beyond their control. Patients can gain control of these mechanisms only when they are conscious of them and perceive them as undesirable.

Restructuring Primary and Secondary Gain

To restructure defenses, the therapist must focus on both primary and secondary gain. The primary gain of avoidance of conflicted feeling needs to be given up with the help of systematic desensitization. Secondary gain—the hidden reward—needs to be given up by discovering healthier, more adaptive, and equally rewarding responses as replacements. Here are two examples.

The Agoraphobic Woman

Defensive action: A woman doesn't leave her house.

Primary gain: She avoids her fears of autonomy.

Secondary gain: Her husband must drive her everywhere, so she feels closer to him or more cared for by him.

The primary gain for the Agoraphobic Woman needs to be restructured by systematic desensitization of her conflicts centering around autonomy and sense of self (remember from Chapter 2 that systematic desensitization includes exposure, response prevention, and anxiety regulation). When the conflict is reduced, she can learn to enjoy going out on her own. To restructure the secondary gain, the Agoraphobic Woman needs to find other ways to feel close to her husband.

The Passive–Aggressive Man

Defensive action: A man passive-aggressively refuses to speak for days if his wife does something to displease him.

Primary gain: He avoids his fear of asserting himself.

Secondary gain: Consciously or unconsciously, he enjoys the power he wields by driving his wife crazy with frustration.

The primary gain for the Passive–Aggressive Man is also restructured by systematic desensitization. As he becomes comfortable with assertion (through exposure), he will be able to talk spontaneously to his wife about what's bothering him. The Passive–Aggressive Man will be able to give up the secondary gain of the defense (response prevention) as he learns how he can feel powerful with his wife in a more constructive, nonwithholding way.

Multiple Types of Primary Gain

Therapists must be vigilant in identifying the many ways patients are profiting from defenses used to maintain their Affect Phobias. For example, the Passive–Aggressive Man may be deriving primary gain from avoiding (1) anxiety about retaliation and (2) shame about being a bad person if anger is expressed. These are just a few examples. There are many more things he may be avoiding (e.g., fear of rejection, fear of his own aggressive impulses, guilt about possibly hurting others, unbearable pain because of the pain he felt when someone was angry at him, etc.).

Multiple Types of Secondary Gain

In addition, there can be multiple examples of secondary gain, because a patient may be rewarded in many ways for employing a specific defense. For example, the Agoraphobic Woman not only (1) gets to feel closer to her husband, but (2) gets to feel like the protected child she never was, and (3) doesn't have to work at a job that she hated. **Each inhibitory affect of primary gain, and each factor of secondary gain, must be dealt with and resolved before the defense will be given up.**

Because identifying secondary gain is so important in Defense Restructuring, many of the forms that it can take are discussed at length in Sections VI and VII at the end of this chapter. Now we proceed with the other methods in Defense Relinquishing.

III. DISTINGUISHING THE ORIGIN OF DEFENSES FROM THE MAINTENANCE OF DEFENSES: THEN VERSUS NOW

Responsibility for Defenses

Distinguishing the origin from the maintenance of defenses is extremely helpful in reducing the shame associated with defensive behavior. This intervention is similar to the validation of defenses (taught in Chapter 5), because it shows the patient how the defense makes sense. But it goes further by describing **how the defenses began—their origin.** Conditioned defensive responses generally begin in childhood, in reaction to early-life caretakers. This is tremendously helpful in teaching patients that they were not responsible for starting their defensive behaviors. However, patients are taught that responsibility for the **maintenance** of their problem behaviors belongs to them. Thus there are two main points to make:

1. **Children are not responsible for the origin** of their defensive patterns. Defensive reactions began in the past, whether desired or not.

Children are enormously dependent, and their behaviors are, to a large degree, responses to their caretakers. Furthermore, the defensive reactions probably made sense and had more benefits than costs, given the past situation.

2. Patients must learn that **they are responsible now** for maintaining or giving up these defensive behaviors that are destructive in the present. The only person who can make changes to these patterns is the patient.

Assigning Correct Responsibility

It is common for patients to blame themselves for having defenses. The goal is not to blame the patient—or the patient's parents—but **to compassionately assign correct responsibility** for where the problem started versus who has to correct it. Assigning correct responsibility allows patients to realize the past origin of the problem behavior rather than blame themselves.

Blame versus Responsibility

Many patients become terrified or guilty for assigning responsibility for the **origin** of their behavior to the parents. They often mistakenly feel that therapists are making them blame their parents instead. It is common for patients to say, "But I do not want to blame my parents." It's important to make clear that blame is a defensive maneuver that keeps the patient in the "victim" role. When patients blame their parents, they do not take responsibility for their actions. When patients don't want to examine parental responsibility, they instead blame themselves for their defensive reactions. Here is an example of how a therapist might address the blame-versus-responsibility issue with a patient:

THERAPIST: We are not here to blame you **or** your parents. Doing either of those would be destructive. We're here to examine how your parents were responsible for the conditions in which the patterns began—even though they may have done the best they knew—and how now only you have the responsibility for keeping them going or changing them.

PATIENT: OK, I can see what you mean, but it's hard to face. It's not fair.

THERAPIST: No, it isn't fair. It's sad, isn't it, that you have to undo things that you had no control over starting.

Patients need to realize that they had no control over the conditions under which they lived as children, but that now they do have the control to be able to change things. Even if their biological makeup made them an anxious or impulsive child, this is not the patients' fault. It was the responsibility of the parents to deal with that problem as best they knew, and it is the responsibility of the patients now to manage those disorders (whether biological or psychological) as well as possible.

To help therapists assign correct responsibility for defensive behaviors, we offer some further examples:

THERAPIST 1: As a child, you were **totally** dependent on your parents or caretakers. They created the home you grew up in. Every home has its patterns of dealing with things, but sometimes these solutions are not the best ones for you. It is sad that you are now left with the responsibility for correcting patterns of behavior that were given to you and that you did not ever choose to have.

THERAPIST 2: Your parents may have had the best of intentions, but no parent is perfect or can predict exactly what a child needs. You may have had special needs that your parents didn't know how to handle. Now it is your responsibility to learn to work with whatever your situation is.

THERAPIST 3: You did not ask for these defenses. You just responded as a dependent child to the conditions around you. The sad thing is that you did not ask for the problems that resulted, and you did not create the problems you have. But now you are the only one who can do anything about it.

THERAPIST 4: Even though you did not start these patterns, now you—**and only you**—are responsible for doing something about them.

Identifying Correct Responsibility Helps to Reduce Shame

Many patients have told us that learning the difference between the origin of the defenses (which was their parents' responsibility) and the maintenance (which is their own responsibility) **was the single most shame-reducing intervention in the therapy,** and helped them to be better able to face what they were doing.

IV. GRIEVING LOSSES DUE TO DEFENSES

Safe Place Needed to Grieve

Therapists need to guide patients in exploring the sadness of all that they have missed due to their defenses—the past costs of the "protection" of defensive behavior. The therapist should reflect on these losses slowly and with feeling, creating a "safe place" where the patient can be encouraged to express his or her grief.

Sadness Indicates Motivation to Change

Patients' sadness over losses incurred by defenses is a strong indicator that motivation to change is increasing:

PATIENT: (*Crying*) I've wasted so many years—so much time without feeling anything! (*Sobbing deeply*) Oh, it hurts so to feel this!

Emphasizing the sadness of a patient's life is often very hard for therapists to do, because it often means bringing up great pain along with the grief. However, only by grieving the loss will patients be activated to change their behaviors. Furthermore, this grief signals the birth of the new sense of self.

PATIENT: [After a long period of grieving] Now that I feel how badly I've treated myself, I **never** want to do that again! I see that I deserve better.

Therapists must pay close attention to regulating patient anxiety and pain. Sometimes the patient so wishes to avoid this process that the therapist needs to provide much support and encouragement.

THERAPIST: I think you'll find that experiencing these feelings here with me will be more bearable than when you were alone. It may be very painful at times, but I will be here to help you bear that.

Anxiety Regulation: Lighten Up, Note Patient's Strengths

At other times the patient's discomfort and grief may become so intense that the patient will be confused, flooded with anxiety, or overwhelmed. Then the therapist will need to lighten up for a while before trying again, gently. There are many ways to do this, but often it can be helpful to offer support and reflect on the patient's strengths.

PATIENT: I feel overwhelmed right now. My heart is racing, and I just want to run. It's too hard to look at some of these things.

THERAPIST: Let's just stop for a while then. You've been doing a great job [strength], and you do not have to go so fast that you feel this uncomfortable. It may help to talk about what is feeling so overwhelming [anxiety regulation] until you feel more in control. We don't have to proceed until you feel able to bear the grief and feel relief doing so.

V. BUILDING SELF-COMPASSION WHEN THERE IS NO GRIEF

There are many times when the interventions outlined above do not move a patient to change because the patient is unable to feel grief. When there is no grief over the costs of defensive behavior, generally the defenses are ego-syntonic (i.e., the patient embraces the defenses as an integral part of his or her personality). In such cases, the sense of self is not strong enough to alter the defenses. Therefore, special work will need to be done to assess and build self-compassion.

PATIENT: Sorry, but I am a passive person, and I will probably stay passive.

THERAPIST: Why would you want to keep yourself so pinned down?

PATIENT: That's who I am, and I feel good that I am not violent or aggressive.

THERAPIST: Are those the only options?

PATIENT: This is who I have always been.

THERAPIST: Well, then we need to help you learn to protect yourself or care for yourself in a way that is in line with your values.

Replace Defenses with Equally Rewarding Responses

Giving up such comforting responses (e.g., always being the good guy, or the dependent child, or the defiant one, or any other form of secondary gain) means that something else at least equally valuable has to occur in its place. Other behaviors or values that are equally reinforcing have to be acquired. For example, patients need to come to deep, self-affirming realizations such as the following:

PATIENT: I can see now that never getting angry [or grief-stricken, or enthusiastic] is not the kind of person I want to be. I just don't respect that any more. And it's so sad that my mother [or father, or other caretaker] couldn't see this (*crying*). But now I'm the only one keeping me in that role.

Thus self-compassion can motivate patients to give up their defenses. When patients are lacking this fundamental capacity, Self-Restructuring is needed. Please refer to Chapter 9 to learn how to build compassion when it is missing.

VI. IDENTIFYING THE SECONDARY GAIN OF DEFENSES: HIDDEN MEANINGS AND REWARDS

In contrast to primary gain (where avoidance of feeling is fairly straightforward), secondary gain presents a much more complex picture; multiple types of hidden meanings and hidden rewards are used to avoid underlying feelings. Affect Phobias maintained by secondary gain can be very hard to desensitize, because defenses are held onto so strongly. In such cases, patients not only are unaware of what they are doing, but also tend to act in unconscious ways to cling to the defenses and obscure the deeper reasons for doing so. Thus the many rewarding factors underlying these more entrenched defenses can be hard to see, and even harder to change.

Questions for Identifying Secondary Gain

Discovering the secondary gain takes a lot of collaborative "detective work" by therapist and patient. Just as with primary gain, it is important to look at costs and benefits of the defenses. Here are some questions that may help identify secondary gain:

- What does the defense give to the patient?
- How does the patient benefit from this defensive behavior?
- What would happen if the patient didn't use the defense?
- What would the patient miss out on?

Discovering Secondary Gain through Hidden Meanings and Rewards

Two helpful ways to decipher secondary gain are: (1) discovering the **symbolic or hidden meanings** of the defenses, and (2) discovering the **hidden rewards** that the secondary gain provides. These are not two separate categories of secondary gain; all hidden meanings have a reward value, and all hidden rewards are embedded in hidden meanings. Examining hidden meanings and rewards simply provides two useful ways of figuring out or decoding the mysterious purposes of secondary gain.

It is also useful to keep in mind that hidden meanings are often rewarding because they contribute to patients' image of themselves or their sense of their value. Questions like the ones above can help to uncover these hidden meanings. Consider this sample patient–therapist exchange:

THERAPIST: What would happen if you just let yourself cry?

PATIENT: I don't know. It makes me cringe.

THERAPIST: Cringe? Why would that be?

PATIENT: I guess it feels like I would be weak . . . not worthy of respect.

THERAPIST: Who taught you that?

PATIENT: I don't know. I guess it was probably my father. Oh, man, now that I think about it, he only respected people who kept a stiff upper lip!

To summarize for this patient: "Never crying means that I am a strong person that my father could respect." Note that this meaning is rewarding, so the patient gains by behaving this way.

Here are some other examples of possible meanings:

PATIENT 1: Staying distant and detached, rather than enthusiastic and involved, **means** that I am safe from others devaluing me [hidden reward].

PATIENT 2: My feeling that God hates me **means** that I imagine God to be as unforgiving as my father, so I don't have to try very hard because it's no use anyway. If I don't risk anything, I never get hurt or disappointed [hidden reward].

Need for Persistent Exploration of Hidden Meanings and Rewards

Because secondary gain is so difficult for patients and therapists to see, it is particularly important to examine **all the many different possible meanings, and the hidden rewards** obtained by them. **Identifying exactly what the patient is getting from the defenses** (other than just the avoidance of feeling) will help to discover the nature of the secondary gain. Once these hidden meanings and their rewards are understood, then it is easier to know how to replace them with a more adaptive reward. This will help the patient be able to give up the entrenched, maladaptive defenses. **Unless all the hidden meanings and rewards are identified, addressed, and replaced, the defenses are likely to remain entrenched and unmovable.** (Also see CC, pp. 170–172, 176–178.)

Common Hidden Rewards or Secondary Gains

The following are common categories of secondary gains or rewards associated with various defenses and Affect Phobias (derived from Davanloo, 1980):

- **Avoidance of closeness:** A defense stemming from an Affect Phobia (fear) about being close, tender, open, vulnerable. The hidden reward or secondary gain is the safety of isolation.
- **False self:** A defense stemming from an Affect Phobia about valuing or revealing the true self. The hidden reward or secondary gain is the protection of the fragile sense of self.
- **Impaired sense of self:** A defense stemming from an Affect Phobia about self-worth/being abandoned or unloved. The hidden reward or secondary gain is avoidance of the pain of abandonment or lack of love.
- **Sabotage of treatment:** A defense stemming from an Affect Phobia about change. The hidden reward or secondary gain is the maintenance of sameness.
- **Lack of motivation for change:** A defense stemming from an Affect Phobia about change, autonomy, or fear of taking personal responsibility. The secondary gain or hidden reward is both the maintenance of sameness and giving someone else the responsibility for change.

Although we call these **hidden rewards** here, in *Changing Character* these secondary gain categories were referred to as the different **functions** of the defenses, because defenses "function" or are "used" in very specific ways that are very rewarding to patients. (See pp. 128–138 of CC.) In this section we examine these defenses, Affect Phobias, and hidden rewards in more detail.

Avoidance of Closeness, Phobia of Closeness, and the Safety of Isolation

Recall from Chapter 1 (Section III there) that **closeness** is not a single affect, but a complex blend of basic affects proposed by Tomkins, including tenderness, care, compassion, interest, and loving feelings. However, since closeness is a crucial focus in clinical work and fits well into the Affect Phobia schema, we put closeness on the Feeling Pole of the Triangle of Conflict, and use systematic desensitization to resolve conflict about the tender or caring feelings involved.

How to Treat Patients with Avoidance of Closeness

Whereas some patients have relatively circumscribed phobias about closeness, others tend to avoid not only closeness or tenderness but all feelings, acting shy and withdrawn. When this is true, it is not necessarily helpful for a therapist to point out defenses against specific Affect Phobias such as anger or grief. Instead, such patients need to be made aware of how they are "walling off" or emotionally isolating themselves from others. When there are problems with or phobias of closeness, the therapist–patient relationship is crucial as a vehicle to change. An Affect Phobia about closeness that is present in the therapy relationship provides a powerful opportunity for exposure and desensitization. It is a unique opportunity for a patient to learn to trust and be vulnerable in a safe setting. It is essential for the patient to learn to feel safe with the therapist first, in order to open up and become more vulnerable with others.

THERAPIST 1: It seems very hard [A] for you to share your feelings [F] with me [T].

THERAPIST 2: Isn't it sad that you come for help with issues that are so painful, and then feel that you can't open up [D] with me [T]?

THERAPIST 3: Could you be putting up barriers [D] here with me [T] by staying silent [D]?

False Self: Phobia of Revealing True Self, and Protection of Fragile Sense of Self

The false self represents a level of defensiveness that is even more complex and difficult to deal with. People who are withdrawn and shy are easy to identify. In contrast, narcissistic individuals will hide their deep insecurity and sense of inadequacy behind false confidence, self-assurance, grandiosity, and charm. Such people often appear to be at ease and without anxiety.

As noted in Section I of this chapter, the active uncovering of STDP is typically contraindicated with patients with narcissistic personality disorder. Confronting defenses that protect a fragile sense of self can be extremely painful and can cause an outburst in the patient, or a serious rupture in treatment. This has been referred to as a **narcissistic injury.**

How to Treat Patients with a False Self

When narcissism is present, building a genuine self-image and establishing an alliance can take months or years rather than weeks—thus often requiring long-term treatment. This process is like tearing down a scaffolding that has sustained the patient throughout his or her life. It is important to build new structures (i.e., new affective, cognitive, and behavioral capacities toward the self and in relationships, via Self- and Other-Restructuring) as the old scaffolding is taken down, so that the patient has a strong and adaptive platform from which to act. With such patients, phobic affects should not be uncovered too precipitously (see CC, pp. 411–415).

Just as closeness is represented as an affect focus [F] on the Triangle of Conflict, issues involving the self are often represented on the Feeling Pole as positive feelings toward the self, self-worth, or self-esteem. Of course, many patients have problems in these areas without having a false or impaired self, but when self-related issues are prominent, it is generally best to concentrate on them first with Self-and Other-Restructuring (see Chapters 9 and 10), which will help build tolerance for more focused affect work.

THERAPIST 1: I'm so glad you were able to tell me that what I said bothered you. Before we get to the specifics, I just want to say that I think it was really courageous of you to tell me, and I know from what you've said before that being this open is not your first impulse. [Support]

THERAPIST 2: You've told me how hard it is for you to let other people see you. I really appreciate your trusting me with your real feelings.

THERAPIST 3: You talked before about how difficult it is for you to "be yourself" with other folks. Now that you've told me a little bit about what it was like to grow up in your family, I can see why hiding your real self seemed like the best option if you were going to survive. [Validation]

Impaired Sense of Self, Phobia about Self-Worth/Abandonment, and Avoidance and Abandonment Pain

Some patients have defenses whose hidden reward is to mask a serious disturbance in the development of identity or sense of self. They may carry diagnoses such as borderline personality disorder, or more complex forms of posttraumatic stress disorder that include Axis II personality disorders. According to the diagnostic criteria for such disorders, these individuals do not know "who they are," what their values are, or whom they want as friends or lovers. In addition, they fear being abandoned or unloved, and often feel empty or bored inside.

How to Treat the Patient with an Impaired Sense of Self

Rapid uncovering treatment is generally not suitable for such individuals until the sense of self has been restructured. This is particularly true for patients with poor impulse control, since addictive or other acting-out behavior can be triggered to manage uncomfortable affects; as mentioned in Section I, Linehan's (1993) Dialectical Behavior Therapy can be helpful to stabilize such patients. Even with patients who act out, however, much time can be saved in treatment by helping the patients recognize destructive defensive behaviors and build self-care and self-compassion.

Therefore, as for patients with a false self, Self- and Other-Restructuring (Chapters 9 and 10) will be needed for patients with an impaired sense of self. It can also be helpful to use aspects of Defense Restructuring (pointing out how their behavior hurts them) and Affect Restructuring (only identifying and labeling conscious feelings as well as feelings of self-compassion) to develop a more adaptive sense of self and others.

THERAPIST: I can see how much distress you're in over not being able to find work that's fulfilling for you. Can you tell me what gives you real pleasure and what you're really interested in?

PATIENT: God, I'm 40 years old and I have no idea. Isn't that pathetic?

THERAPIST: You are really hard on yourself. Maybe instead of focusing on your work, it would help us to focus on you, the person—your values, your hopes, your dreams, what you like, what you hate. If we can get a little clearer about your positive feelings and what interests or excites you, the job question might be easier to solve.

Sabotage of Treatment, Phobia of Change, and Maintenance of Sameness

Patients in this category and the one that follows (lack of motivation for change) cause therapists the greatest frustration by never changing or by taking a few steps toward change and then undoing it. Individuals who sabotage treatment tend to come to therapy with most of the hidden rewards or secondary gains of the defenses listed above. For example, such patients have many Affect Phobias, which are held in place because they operate to avoid closeness with isolation or alienation, and they work hard to hold onto their old destructive patterns in a dependent, "victimized," or immature manner. Because of their fears of giving up defenses, these individuals may work hard (generally unconsciously) to preserve the same old maladaptive patterns.

How to Treat Patients with Self-Sabotage

If the therapist misses the patient's often subtle sabotage of treatment, the therapy process can become frustrating and often futile. Here are some examples of sabotaging behaviors:

1. Some patients continually dabble with change (after all, they **have** sought therapy), but repeatedly revert to the old, destructive patterns.

2. Some patients appear to work hard in the therapy session, but do not remember anything that was said the following week.

3. Other patients seem to be motivated, but months go by without their earnestly attempting to make changes in their lives.

To identify such deep Affect Phobia patterns, the therapist must take a step back and look at the broader perspective of whether or not change is occurring. When change is not evolving over time, this needs to be pointed out to the patient compassionately.

THERAPIST: I'm struck by the contrast between how much you seem to want to change while we talk here and how completely our work seems to disappear between sessions—almost as though you completely forget about it [D]. Even though we've identified some pretty destructive patterns of behavior, it seems like it's almost impossible for you to make headway against them.

PATIENT: [After much discussion on this topic] Yeah, part of me is going through the motions without believing I can be different.

THERAPIST: Well, something very powerful [secondary gain] must be going on to keep you locked in behavior patterns [D] that cause you so much pain [A]. There must be something terrifying [A] about letting go of these patterns [D]. What's the hardest part [A] about making some of these changes? [Anxiety regulation]

Lack of Motivation for Change, Phobia of Personal Responsibility, and Maintenance of Sameness/Refusal of Responsibility

The most resistant patients even lack the motivation to engage in therapy. They take a passive stance in treatment and inwardly hope that the therapist will have the power to make them change. It is pointless for the therapist to use energy to restructure defenses that block specific feelings when the patient has no real desire or intent to change, as in this example:

PATIENT: Doc, when are you going to do something for me? Nothing is changing. I thought you would have made me better by now. This isn't helping me. I've been here for 5 weeks, and I don't feel better. When are you going to do something that helps me?

The patient may be saying, in effect, "It's the therapist's responsibility to make me change." Some patients do not want to do the work of therapy, but want to have the therapist make them better without any effort on their part. Or, as with sabotage, they may seek to preserve sameness at almost any cost.

How to Treat Lack of Motivation

If the therapist has made active, involved interventions and pointed out the patient's destructive patterns, but no improvement has occurred, the therapist needs to address the patient's strong resistance to change. This has to be pointed out to the patient compassionately, but honestly and directly.

THERAPIST 1: I wish I could wave a magic wand, or flip a switch and take your suffering away. If I could, I would do it in a second! But, unfortunately, I don't have that power.

THERAPIST 2: I've been thinking that you've been coming here and spending your hard-earned money, but it doesn't look like your heart is in it. We need to find something you really feel able to work on—or maybe we should consider ending treatment until a time when you'd feel more motivated. What do you think?

The suggestion of termination is only used as a last resort. However, it can often serve as a powerful motivator for a patient. If the patient remains unmotivated, termination—or a move to a purely supportive form of treatment—may be a worthwhile consideration.

VII. REPEATING INTERVENTIONS TO ENHANCE MOTIVATION TO GIVE UP DEFENSES

Repeat Interventions until Change Happens

The constant question in the STDP therapist's mind—before, during, and after every session—should be this: **"Is there change, and if not, why not?"** If defensive patterns are not shifting, then something is not being attended to. Excessive inhibition (primary gain) and/or hidden rewards (secondary gain) are continuing to hold the defenses in place.

Tenacity in Exploration of Secondary Gain

Secondary gain requires special persistence and tenacity on the part of both therapist and patient, in repeatedly going over the patient's possible reasons for holding onto the defenses. We have said this before, but it bears repeating: **unless all the hidden meanings and rewards are identified, addressed, and replaced, the defenses are likely to remain en-**

trenched and unmovable. When defenses are not being given up, even after much secondary gain has been worked through, there is probably some additional meaning or reward that has not been discovered. It is helpful to use the list of categories of secondary gain listed in Section VI to guide your search. Sabotage of treatment and lack of motivation for change are particularly important possibilities to consider when patients stubbornly cling to maladaptive defenses. (For more detail on the hidden rewards of defenses—or "functions" of defenses, as they are called in that text—see CC, pp. 128–138, 170–172, and 176–178.)

A therapist must stay resolutely focused on understanding why defenses are not changing (i.e., must analyze the resistance, the anxieties, and the costs and benefits of primary and secondary gains) session after session, week after week, until the structure underlying the defenses is clearly seen and altered. Again, the therapist should try to achieve at least some small increment of change (whether cognitive understanding of defenses or affective shifts) each week.

THERAPIST: How are you doing with the problem we've been focusing on?

PATIENT: I'm no better. I still do the same old thing, like a broken record [D].

THERAPIST: So let's look at it again and again—until we get to the core of it. There must be strong forces holding these defenses in place. [Therapist holds the focus and validates the need for the defenses.] We know that intellectually you want to change it, but emotionally you seem to fall back in the same patterns. [Empathy]

PATIENT: That's right!

THERAPIST: Let's look again at what are the hardest things about giving it up? [A—primary gain] . . . [After much discussion] Besides all the things we have already discovered, let's consider **what else** might you lose by stopping these defenses? [multiple secondary gains—refer back to the list of categories in Section VI above.]

Although the process may seem tedious at times, only when patients are helped to increase their motivation for change in this way can they go to the heart of treatment for Affect Phobia—Affect Experiencing, which we turn to in the next chapter.

Summary of Defense Relinquishing Steps

The basic steps of Defense Relinquishing are summarized in Table 6.1.

TABLE 6.1. Steps in Defense Relinquishing

- Actively and energetically point out defenses to the patient.

  Point out costs and benefits of the defenses.

  Turn ego-syntonic defenses into ego-dystonic defenses.

- Distinguish the origin from the maintenance of the defenses.

- Motivate change by emphasizing negative effects of defenses.

- Demonstrate concern.

- Dramatize what is at stake—highlight the patient's indifference.

- Work to understand why the patient is doing what he or she is doing (primary and secondary gain).

- Point out or help build more adaptive behaviors or more mature defenses.

- Be vigilant for the sadness (grief) due to the defenses, signaling motivation to change.

- Work on Self- and Other-Restructuring if there is no sadness over defenses.

CHAPTER 6 • EXERCISES

EXERCISE 6A: IDENTIFY THE BENEFITS AND COSTS OF DEFENSES

Directions: For each of the following clinical vignettes, try to imagine possible costs and benefits, based on your own clinical and life experience in addition to your reading here and elsewhere.

Remember that there are many possibilities; speculate and form a tentative hypothesis for the reasons for the defenses.

Example: **Defensive behavior:** A 55-year-old woman prevents herself from feeling grief and thereby avoids shame over feeling weak. She says, "It's wrong to feel sorry for myself."

Answer: **Possible benefits:** Her primary gain is the avoidance of the shame she has associated with grieving. She also avoids the common anxiety that feelings of grief, once entered into, will be unending. Her secondary gain is the resulting sense of herself as tough and independent.

Possible costs: Ironically, by working so hard to avoid grief, she actually keeps herself stuck in low-level, ineffective grieving and deprives herself of the relief of unfettered grief. This sort of unresolved grief often directly relates to patients' problems that bring them into therapy: depression, anxiety, and difficulties with closeness. Avoiding grief also prevents the patient from developing a sense of compassion for others as well as herself.

Exercise 6A.1. **Defensive behavior:** A schoolteacher generally shows a passive acceptance of others' unreasonable demands, but every few weeks he has an outburst of temper. He comes to therapy complaining of these outbursts, saying he has a "problem with anger." (Temper outbursts can be a discharge of bottled-up frustration [a defensive form of anger], which blocks the expression of assertion [an adaptive form of anger].)

Possible benefits: _____

_____

Possible costs: _____

_____

Exercise 6A.2.

Defensive behavior: A single young woman who was the oldest of five children tends to "take care" of her therapist by minimizing her problems and not speaking up when she feels misunderstood or slighted.

Possible benefits: _____

_____

Possible costs: _____

_____

Exercise 6A.3.

Defensive behavior: A 30-year-old chemical engineer feels "stuck" in his career and is unable to work productively; he does not see any relationship of his job problems to the fact that his mother and siblings were killed in a house fire when he was in college 8 years prior.

Possible benefits: _____

_____

Possible costs: _____

_____

Exercise 6A.4.

Defensive behavior: A 32-year-old woman says that she wants very much to get married and have children, but feels ashamed and mystified when she finds herself being "a witch"—angrily picking fights with her boyfriend, who is devoted to her and whom she describes as "perfect . . . he's just the kind of guy my parents always tell me I should marry."

Possible benefits: _____

_____

Possible costs: _____

_____

Exercise 6A.5.

Defensive behavior: A 26-year-old peace activist has difficulty getting sexually aroused with his girlfriend. In exploring this problem, he vividly recalls the shame he felt as a young adolescent when he became aroused by seeing his older sisters when they were partially clothed.

Possible benefits: _____

_____

Possible costs: _____

_____

EXERCISE 6B: IDENTIFY THE ORIGINS AND THE MAINTENANCE OF THE DEFENSE

Directions: For each set of defensive behaviors, imagine (1) how it might have originated and (2) how it might be maintained. What would you say to explain each of these to the patient? (Again, there is no "right" or "wrong" answer to these. The point is to come up with a plausible scenario and practice presenting it to the patient.)

Example: **Defensive behavior:**

THERAPIST: Now we've seen how quickly you become passive when you get angry. [History: The family fought viciously throughout the patient's childhood, and he hated it.]

Answer: **What the therapist might say about origins of the defenses (early-life costs and/or benefits):** It was probably helpful [benefit] for you to stay silent and withdrawn in your angry, fighting family while you were growing up.

What the therapist might say about maintenance of the defenses (current costs and benefits): Yet you continue this pattern even though you're not living in the same situation. Being silent used to keep you safe [original benefit], and even now it lets you feel like you're a "good person" [secondary gain]. But actually it keeps you desperately lonely [cost]—and, in fact, it seems to make some people mad at you [cost], because they want you to speak up.

Exercise 6B.1. **Defensive behavior:**

THERAPIST: It seems as though these home improvement projects are most pressing when your wife or children want to do something with you. [History: This patient came from a cool, distant family. The members of the family kept to themselves and had their own private interests. There was very little personal sharing of any kind.]

What the therapist might say about origins of the defenses (early-life costs and/or benefits): _____

_____

What the therapist might say about maintenance of the defenses (current costs and benefits): _____

_____

Exercice 6B.2.   **Defensive behavior:**

THERAPIST: Have you noticed that when we get close to those sad feelings [F] over your brother's death, you tend to make a joke [D] or change the subject [D]? [History: The patient's family always lightened up feelings. No one was ever allowed to cry; anyone who did would be teased as a "sissy."]

What the therapist might say about origins of the defenses (early-life costs and/or benefits): _____

_____

What the therapist might say about maintenance of the defenses (current costs and benefits): _____

_____

Exercice 6B.3.   **Defensive behavior:**

THERAPIST: It's so striking to me how your depressed feelings seem to come up exactly when we're talking about situations in which another person might well get angry. [History: This patient's mother was depressed and passive. She taught her son that he was to be "saint-like." He was forbidden ever to get in a fight with boys at school. He was also taught that he should always put others' needs above his own.]

What the therapist might say about origins of the defenses (early-life costs and/or benefits): _____

_____

What the therapist might say about maintenance of the defenses (current costs and benefits): _____

_____

EXERCISE 6C. HELP PATIENTS GRIEVE THE COSTS OF DEFENSES

Directions: What might you say in the following examples to do the following:

- Intensify the grief over the costs of the defenses?
- Lighten things up if the patient starts to feel overwhelmed?

Again, remember that there is no "right" answer. We are looking for possible responses. A tip for intensifying feeling is to present a variety of details to the patient to give your responses more vitality.

Example: **Defensive behavior:**

THERAPIST: We've seen how difficult it's been for you to ask for what you want, that you've had a tendency to be passive.

Answer: **What the therapist might say to intensify:** There have been so many things you have let go by without even asking. You've missed out on so much that it's tragic.

What the therapist might say to lighten up: Everyone in your family was so overwhelmed that you got the message that the only possible result of asking for what you wanted was disappointment. [Validation] So you have learned to be incredibly self-reliant, and in spite of these obstacles, you've achieved a lot. [Pointing out strengths]

Explanation: Each of these responses might be appropriate, depending on whether the therapist was trying to deepen the grief to increase motivation for Defense Relinquishing or to reduce shame over the defenses.

Exercise 6C.1.

Defensive behavior:

THERAPIST: You've really been holding the grief over your mother's death at arm's length for years by numbing yourself, haven't you?

What the therapist might say to intensify: _____

_____

What the therapist might say to lighten up: _____

_____

Exercise 6C.2.

Defensive behavior:

THERAPIST: You know, when you avert your eyes from me in this way, I can't help but think you may well do the same thing with other people, and there may be other ways you hold people at a distance. [One of this patient's chief complaints is about failure to find a long-term relationship.]

What the therapist might say to intensify: _____

_____

What the therapist might say to lighten up: _____

_____

Exercise 6C.3.

Defensive behavior:

THERAPIST: It seems as though the times when you spend excessive amounts of time cleaning, there might be a chance that things may become sexual with Elaine [the patient's lesbian lover]. [This patient's family was very uptight about sexuality and very rejecting about her homosexuality.]

What the therapist might say to intensify: _____

_____

What the therapist might say to lighten up: _____

_____

EXERCISE 6D: IDENTIFY THE HIDDEN MEANINGS OF DEFENSES

Directions, Part I: Imagine a possible hidden or symbolic meaning behind these defensive **thoughts**.

Example: "I must do every job perfectly."

Answers: Some of the many possible meanings of this thought are as follows: (1) "If I do every job perfectly, it means I'm not stupid." (2) "If I do every job perfectly, it means people will like me." (3) "If I do every job perfectly, it means I'm competent and valuable."

Exercise 6D.1 "I absolutely must look my best."

Possible meanings: _____

_____

Exercise 6D.2. "Those people are talking about me."

Possible meanings: _____

_____

Exercise 6D.3. "Why don't they realize how great I am?"

Possible meanings: _____

_____

Directions, Part II: Imagine a possible hidden or symbolic meaning behind these defensive **behaviors**.

Example: Excessive collecting of things.

Answers: Some of the many possible meanings of this behavior are as follows: (1) "Excessive collecting of things means I'll be ready for anything." (2) "If I have everything on hand, it means I won't look stupid." (3) "Holding onto things from the past means I do not have to grieve for what I lost."

Exercise 6D.4. Inability to start tasks on one's own.

Possible meanings: _____

_____

Exercise 6D.5.   Inability to throw things away.

           Possible meanings: _____

_____

Exercise 6D.6.   Kicking the dog,

           Possible meanings: _____

_____

Exercise 6D.7.   Sarcasm, cynicism.

           Possible meanings: _____

_____

Exercise 6D.8.   Stinginess.

           Possible meanings: _____

_____

Exercise 6D.9.   Mood swings.

           Possible meanings: _____

_____

EXERCISE 6E: WHAT IS THE HIDDEN REWARD (SECONDARY GAIN) OF THE DEFENSE?

Directions: Each exercise below presents a possible patient response to the following observation of a patient's defense. For each patient response, please do the following: First, identify the hidden reward of the defense (see Section VI of this chapter). Second, imagine what a therapist might say to direct the patient's attention to this hidden agenda.

Example: PATIENT: So what if I smile all the time? That's just who I am. I'm a cheerful person. What should I do, be nasty? I couldn't. Besides, the only reason people like me is because I'm cheerful.

Answer: **What is the hidden reward of the defense?** The first obvious reason for the avoidance of feeling is the discomfort with the feeling of anger. But the last statement that the patient makes give a clue that there is secondary gain in avoiding interpersonal anxiety or distrust about closeness ("the only reason people like me is because I'm cheerful"). It also suggests a problem with her sense of self and her relationships to others.

What might the therapist say to point this out to the patient? Are you sure that people only like you if you're cheerful? What makes you think that? Isn't it unfair to ask someone always to be cheerful?

Exercise 6E.1.

PATIENT: I don't know, I guess she was unkind, but what good would it do to get angry? What's done is done, and it's better to laugh it off than spend time moping.

What is the hidden reward of the defense? _____

_____

What might the therapist say to point this out to the patient? _____

_____

Exercise 6E.2.

PATIENT: I'll be darned if I'll let her know what's really going on inside **my** head! She'd have something on me!

What is the hidden reward of the defense? _____

_____

What might the therapist say to point this out to the patient? _____

_____

Exercise 6E.3.

PATIENT: Last month, when my girlfriend wasn't even being that mean to me, I got totally furious and just started screaming at her. Looking back at it now I feel kind of bad about it, but it made total sense to me at the time. For weeks, when she was acting OK to me, I just felt irritable every time I saw her.

What is the hidden reward of the defense? _____

_____

What might the therapist say to point this out to the patient? _____

_____

Exercise 6E.4.

PATIENT: I have no idea what to talk about today. I haven't given a moment's thought to therapy since I walked out of here last week.

What is the hidden reward of the defense? _____

_____

What might the therapist say to point this out to the patient? _____

_____

Exercise 6E.5.

PATIENT: (*Furious*) How **dare** you suggest I might have some hidden agenda here! I have been completely honest with you! Completely! I wonder if I should even continue therapy if you are so unable to understand me.

What is the hidden reward of the defense? _____

_____

What might the therapist say to point this out to the patient? _____

_____

Affect Restructuring, Section 1: Affect Experiencing

Chapter Objective
To demonstrate how to desensitize Affect Phobias by helping patients experience adaptive but warded-off affects until anxiety subsides,

Therapist Stance
Encouraging feeling and sharing the experience.

Anxiety Regulation
Desensitizing fears (phobias) over experiencing affects, and titrating the exposure.

Topics Covered

I. Overview of Affect Experiencing

II. Exposure to Phobic Feeling/Feared Affect

III. Response Prevention: Defense Restructuring as Needed

IV. Identifying Pitfalls in Affect Experiencing

V. Repeating Interventions Until Affect Phobia Is Desensitized

VI. Some Frequently Asked Questions

Indications for a Focus on Affect Experiencing

- The patient's Global Assessment of Functioning (GAF) score is above 50.
- There is no history of acting out.
- Impulse control has been maintained for 1–3 years.
- The patient feels able to contain the affect to be experienced.

I. OVERVIEW OF AFFECT EXPERIENCING

Affect Experiencing is the heart of Short-Term Dynamic Psychotherapy (STDP). It means desensitizing Affect Phobias and helping patients to experience adaptive affect (the Feeling Pole, or F, on the Triangle of Conflict) without the punishing inhibition (the Anxiety Pole, or A). The most effective exposure occurs when patients can eventually experience moderate to high levels of affect—for example, full sobbing or (in fantasy) murderous rage. However, if affect is experienced too intensely and too quickly, it is harder to process cognitively and in a controlled way.

Proceed with Graded Steps

It is therefore important to help patients achieve higher levels of affect in a stepwise, anxiety-regulated manner. Otherwise, there is a risk of sensitizing (increasing) rather than desensitizing the conflict (see Section V of Chapter 1).

Guided imagery is the main technique for helping patients experience feeling. In imagery, patients can experience the affect cognitively (in thought) and physiologically (in the body), and imagine the actions and behaviors that flow from the affect—all of which are necessary for desensitization. Desensitization in imagery also teaches the patient how to contain the feeling, which allows time to reflect on the best course of action. In fantasy, the patient's deepest needs and longings can be identified, validated, and experienced as fully as possible.

Understandably, loss of control is one of the greatest concerns that therapists have in eliciting such intense feelings. However, the process is not dangerous or destructive if done in a graded manner, with appropriately selected patients **who understand that thoughts and feelings are not the same as actions.**

When to Focus on Affect Experiencing

As noted above, to proceed with Affect Experiencing, the therapist must make sure that the patient (1) has a GAF score above 50, as discussed in Chapter 3; (2) feels able to contain the affect to be experienced; (3) has maintained good impulse control (e.g., recovery from substance misuse) for at least 1–3 years; and (4) has not had a history of destructive acting out. Patients who meet these criteria for good impulse control should be able to proceed directly to Affect Experiencing if they also:

- Are aware of their defensive avoidance behaviors (Defense Recognition).
- Feel ready to change (Defense Relinquishing).
- Have an adaptive sense of self and others.

Because impulsive behaviors (e.g., substance use disorder, assault, etc.) can be deployed as defenses against high levels of affect, patients' control over their impulses must be assessed before any deep exploration of affect begins. It is important that the patient feel able to contain the affect in question—that is, to experience the affect without a need to act out impulsively.

Many patients worry that they might act out impulsively, when they are actually extremely inhibited. This excessive anxiety needs to be assessed and, when appropriate, regulated. However, when such patients' concerns have some grounding in reality (i.e., a history of impulsivity or acting out), they need to be taken seriously. This is a signal to proceed slowly and with more than the usual caution.

In addition to patients' subjective sense of the risk of experiencing affect, it is important to assess patients' history of impulsive behavior. As noted above, patients with a history of substance misuse should be in stable recovery with good supports for at least 1–3 years. Since past behavior is the best predictor of the future, it is important to ask patients whether they have ever acted out or lashed out physically or in other destructive ways when angry.

When Not to Focus on Affect Experiencing

When a patient has a prior history of impulse control problems, exposure to feeling must be combined with learning of cognitive skills to control outbursts. Proceed slowly, cautiously, and with very small increments of feeling until self-control is built up and assured at each step, as in this example:

THERAPIST: In here it's safe to explore any feeling you want to, to whatever degree you want to. We are talking about feelings, only feelings, and not behaviors. We might let ourselves feel murderous toward someone, but we would never act on it. But since you have had trouble controlling your temper, let's begin with very small doses of feeling angry, and then build up little by little as you become sure you can control it. [Anger management strategy]

Which Affect to Focus on First?

When a patient is ready to proceed, the therapist also needs some guidance on these questions:

- "Which affect or affects should I pursue?"
- "If more than one, what order should I follow?"

The core conflict formulations of the presenting problems identified in the initial evaluation (see Chapter 4) should reveal the patient's main Affect Phobias, such as

- Grief
- Anger
- Tenderness/Closeness
- Positive Feelings about the Self

However, it is possible for new affect conflicts to emerge during the course of treatment, so therapists need to be open to this possibility. When the core conflict formulations reveal more than one Affect Phobia, therapists may be confused over which affect to start with. For example, when both grief and anger are conflicted, which one should be focused on first?

There is no hard-and-fast rule, but general guidelines have been discussed in the Introduction to Part II of this book, and you may want to review them at this point. Because of such individual differences, the therapist must use intuition and skill to determine the affect focus. Here are some additional guidelines for determining affect focus during a particular session:

- The affect focus can be determined by the problem the patient wants to work on during that session.
- The focus can be on the most prominent or salient conflicted affect in the problem being discussed.
- If undecided, the therapist can use trial and error—focusing first on one feeling, then another—until the patient becomes engaged in a specific conflicted affect.
- The therapist can ask the patient which feeling is the most readily available to be worked on. There are times when the patient can sense the necessary affect focus better than the therapist can.

Make Sure the Focus Is on Adaptive Affect

Recall the importance of distinguishing defensive/maladaptive affect from adaptive affect (see Section IV of Chapter 1, and Section III of Chapter 2). In proceeding to desensitize affects, it is extremely important for the therapist to distinguish carefully whether the affect is adaptive or maladaptive—**and to desensitize only the adaptive affect.** It is very easy for a therapist to focus mistakenly on defensive feeling, which can result in the patient's becoming more and more regressive.

Remember, adaptive versions of the affects are those that have an **outward-flowing,** opening, relieving quality, and result in behaviors that are the most constructive solutions possible for the self and for others involved. In contrast, maladaptive versions of the affect have an **inward-drawing** reaction, often with a helpless, "victimized" quality—a feeling of "Boo-hoo, poor me," representing an unconstructive complaining, rather than genuine sorrow or compassion for the self. There is generally a tightening, closing-off, shutting-down response. In more regressive versions of maladaptive affects, there is a tendency toward acting out of feeling or explosive venting, which is hurtful or destructive to self or others.

Key Steps in Affect Desensitization

Once the conflicted adaptive affect has been identified, the therapist uses guided imagery to start the exposure process. This process is designed to desensitize the conflict about the feeling. Desensitization involves the following steps (see Section V of Chapter 1), each corresponding to a pole on the Triangle of Conflict:

1. **Exposure to the feared affect (F Pole):** Exposing patients to warded-off affects in bearable but increasing doses. This is done primarily through guided imagery.
2. **Response prevention (D Pole):** Preventing the defensive or avoidant responses as needed during exposure (i.e., Defense Recognition and Relinquishing, as covered in Chapters 5 and 6).

3. **Anxiety-regulation (A Pole):** Regulating the anxieties as they arise; briefly shifting focus to exploration of the anxiety until the patient feels more in control or able to cope.

During desensitization, therapists need to move deftly among these three steps.

Keeping the Triangle of Conflict in mind during Affect Experiencing can help therapists strike an appropriate balance among these elements. Figure 7.1 illustrates the motion back and forth between exposure to affect (F Pole) and anxiety regulation (A Pole) while blocking defenses (response prevention, D Pole).

These procedures must be repeated until the feeling can "flow" adaptively and the patient can freely experience it with relief and satisfaction.

Titrating Anxiety

Thus, during desensitization, the therapist delicately shifts among exposing patients to affect in a graded way, encouraging them not to defend against or avoid the process, and helping them cope with the anxieties that exposure creates. It is this systematic desensitization process that resolves Affect Phobias.

After discussing the therapist stance in Affect Experiencing, we examine the components of systematic desensitization in more detail. Because of the importance of keeping anxiety within adaptive limits, we first discuss anxiety regulation (with emphasis on various fears about eliciting affect, and on some specific techniques for anxiety regulation). We then cover exposure in Section II and response prevention in Section III.

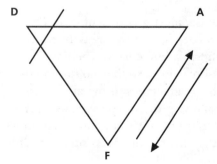

FIGURE 7.1. The process of affect desensitization. The directional arrows between the Anxiety Pole (A) and the Feeling Pole (F) illustrate how the therapist moves back and forth between exposure to feeling (F) and the regulation of anxieties (A) about feeling in order to proceed smoothly through a step-wise systematic desensitization. The solid line cutting off the Defense Pole (D) illustrates how the therapist helps the patient block the defenses (response prevention).

Therapist Stance: Encouragement and Shared Affect

Affect Experiencing presents a major emotional challenge to therapists, because in staying attuned, therapists must share the patients' experience of the feelings as much as is professional and reasonable. This can be quite difficult, especially if therapists are not comfortable with the feelings themselves.

No one attitude will be optimal for all patients. The therapist must be involved and authentic, especially in cases where the patient's parents were distant or neglectful. At the same time, the therapist must allow the patient enough space to feel safe and develop greater autonomy, especially in cases where parents were intrusive.

Share Feelings

Therapists may decide to make their feelings explicit, depending on the needs of their patients. One guideline is for the therapist to acknowledge the shared feelings, while also making explicit the boundaries or the limits in the relationship—sometimes in the same sentence.

THERAPIST 1: [Anger] As you speak of the abuse, it brings up anger in me on your behalf . . . but my anger must be small compared to yours.

THERAPIST 2: [Closeness] Yes, there are warm feelings here. Therapy is a safe place to discuss both positive and negative feelings—for, as you know, there are clear boundaries. We know that talking is all that will happen.

Transference and Countertransference Issues

Due to the challenge to the therapist in Affect Experiencing, transference and countertransference issues often come to the forefront. Patients are often afraid that their openness will elicit ridicule or devaluation from the therapist—which then leads them to create distance. The empathic connection is crucial in providing a safe and protected place for inhibited affect to be experienced and expressed. Affect is contagious. The intense emotions of the patient present an emotional challenge to the therapist.

Therapists must guard against overinvolvement, as well as the more common tendency to move away from feeling and lighten up, thereby losing the affective immediacy. Therapists also need to work to recognize and control reactions, so they do not interfere with the richness of the session. Watching videotapes of therapy sessions is an excellent way to study reactions and to grow and develop as a therapist—not to mention desensitizing a therapist's own Affect Phobias. For more on how to use videotape to evaluate therapy, see our Web site, www.affectphobia.org.

It is not realistic to expect therapists to have all their affective conflicts resolved. But in order to know whether a sobbing patient will ever stop crying, the therapist needs to have navigated these emotional waters first. Therapists who have the capacity for vulnerability and tenderness will be better able to tolerate experiencing it in others, and know what general forms it may take. For example, in order to feel comfortable with anger, a therapist needs to be able to tolerate a strong but controlled inner sense of anger as well.

Compassion for Therapists, Too

Optimally, therapists should be able to promote and not impede their patients' ability to face feelings. Nevertheless, therapists' own struggles to deal with patients' feelings should be treated with the same compassion as the patients' struggles (see CC, pp. 199–201).

Anxiety Regulation: Titrating the Exposure to Feeling

Anxiety regulation is a key component of desensitization that focuses directly on the phobic reactions (i.e., the mounting anxiety, shame/guilt, or pain). It reduces the inhibition of the adaptive feeling, allowing desensitization to continue by breaking the conditioned connection of adaptive affect and inhibitory affect. Moderate amounts of anxiety need to be evoked to keep the affect exposure process unfolding; too much anxiety, however, can be traumatizing and actually increase Affect Phobia (due to sensitization rather than desensitization; see Section V of Chapter 1). Affects and the anxiety they evoke should both be experienced repeatedly in small doses until patients are comfortable with their ability to control them.

To Calm a Flood of Anxiety

If a patient becomes flooded with anxiety or begins acting out between sessions, calm the patient by offering support and reassurance, and by exploring the fears, shame, or pain. For example, if a patient feels that he or she is starting to have a panic attack, here are some possible responses:

THERAPIST 1: Then let's not go any further with the tender feelings right now. Why don't we stop for a moment and see what's the scariest thing about this? (*Pause. A few minutes later:*) Can we look at the tender feeling again?

THERAPIST 2: You will feel some anxiety in the course of this therapy, but it's important that you are not overwhelmed by it. Let's better understand the fear. (*Pause. Then, when the panic episode is over:*) Now can we return to the feeling that scared you, and see if you can tolerate it better?

This "imaginal" desensitization of the feeling (i.e., exposure in imagery) brings anxiety, guilt, shame or pain to within normal limits. "Normal limits" means that there should always be enough inhibition to modulate or regulate feeling, but there should be flexibility and freedom in responding. (Also see CC, pp. 201–202, 209–215.)

Repeatedly Regulate Anxiety

Over many repetitions, the exposure to the feelings in the fantasy should be titrated (given in small amounts) from bland to moderate to strong as the patient demonstrates the capacity to control the expression outside the session. Anxiety, shame, or pain can be resolved by focusing on the inhibitory feeling until the patient gains some perspective and feels better able to cope with the fears:

PATIENT: It's so painful to remember this! I shut it all out after Granny died. There was no one else there.

THERAPIST: What's the most painful part of remembering her?

Return to Response Prevention If Necessary

Throughout anxiety regulation, there may be a tendency for the patient to return to the defensive response. Defenses are always present to some degree. However, if the defenses become so strong that the patient cannot proceed with the exposure, return to Defense Restructuring or Self- and Other-Restructuring to reduce the resistance.

PATIENT: I never let anyone close after that. I was so lonely I can hardly bear to think about it [D], even now.

THERAPIST: Try to stay with these feelings a little longer [Preventing defensive avoidance]. The feelings will be less painful over time [Anxiety regulation—reassurance]. Let me hear what made it so bad for you [Continued anxiety regulation].

But return to exposure as soon as the anxiety is reduced, to see whether the feeling is now better tolerated and more easily experienced.

PATIENT: Yes. Part of me longs to have her with me again. Her softness and gentleness soothed me so. When I go home, I think I'll get out some pictures of her that I put away in the attic.

Anxiety Regulation and Fears about Eliciting Affect

Patients and Therapists Fear Feelings

While working hard to elicit affect, therapists will inevitably encounter fears emerging—both patients' and their own. The main pitfall is that therapists will collude with patients' defenses in wanting to get away from the affect. The following discussion covers common fears about opening up to feelings. In the next subsection, we discuss some additional ways to help regulate the anxieties.

Shame of Having Feelings

"Why can't I just get over it?" One of the main problems in eliciting affect is that patients are told—or tell themselves—to "put the past away and just move on." This is unfortunate, because healing actually requires remembering and reintegrating past experiences, including painful feelings. Of course, we do not mean chronic blaming or complaining about the past, which is a defensive position.

PATIENT: What good is it going to do me to let myself cry about it? What's done is done, I just want to put it behind me!

THERAPIST: Of course you do. [Validation] But the irony is that what is keeping you stuck [cost] is how hard you work to avoid [D] crying [F]. If you let yourself have your feelings, it will **help** you move on, because it will free up all the energy that you're using to push those feelings away. [Defense Relinquishing]

The goal is the resolution of the Affect Phobias so that the patient can "move on" and face the future in a new and adaptive manner (see also CC, pp. 215–216).

Lack of Entitlement to Feeling

"Are my feelings justified?" As discussed in Chapter 1, feelings are vital signals that need to be attended to. Many patients wonder whether their feelings are "justified" or "correct" or "right." In the first example below, the patient has a phobia about joy. In the second, the phobia is about sexual desire.

Phobia of Joy

PATIENT: Is this feeling right? I mean, am I supposed to want to burst out crying because something good has happened? It feels stupid.

THERAPIST: Right now, try not to judge what you are feeling [Response prevention]. Just explore it to understand what the feeling is telling you.

Phobia of Sexual Feelings

PATIENT: As we started making love, I suddenly wanted my boyfriend to be rough with me. This goes against my feminist philosophy. Am I sick or something?

THERAPIST: Feelings aren't "right" or "wrong"—they're just feelings. It's important to listen to them, because you can learn from them.

Patients need to learn to always pay attention to their vital inner signals and ask, **"What are my feelings telling me?"** Even if the feeling is defensive, destructive, or self-attacking, it does not create a problem if it is **contained in fantasy** and not acted upon. The patient needs to understand the true underlying want or need, and take action accordingly. One of the reasons why so much effort in this approach is put into experiencing feelings in fantasy is so that feelings can be sorted out cognitively at a later time.

Fear That Affect Will "Take Over"

"What if I lose control?" One of the greatest barriers encountered in eliciting feeling is that patients fear the feeling will take complete control of them and destroy everything. The following list gives some examples of these fears. (For more on a patient's fear of losing control, see CC, pp. 220–227.)

Affect (F Pole)	**Fears of the Affect (A Pole)**
Anger	"I will destroy relationships, or turn into a violent monster who will kill and be abandoned. Once angry, I will never stop being angry."

Affect (F Pole)	Fears of the Affect (A Pole)
Grief	"I will never stop crying, the world will feel empty, and I will never experience happiness again."
Closeness	"I will be swallowed up, controlled, or unable to protect myself."
Positive feelings toward the self	"I will become arrogant and selfish, and no one will want to be with me."
Sexual desire	"I will become uncontrollably promiscuous or perverted."
Joy	"I will soon lose good feeling or 'burst,' 'the ax will soon fall,' or some kind of punishment will soon follow."
Shame	"I will appear disgusting and thus be abandoned."
Fear	"I will have overwhelming panic or feelings of impending doom."
Contempt/disgust	"I will seem like I am arrogant and mean, if I show how appalled I am by what he did."

Some Techniques to Regulate Anxiety

Small Steps for Fearful Patients

Desensitization should be done slowly and in small doses until patients feel confident in their ability to control their feelings. Consider this exchange:

THERAPIST: Do you feel comfortable with the intensity of these feelings, or are you worried you might lose control after this session?

PATIENT: I don't want to [D] cry [F] here. I don't know if I could stop [A].

THERAPIST: There's so much sadness in you that it feels like it would go on forever. [Reflecting both adaptive affect and the anxiety]

PATIENT: There's so much.

THERAPIST: Let's look at what seems to be your anxiety about crying. [Anxiety regulation] What's the longest you've ever cried? When you cried at home this weekend, how long did it last?

PATIENT: Probably only moments, and it was such a relief.

THERAPIST: So in fact, it wouldn't really go on forever, even though it feels that way.

PATIENT: I see what you mean (*looking as if wanting to cry*).

THERAPIST: What if you really allowed yourself to feel what you're feeling, without holding it back? [Return to exposure]

Encouragement and Reassurance

Encouragement and reassurance can help regulate anxiety:

THERAPIST: It may feel like you will never come through it, but you will. You won't be swallowed up. In fact, the real difficulty is to stay with the sadness until it is worked through. The problem is that it can feel so bad that most people want to run from it, rather than stay with it.

Use of Humor

Humor can sometimes help a patient bear difficult affect:

THERAPIST: I know it feels like you'll never stop crying. But the truth is, you'll get hungry or have to go to the bathroom at some point!

Use caution, however, since mistimed humor can be experienced as insensitive or belittling. Humor works only in the context of a strong alliance and positive therapist regard.

With this thorough grounding in anxiety regulation and its various aspects, we are ready to turn to exposure.

II. EXPOSURE TO PHOBIC FEELING/THE FEARED AFFECT

Three Dimensions of Affective Experience

Exposure to adaptive affect is the heart of this therapy. The more the patient is able to experience affect **verbally, physiologically,** and **in the imagined action of fantasy,** the more thorough the desensitization of conflict will be. Therefore, the therapist must work to elicit these three dimensions for full affective experience. Using guided imagery (while carefully monitoring the physiological signs of feeling and anxiety), the therapist must help the patient do these three things:

1. Verbally label the affect—correctly.
2. Identify the physical feeling of the affect in the body.
3. Imagine desired action in fantasy.

Verbally Label the Affect to Heighten Cognitive Awareness

The patient must first be able to label correctly the specific affect being avoided (e.g., must not mistake anxiety for anger or depression for sadness). It is common for patients to mislabel their inner feelings. Patients often confuse anxiety with anger, mistake depression for grief, confuse neediness with longing for tenderness—or have no idea what words to put on their internal sensations.

THERAPIST: When your friend refused to help out, what did you feel?

PATIENT: I don't know.

THERAPIST: Well, did you like it or not like it?

PATIENT: I didn't like it.

THERAPIST: So what feeling is that?

PATIENT: I guess it's anger.

Thus the therapist can help sort out this confusion and guide patients to the correct identification of feeling by getting them to assign **a specific word** to the inner experience (anger, sadness, joy, etc). This is a preliminary exposure to the awareness of the feeling—first on a cognitive level—which can be anxiety-provoking in itself.

PATIENT 1: I'm ashamed to see myself as an angry person!

PATIENT 2: It frightens me to think I've been carrying sadness all these years.

PATIENT 3: I feel joyful and calm now, but sometimes it terrifies me to be so relaxed!

(For more information on labeling affects, see CC, pp. 138–139, 202–204.)

Blends of Adaptive and Maladaptive Feeling

It is common that feelings can be blends of adaptive and maladaptive feelings—for example, excessive anger at an abusive parent that needs to be better modulated, or exaggerated crying that includes genuine grief but is mingled with a "victimized" response. **Both maladaptive and adaptive feelings need to be desensitized enough to tolerate facing them and exploring them. But only adaptive feelings should be desensitized enough to act upon them.**

Healing Potential of Acceptance of Feeling

It is vital for people to be conscious of the full range of inner emotional experiences, for we all have them. They guide and control our actions. To know and understand oneself fully, one needs to be able to give feelings free rein—something that is not always possible in reality, but is always possible and available in fantasy. It can be enormously self-validating to accept this previously warded-off part of the self by the use of fantasy or imagery.

Experience the Physical Feeling of the Affect

Therapists must help patients experience the physiological or bodily feelings of affect by helping them connect the verbal label for the affect with the correct physical feelings in the body.

THERAPIST 1: How do you experience tenderness in your body?

PATIENT 1: I feel a warm feeling in my chest. And I want to show that—a feeling of wanting to cuddle up and hold her.

THERAPIST 2: How do you experience that anger in your body?

PATIENT 2: My arms feel like they have to strike out, and I get a rush of energy flowing up and out.

THERAPIST 3: How do you experience the joy in your body?

PATIENT 3: Well, now that I focus on it, I feel relaxed, my stomach is soft, and I'm breathing slowly and easily.

THERAPIST 4: How do you experience the excitement about that in your body?

PATIENT 4: Oh! I'm so focused. All my attention is there, and my heart is pumping. I'm drawn to it. I feel eager and good inside.

Always Monitor Bodily Arousal

Having the patient experience visceral bodily sensations of feeling is essential to the desensitization process. With affective arousal, there may be signs of activation, or there may be signs of withdrawal, tension, tightness, cowering, or pulling away—which signal inhibition and anxiety, not activation. Desensitization will not work if the patient only **thinks about** a feeling but does not **experience it viscerally**. That would be like having a patient with a bridge phobia only think blandly about crossing a bridge, but never actually feel the anxiety of doing so. Consider this exchange between a therapist and an inhibited angry patient.

THERAPIST: How does your body feel?

PATIENT: I feel butterflies in my stomach, tightness in my chest, and a buzzing in my head.

THERAPIST: Is that anger or anxiety? [Helping make the distinction]

PATIENT: I guess that's anxiety. That's funny, I always thought of this as anger.

THERAPIST: Many people confuse anger and anxiety signals, so let's focus on what anger really feels like. Let's look at a time when you were really furious.

PATIENT: I remember once I felt really angry, and there was a rush of energy in my arms and legs!

The phobia about the feeling is not only linked to **thinking** about the feeling. The phobia is most strongly linked to the actual **arousal** of the feeling.

Having patients monitor their bodily sensations helps pinpoint Affect Phobias. When patients have Affect Phobias, they exhibit excessive amounts of bodily tightness, tension, withdrawal, panic, fear, and inhibition whenever they are exposed to the affective arousal.

PATIENT 1: Whenever I get the least bit sexually aroused [F], my body feels deadened and lifeless [D].

PATIENT 2: The last few times I've felt like crying [F], my throat tightened up and nothing happened [D].

PATIENT 3: I started to relax and get a massage [F—enjoyment/joy], and then I just freaked out [D, A].

Imagine Desired Actions in Fantasy

In addition to labeling the specific affect verbally, and linking the label with accurate bodily sensations (i.e., not confusing adaptive feelings with inhibitory feelings), the next step is to explore what the feeling makes them want to do—in fantasy, of course. Affect Phobias are not only fears of feeling; they are also fears about what the feeling might move one to do—and the fear of those actions can increase the avoidance of the feeling itself (see also CC, pp. 205–208).

Sustained Exposure Should Be Repeated in Multiple Sessions

There is another reason why exposure in fantasy is necessary: For desensitization of Affect Phobias to be effective, there must be sustained bodily arousal. While conducting the imagery, it is generally necessary to **sustain the exposure to the visceral experience of the feeling (e.g., 5–40 minutes) in repeated sessions,** to help patients become comfortable with the affect and to diminish the inhibitory feelings. Exposure by using imagery is one of the easiest ways to achieve such sustained experience of affect. As we have frequently noted, to sustain the exposure in those sessions, anxieties need to be regulated and defensive responses must be prevented as the affect is experienced (see Sections II and IV of this chapter).

Fantasies Are Not the Goal of Therapy

Of course, these fantasies are not the goal of therapy. Imagery, though it can be gratifying in itself, is employed as a means to feel comfortable with and understand previously avoided feelings. It is a means of accessing, containing, and desensitizing conflict around feelings that later must be expressed or acted upon in adaptive ways—so that patients can achieve authentic, mature, well-guided expression of feeling, and thereby resolve problems in living (see Chapter 8 on Affect Expression).

It bears repeating that therapists must emphasize to patients that they can't face feeling solely by thinking. Desensitization means that patients must do the following:

- Feel the bodily arousal of the specific affect.
- Examine how the feeling might propel them to act.
- Face the fears that are elicited by the fantasy.
- Master or cope with the associated fears until the feeling is freed up.

Yet, throughout Affect Experiencing, patients need to be reminded that **feelings are not actions** and that extreme feelings experienced in fantasy are not to be acted upon in destructive ways.

Exposure as "Benign Regression"

Affect-laden imagery provides a safe place for such feelings, desires, and wishes to be explored and gratified, while remaining contained and thus not destructive. In his book *The Basic Fault,* Michael Balint (1968, p. 32) referred to such immersion into and exploration of deep feelings as "regression in service of the ego" or "regression to foster progression," because it can be thought of as returning to an earlier developmental stage to foster the patient's growth. In the "benign regression" of fantasy, abusive authority figures can be murdered; one's lust can be fulfilled with whomever one pleases, however one pleases; and one can be held and caressed tenderly and lovingly by anyone, for as long as one wishes. **But once again, it is crucial to remind the patient that regressive feelings are safe to experience as long as they are not acted upon in real life.** (See CC pp. 206–208, for a further discussion of regression.)

Example: Exposure to Anger

PATIENT: I'm getting angrier and angrier at my boss.

THERAPIST: How do you experience that anger? Where is it in your body?

PATIENT: My chest feels tight, constricted. It feels awful.

THERAPIST: Is that the anger, or is it something else?

PATIENT: Maybe I'm just keeping a lid on the anger.

THERAPIST: What would happen if you let the lid off a little bit? If you allowed yourself to be really furious at him rather than feel anxious?

PATIENT: I'd just want to tell him off really well. (*Becoming more animated*) I could just slap him [action tendency], I feel so mad [label]. Not that I'd really do it.

THERAPIST: Of course not, but what does that feel like in your body [physiological sign of anger]?

PATIENT: It's like there's all this energy. It starts in my chest, but then it's flowing out into my arms and legs. It's a powerful feeling—my anger.

Acceptance of All Parts of the Self

Regression in fantasy permits patients to explore—and come to accept and understand—the most disturbing parts of themselves. Such fantasies can be disturbing for therapists to listen to. But for patients, sharing fantasies like these in a nonjudgmental atmosphere can provide a corrective emotional experience. Here are some examples of potentially disturbing fantasies:

• **Violent or sadistic angry images.**

PATIENT: I wanted to drag my fingernails through her flesh and watch her scream!

THERAPIST: She must have hurt you so.

Sadistic feelings arise from the enormous pain of being abused, and need exposure to both anger and grief.

• **Perverse or wanton sexual feelings.**

PATIENT: I wanted to have sex with as many partners as I wanted, in a violent or aggressive way, and have people watching.

THERAPIST: What do you think you are longing for the most in that scene?

Disturbing sexual desires are often a defensive way of seeking love and acceptance—or a way of punishing oneself.

• **Dependent and childlike fantasies.**

PATIENT: I just long to live with you and have you take care of me.

THERAPIST: What would be the most soothing part of that image? What would you long for from me that you have trouble doing for yourself? (*Later*) How can we help you find that in your life?

Cravings for dependency often cover a lack of confidence in one's own capabilities.

By addressing and developing such warded-off capacities, patients come to accept and work with parts of themselves that they may previously have had to block or deny.

Capacity to Tolerate Feeling Reduces Need to Act Out

The ability to tolerate such material in fantasy allows patients to reduce their shame about such reactions, and to come to understand their underlying adaptive wishes. Processing these images in fantasy also reduces the tendency to act them out. However, perpetrators of violent acts often ruminate about the violence that they would like to do to someone. This is an example of defensive anger, and is often insufficiently inhibited by appropriate shame or guilt, so that it is easily acted upon in real life. Obviously, in such cases, a therapist would not focus on eliciting more angry impulses. When anger is used in this way as a defense, the truly avoided affect is usually positive feeling about the self, or closeness and vulnerability to trust of others. It is important to remember that in order to tolerate and appropriately modulate the desensitization of blocked anger, a patient must be well connected interpersonally and well controlled.

Here are more examples of exposing patients to affects with regressive fantasies:

Exposure to Anger in Regressive Fantasy

THERAPIST: What would you want to do if you let those feelings out? Of course, we are not talking about acting here; we are only exploring these feelings in fantasy.

PATIENT: Well, I was so mad that I really wanted to punch him. Oh! How I would have loved to take a crack at him! I can feel myself doing it . . . and I wouldn't want to stop pounding on him for a long time!

THERAPIST: What do you imagine doing to him next?

Exposure to Phobia about Sexual Feelings

A happily married accountant is distressed by her intense sexual desire for her coworker. Imagery can be used to uncover unconscious wants and needs:

PATIENT: Every time I see him, I just long to make love to him.

THERAPIST: How do you imagine that happening? And what would you long for the most? What would be the most compelling thing about this person?

Allowing her the full exploration of that sexual arousal in fantasy can (1) provide some relief (at least in the short run), and (2) lead to greater understanding about what might be missed and longed for from her partner, without her having either to deny the feelings or to enact them. As with other imagery, it is essential that the patient be able to contain the fantasies rather than act on them, so that the material that is uncovered can be used to improve her real relationship. (For more on regression in fantasy, see also CC, pages 206–208.)

More Examples of Exposure to Specific Affects

Here are further examples of exposure to affect, using imagery:

Exposure to Sadness/Grief

THERAPIST: How do you feel when you remember being with your grandmother? [Exposure]

PATIENT: Granny would take me everywhere with her. It was wonderful. She would look at me a lot and smile at me, and I'd glow inside.

THERAPIST: That sounds wonderful.

PATIENT: Actually, I find myself not wanting to remember her. My body feels tight. I guess that's me trying to hold back crying [D].

THERAPIST: What would happen if you didn't hold back? [Response prevention and anxiety regulation]

PATIENT: I'd feel more sad. I get a heavy feeling in my chest and . . . yeah, if I relax a little and think about how it was to be with her, my eyes feel teary and I want to cry my heart out [F]!

Exposure to Sadness/Grief

THERAPIST: Can you remember the moment when you were the saddest about your friend moving away? Are there words you would put on the sadness?

PATIENT: I would want to say how much I will miss her [the adaptive part of the feeling] (*tearing up*), and how I feel I will be miserable all the time now that she's gone [the more regressive part of the feeling].

THERAPIST: Can you imagine how it was when your friend was here, to see what you miss so much that it feels irreplaceable? [Imagery to continue the exposure and exploration]

Exposure to Excitement

THERAPIST: You said you loved to sing. Did you let yourself do it at the party?

PATIENT: No. I stood over to the side and watched. I would have been mortified to get up there with them, and mess things up with my voice.

THERAPIST: How sad you missed out! Now can you let yourself imagine singing wholeheartedly at the party, and tell me what would be the hardest part of it for you?

Exposure to Anger

THERAPIST: What do your angry feelings make you feel like doing? Let's explore these feelings here in the office where it is safe.

PATIENT: The other day I was so mad about his jumping all over me [the adaptive part of the feeling] that I just felt like grabbing him by the throat and choking him [the more regressive part of the feeling]. It made me feel like a monster.

THERAPIST: Maybe if you could just stay with all those feelings for a while, you could find out what part of your anger is justified, and what part is the hurt part. We can talk later about how to handle this difficult person. [Affect Expression; see Chapter 8] But now let's just stay with how hard that hit you and what the feeling means. [Continuing the exposure and exploration]

Exposure to Joy

PATIENT: I was relaxed for the first time—maybe in years. Just sitting at my kitchen table, in the sunlight, sipping some coffee. There was a lightness that was so new. Then I panicked!

THERAPIST: Could you try to relax right now and remember that? Let's try to see what is so scary about something so tranquil and safe.

Exposure to Closeness

THERAPIST: Can you imagine going to your father's house, and telling him some of the things you've told me . . . about how much he meant to you?

PATIENT: Yes, I can, and it feels wonderful to think about doing that.

THERAPIST: Can you imagine letting yourself give him a hug?

PATIENT: Oh that would be a first! But let's see . . . yes, I can. I think I want to do that. I do want to give him a hug [the adaptive part of the feeling]. In fact, when I think of it I just want to hold on so tight I never want to let go [the more regressive part of the feeling]. And then I get scared, because sexual feelings start to come up [another conflict that need desensitizing].

Sexual feelings often arise along with closeness. The fear of that response is often far more difficult to bear than the sexual arousal itself. The goal in such a case is to learn to tolerate sexual feelings without having to act on them.

THERAPIST: Well, these are just feelings that everyone has to a greater or lesser degree. [Anxiety regulation] Let's explore them here where it feels safe to help you understand them and manage them better. How do you imagine yourself hugging him? And let's look at all the feelings that come up. [Continuing the exposure and exploration]

(For more on exposure to specific affects, see CC, pp. 191–192 and 223–224.)

Ways to Deepen Patients' Affect Experience

It is common for patients to need much help eliciting emotional arousal. They often have spent a lifetime running away from certain feelings. This is new and strange territory. In our discussion of anxiety regulation, we have focused on ways to help with exposure by reducing the barriers to feeling. This section focuses on methods to **directly intensify exposure**.

The therapist needs to emphasize to the patient that feelings need to be explored initially, without being acted on, until the feelings are well controlled and actions are the most constructive. With practice, finding constructive action can become automatic—like riding a bicycle. But at first, adaptive affective responding takes contemplation. As patients come to recognize and acknowledge their desires, bear them, and learn how to adaptively and realistically respond to them, problems become resolved and healing occurs.

Full Inner Experience During desensitization, greater intensity of feeling is experienced when the body is still, because this allows the patients to attend deeply to inner experience. Although acting out the feeling through bodily motion can sometimes "jump-start" the process, it can ultimately be distracting and can actually diminish the fullness of inner experience. Therefore, if a patient has the capacity to experience a particular feeling—even slightly—it is generally advisable to build the inner awareness of the experience in imagery ("imaginal desensitization") with the body remaining fairly still. When patients are unable to experience feeling, bodily movement may be essential; this is discussed below.

Here is a list of specific techniques to help patients access fuller arousal of feeling during the process of exposure; we then go through them in more detail below. When you are applying these methods, watch patients closely to monitor the deepening of their feeling as well as their self-control.

- Stay relentlessly focused on the feeling.
- Use empathic phrases.
- Reflect back the patient's words.
- Focus on details.
- Explore bodily sensations.
- Imagine what might have been.
- Share your own feelings.

- Encourage benign regression to intense feelings in fantasy.
- Use Eye-Movement Desensitization and Reprocessing (EMDR).
- Use bodily movement when feeling is blocked.

Different techniques have differing impacts across patients. If one approach doesn't appear to help, try another. You can add techniques from your own therapeutic repertoire.

Relentlessly Focusing on Feeling

Stay focused on the feeling—the bodily sensations, the action tendencies. Avoid intellectualizing or pursuing your own questions or curiosities when the patient is full with feelings. Stay doggedly with the emotion! You can discuss the meaning later in the session, after the experiencing. Here is an example in which the patient appears choked up with emotion but is holding back:

THERAPIST: You want so much to cry. . . . What is your body feeling now? What words come up with the feeling? [The therapist is not trying to elicit intellectual insight, but the simple phrases that come with sorrow— e.g., "I miss him so!"]

Sometimes simple encouragement is enough to handle residual defensiveness:

THERAPIST: It feels like there's still a part of you that's holding back the tears.

PATIENT: It's habitual—putting the emotional brakes on. I'm not trying to hold back.

THERAPIST: What if you allowed yourself to really have your sadness? To let the brakes off a little more?

Empathic Phrases

Use empathic phrases to deepen affect. Many of these phrases are time-tested responses familiar to most therapists in empathizing and validating emotional experience.

- "Mmm" or other empathic noises.
- "Stay with that."
- "Tell me more"
- "That sounds sad [upsetting, infuriating]."
- "This must be very difficult to go through."
- "Of course you're angry!"
- "This experience has been terribly painful for you."
- "No wonder you become angry with him when he treats you this way!"
- "You seem much more capable to me than you let yourself to take credit for."

Reflect Back the Patient's Words

There is great power in exact repetition of the patient's words, though care must be taken to use an empathic intonation.

PATIENT 1: My mother never loved me.

THERAPIST 1: Your mother never loved you.

PATIENT 2: All my childhood I longed for my father to pay attention to me.

THERAPIST 2: You longed for your father to pay attention to you.

Focus on Details

The more textured the image, the more powerful the affective arousal. Ask for vivid descriptions of the circumstances: the room the patient was in, the color of the walls, the patient's age, the way the body felt sitting next to the grandfather, sights, sounds, smells, and so on.

PATIENT: My mother used to sit around alone in a dark room, smoking.

THERAPIST: Did she have a particular place where she used to sit?

PATIENT: I remember her sitting in a rose armchair all day and not moving. The cigarette smoke hung around her head.

When patients are not able to generate images themselves, therapists can suggest tentative images based on previous data. The therapist needs to help the patient paint a picture of what happened in vivid detail. For example, in a death scene, the therapist might ask, "How was it sitting on the bed?" or "Did you put your hand on his arm?" or "How did his face look?" or "How long did you stay?" Be mindful of pacing, however. "Peppering" patients with questions can pull them out of the affect.

Explore Bodily Sensations

As discussed earlier, the bodily sensations of affect are an integral part of Affect Experiencing. Checking the patient's bodily sensations periodically can help the patient stay in touch with the affect.

THERAPIST: What are you feeling in your body right now?

PATIENT: Nothing.

THERAPIST: Just a little while ago, you said you were feeling energy in your arms and chest. Let's see if we can figure out where that energy went.

Imagine What Might Have Been

Asking the patient to imagine what might have been can be a powerful way to elicit affect, especially grief or longing. Here are some questions the therapist can ask:

- "What was in your heart that you longed to say but weren't able to?"
- "What would it have felt like to look in his eyes?"
- "What did you most long to hear him say to you before he died?"

Sharing Your Own Feelings

Self-disclosure can profoundly intensify the affective experience, though it needs to be done wisely and professionally, as discussed above in connection with therapist stance (see Section I).

In the following example, the patient has just told a story about getting a shoeshine—a symbolic act of self-nurturance that signifies his desire to treat himself better. It is a small step, but it represents his first important move toward a change in his relationship with himself.

PATIENT: I'm crying partly because it was such a kick to do this for myself, and partly because of the years I have spent not providing these kinds of things for myself. For all the times I've been so hard on myself. But mostly it's a happy thing.

THERAPIST: It's such a moving story. And it captures so much of what you've been doing here in therapy. It brings tears to my eyes as well. I'm feeling very happy for you, and I also feel sad for all the times you weren't able to care for yourself.

Encourage Regression in Fantasy

As discussed above, regression in fantasy can be an extremely powerful tool for therapeutic change in patients who are able to contain the affect in fantasy without acting on it. Because of the strength of patients' defenses, it can take a great deal of encouragement to get them to a full fantasy experience of a regressive affect such as murderous rage.

THERAPIST: We've seen over and over how you turn your anger on yourself, and how you suffer for it: with depression, with feeling bad about yourself as a person [costs]. I've seen this in many people, and one thing that really helps is to imagine, as vividly as you can, what your body would like to do to the other person, understanding that this is a fantasy so it can't have any negative consequences—for you or for them. In fact, the goal is to help you feel better in a harmless way [benefit]. Your thoughts and feelings hurt no one, but learning to accept these feelings can greatly help you—by making peace with them.

Use EMDR

Eye-Movement Desensitization and Reprocessing (Shapiro, 2001) is a promising and empirically supported therapeutic approach that uses eye movement (or various other means of bilateral alternating stimulation) to help patients reprocess traumatic or disturbing memories. Though EMDR was originally employed in the treatment of posttraumatic stress disorder (PTSD), our experience has been that EMDR can also be helpful in eliciting warded-off feelings and in facilitating affective change. Several of the authors have been trained in EMDR and have found it to be a useful adjunct in Affect Experiencing work, particularly at moments in therapy when affect appears to be blocked. (For a more detailed discussion of integrating STDP and EMDR, see McCullough, 2002).

Use Bodily Movement When Feeling Is Blocked

Therapists frequently ask whether it helps to have patients use body movement (e.g., punching pillows) to access feelings. The answer depends on the needs of the patient. When patients (especially those who are alexithymic—see Sifneos, 1973) are not able to access feelings, **sometimes bodily movement is a very helpful and effective way to begin to identify inner feeling states.** Acting out the feeling in a symbolic manner can sometimes bring warded-off feeling into consciousness. Punching pillows, pounding nails, slamming tennis balls, or wringing washcloths can "jump-start" the process of bringing the sensations of anger into awareness. Martial arts classes can help some people get in touch with their sense of bodily power. Also, "batacas" made from a thick pad of dense foam rubber ($6'' \times 1' \times 3'$ is a recommended size) covered with heavy cloth are safe objects to pound with—or to pound **on** with fists or a heavy object. Sometimes patients need to use these external methods for weeks until the feelings are easily accessed and experienced. However, as noted above, the eventual goal is to have the patients learn to experience all feelings in fantasy.

Only in fantasy do patients have full freedom to come to know what the feeling is signaling, and how best to act on it. The practice of inner containment of feeling is important, because when one is angry, it is not productive to have to "get it out" by acting out the feelings on the spot! **Quiet contemplation of intense inner experience is empowering and can lead to more mindful responses.** (For more on how to encourage affective experience, see CC pp., 223–228)

III. RESPONSE PREVENTION: DEFENSE RESTRUCTURING AS NEEDED

When patients have conflicts over feelings, exposure will inevitably elicit anxiety; as a result, there is often a tendency to return to defensive avoidance.

PATIENT: How I dread [A] talking about this. I just want to run [D].

THERAPIST: I know this is difficult, but can you try not to run away [D]? Can you stay with the feeling? [Response prevention with encouragement to return to exposure]

PATIENT: I was so furious with her [F] that I never told her I loved her [F] before she died (*crying*) [F].

If defenses continue to block the experience of feeling, return to the Defense Restructuring procedures discussed in Chapters 5 and 6. Generally, however, it's best to take the briefest possible detour into Defense Restructuring and then return to Affect Experiencing.

PATIENT: When I imagine getting angry at him, I feel like such a jerk!

THERAPIST: So do you see how—just like we talked about before—as soon as angry feelings come up, you turn them around and attack yourself [D]? Do you remember what you said about all that self-attack the last time we talked about it?

PATIENT: Yeah—it's killing me [cost].

THERAPIST: I think that's right. So I'm going to ask you to just put all that aside for now and let yourself have your feelings. We'll come back later and work on how it makes you feel about yourself. [Note: A therapist would do this only if the self-attack is not too severe.]

IV. IDENTIFYING PITFALLS IN AFFECT EXPERIENCING

This section addresses some common problems and misconceptions about Affect Experiencing.

The Fallacy of "Getting Anger Out"

The ultimate goal of Affect Experiencing is **never** to "get feelings out," but to process feelings insightfully and responsibly. The concept of "getting the anger out" is greatly misunderstood. Explosive bursts of anger outside of sessions may be initially relieving, but they usually do not resolve the problem. Instead, things are often made worse. In contrast, assertive responses—responses that state one's needs or limits—can and do bring relief. Similarly, when a patient is justifiably angry in a therapy session, the goal is **not** to have the patient "get the anger out" by exploding, venting, screaming, or yelling. Such behavior may at times help "jump-start" the experiencing of anger, as noted earlier; if it persists, however, it will just maintain a helpless, frustrated—and thus defensive—stance.

In therapy, imagery is used to help the patient experience the intensity of the anger inwardly in a safe place for desensitization, exploration, and understanding. Following this, the patient and therapist decide on the actions that need to be taken to resolve the problem.

PATIENT: I was so mad that I really wanted to kill him! I was astonished at the degree of the fury I felt.

THERAPIST: If your reaction was that strong, there must have been some reason for it. Let's explore it to see what part of it comes from your past relationships, and what part may be justifiable anger toward your coworker. Can you go back to that scene and describe to me what you felt, without taking any action outside of the session until you feel comfortable and in control? Later we'll talk over what needs to be done in reality to make the situation better.

Ultimately, the objective is **how** to express the anger in the real relationship in a way that brings the most possible constructive solution and lasting relief (Affect Expression; see Chapter 8).

Impulse Control Problems

When impulse control is difficult for a patient, then cognitive work should be used to build (1) **adaptive defenses of self-control,** and/or (2) **a positive sense of self** that is not so reactive. These capacities must precede desensitization of affect.

Help the patient identify and control the earliest physiological signs of emotion—for example, minor irritations that precede temper outbursts, or small disappointments that build impulsive action. It is easier to control small arousals of feelings than full-blown ones.

THERAPIST: Can you go back again to when your boss criticized you in front of the clients, and let yourself feel just a little of your anger? How do you feel in your body, and what would be a better thing to do with it?

With each repetition, the patient is put through exercises or "emotional push-ups" until mastery of that particular amount of the feeling is achieved. **Only when the patient feels fully in control of the feeling level being focused on should the therapist return to exposure to the next increment of feeling.**

Acting Out with No Prior History

Sometimes an otherwise well-controlled patient may act out in small ways after an intense session. The more repressed an individual is, the greater the tendency to do so may be (e.g., to yell or lose temper). The solution is to alert patients to this possibility during the session, so they can build cognitive controls over their feelings.

THERAPIST: You may have a tendency to respond more strongly during the coming week because you have started to experience how angry you are at your father during this session. If you feel that beginning to happen, try to stop and think of what might be the best course of action.

Note, however, that most patients with a GAF score over 50 and a history of good impulse control have more current control over their impulses than they may give themselves credit for. (For a more complex discussion of patients' acting out, see CC, pp. 61–62, 217–218.)

Danger of Self-Attack

There is a danger that eliciting feelings too quickly may intensify self-attack, or "acting-in." When strong feelings uncovered in therapy bring with them a painful amount of inhibition (anxiety, guilt, shame, or grief), patients can then become the targets of their own self-attack. The more masochistic patients are, the more they are in danger of causing themselves real discomfort by feeling anxious, guilty, ashamed, or miserable because of the "unacceptable" feelings that have been brought into consciousness.

PATIENT: I felt so pathetic about discovering how I long for my mother's care that I spent the weekend feeling just miserable.

THERAPIST: The point of exposing you to these feelings is to relieve you, not cause you more suffering. So we need to help you reduce that shame until you're not tormented any more. After all, these are only feelings. [Anxiety regulation]

(For more on how to work with self-attacking patients, see Chapter 9; see also CC, pp. 218–219.)

Eliciting Feelings Too Slowly

Often therapists avoid patients' emotional issues because (1) they feel protective and do not want to cause the patients more pain, or (2) the feelings are too painful for the therapists to bear. However, it does not "protect" a surgical patient to let a wound fester because cleaning it would be uncomfortable. Similarly, **our patients are not protected by attempting to keep them anxiety-free.** Suffering can be unnecessarily prolonged by therapists' being overly "protective" and "concerned" about upsetting the patients or causing them pain by facing difficult issues. If a patient is functioning moderately well (GAF score above 50), exposure can usually be tolerated.

Anxiety-Regulating Interventions

Anxiety must be evoked to some degree before it can be reduced and the patient's pain can be lessened. This book has described a number of anxiety-regulating and shame-reducing interventions that help patients bear painful feelings. These interventions include cognitive techniques, Self- and Other-Restructuring, support, and reassurance. Here are a few examples:

THERAPIST 1: What's the worst [scariest, most difficult] thing that could happen if you felt that? [Cognitive/anxiety-reducing technique]

THERAPIST 2: Do you fear that I might think badly of you because of feelings you might have? [Self-Restructuring]

THERAPIST 3: You didn't ask for these defenses—you learned them growing up. [Shame-reducing technique]

THERAPIST 4: Remember, these are only feelings. They hurt no one and can help you. [Teaching, reassurance]

THERAPIST 5: Let's slow down and back off the feelings for a while. You do not have to force yourself through change if it is overwhelming. [Anxiety regulation]

Therapists' Coping with Their Own Fears

When a therapist is having difficulty bearing a patient's feelings, some supervision (including peer supervision) or personal therapy should be obtained. Like patients, therapists need support in tolerating strong levels of feelings. Therapists do not have to be perfect or have all their issues resolved. Therapists need only to be "good enough" and try to stay a bit ahead of their patients in leading them out of Affect Phobias into adaptive functioning.

Training Therapists with Videotapes

Training programs are very much needed to help prepare therapists in how to handle emotion effectively. As noted earlier in this chapter, such training should include watching videotapes of successful high-affect therapy sessions, which is very helpful in reducing therapists' anxieties about intense feelings. (Again, for more on the evaluation of videotaped sessions, see our Web site, www.affectphobia.org.)

V. REPEATING INTERVENTIONS UNTIL AFFECT PHOBIA IS DESENSITIZED

Exposure in imagery must be repeated until desensitization of the conflicted feeling occurs—that is, until the patient is able to fully experience but also contain the feeling. As the patient becomes more and more comfortable with the feeling flowing freely (e.g., crying over long-held grief), then the therapist needs to do very little active intervening, but should stay quietly beside the patient and remain attuned to the feeling.

Stopping a long-standing problem will generally take many presentations of conflicted affect scenes, not just one or two. As noted earlier, repeated exposures are like "emotional push-ups" to develop patients' "emotional muscles." Grief and anger often need 6–10 full sessions devoted to desensitization for deep change to occur.

Affect Must Be Felt Repeatedly

The more often a person accesses an emotion, the easier it becomes to experience it. This does not mean that intense levels of feeling are required, but just as much as the patient can bear. The point is that for behavior change to occur, affect needs to be repeatedly felt in the body, not just in thought or speech. As long as patients feel secure that the affect can be well controlled, they should be encouraged to "practice" these imaginal scenes repeatedly between sessions. Repetition of Affect Experiencing in graded steps helps patients build the capacity to reflect on feelings without having to act on them. This is the heart of "having emotions" without "emotions having you."

Example: The Lady Cloaked in Fog

The following transcript of a session shows a patient slowly beginning to make peace with unpleasant feelings, through the process of Affect Experiencing. The patient who has felt lost in a "fog" of defenses has expressed considerable reluctance about this, but she finally begins:

Learning to Bear Feeling

PATIENT: I want to say to my boss, "Don't bother me with your petty stuff."

THERAPIST: Where do you feel that?

PATIENT: I feel a hot something up and down my body [F]. I want to punch her [F] . . . but part of me wants to run away [D]. [She can identify both the affect and the defensive avoidance.]

The therapist holds the focus—preventing the avoidant response—but the struggle continues for about 30 minutes. The patient is in visible pain from the impact of the violent feelings and wants to run away. The therapist helps her with handling the discomfort.

THERAPIST: What's hurting you now? [Anxiety regulation]?

PATIENT: I want to keep doing it [F]!! (*Sighing heavily*) If I started, I wouldn't stop . . . I'd want to keep on slapping her [F]. (*Wincing*) [A]

THERAPIST: What's hardest for you? [Anxiety regulation]

PATIENT: Recognizing it! That I could do this! I feel something about having a shoe . . . to smash her fingers [F] . . . I could smash her to a bloody pulp [F]. I think I could go on for a very long time. It's so scary to have these feelings [A]!

THERAPIST: We all have these feelings. Remember, these are not actions. [Anxiety regulation]

This reassurance calms the patient somewhat, and she continues the violent fantasy.

PATIENT: I could have boots on and be stomping all over her [F] . . . it feels kind of satisfying.

THERAPIST: That's the truth of it. [Anxiety regulation]

It can be a tremendous relief to feel the depth of one's fury. That is the goal of such imaginal scenes—to accept and to contain the force of the feeling.

PATIENT: (*Later, reflecting on the session*) This is a horrible way for people to feel. It's frightening in its newness [A]. Scary to think of this within me [A] . . . but it's part of me. You really know me.

THERAPIST: It's important to make peace with these urges and know how to control and guide them.

The patient's remark that "You really know me" illustrates the key role of the therapist's nonjudgmental acceptance in the healing process.

VI. SOME FREQUENTLY ASKED QUESTIONS

To conclude this chapter, here are some questions that therapists frequently ask about Affect Restructuring.

"How Do You Know When Affects Are Desensitized and the Phobia Is Resolved?"

Affect Phobias can be considered resolved when patients can do the following:

1. Experience the affective imagery at a moderate to strong level, without running into defenses or feeling bad about themselves.
2. Put the feelings into appropriate action (see Chapter 8).

"Can The Pain Ever Go Away?" or *"Do Painful Feelings Ever Disappear?"*

Desensitization of affect phobias has the potential to put many painful feelings "to rest." Although patients may remember their past with less than happy memories, past grief, anger, and longings do not have to generate endless inner turmoil and suffering.

Taking the Sting Out   Desensitization of Affect Phobias can take the "sting" (the anxiety, shame, pain, or self-attack) out of the anger or the grief or the closeness. As in the example of the Lady Cloaked in Fog, **taking the "sting" out means that the conflict about the feeling is gone.** Then these feelings (F) can be experienced without the painful inhibitory feelings (A) that led to suffering. (For more on trying to "stop the pain," see also CC, pp. 228–232.)

"Once Affect Phobias Are Desensitized, Then What?"

Ultimate Goal of Authentic Functioning   In the next chapter, we will discuss how to apply these newly-desensitized feelings toward the final goal of STDP—putting feelings into authentic, mature, well-guided action, which we call Affect Expression. **As we have said repeatedly, people can't change the past, but they can change the way they react to the past, and build a better future.**

Summary of Affect Restructuring Steps   Before we proceed, however, the basic steps of Affect Restructuring are summarized in Table 7.1.

TABLE 7.1. Steps in Affect Experiencing

- Conduct exposure to the feared affect (F) in guided imagery.
  - Have patient verbally label the affect correctly.
  - Have patient identify the physical feeling of the affect.
  - Have patient imagine desired action in fantasy.
  - Encourage benign regression in fantasy to heighten feeling.
- Engage in response prevention (D).
  - Point out defense/avoidance.
  - Encourage patient to stay with the feelings a little longer.
- Engage in anxiety regulation (A).
  - Calm patient by offering support, reassurance.
  - Explore the patient's fears, shame, pain.
- Return to exposure as soon as anxiety is reduced.
  - Constantly monitor bodily signals of feeling.
- Return to response prevention if necessary.
- Return to anxiety regulation repeatedly

CHAPTER 7 • EXERCISES

EXERCISE 7A: IDENTIFY MALADAPTIVE VERSUS ADAPTIVE VERSIONS OF SPECIFIC AFFECTS

Directions: This exercise highlights the importance of selecting the correct affect focus for exposure. For each of the following affect-based behaviors, check whether these expressions are predominantly maladaptive or adaptive. Remember that maladaptive affects are typically used as defenses and block other more adaptive feelings. Some of these answers may be obvious, while others may be ambiguous and depend on the context in which they occur, especially the cultural context. Our goal here is just to encourage you to begin thinking in terms of whether a given affect may be adaptive or not.

Example:	**Closeness/tenderness**	**Maladaptive**	**Adaptive**
Answer:	• Clinging, neediness	X	___

Explanation: "Clingy" neediness signifies an insecure and maladaptive attachment.

Exercise 7A.1.

	Closeness/tenderness	**Maladaptive**	**Adaptive**
	• Idealized, perfectionistic image of other	___	___
	• Self-absorption blocking empathy	___	___
	• "I–thou"; other is cherished	___	___
	• Envy	___	___

		Maladaptive	Adaptive
• Acceptance of people's strengths and weaknesses, unexaggerated		⸺	⸺
• Comforting, hugging, and holding		⸺	⸺
• Gratitude		⸺	⸺
• Empathy for other		⸺	⸺
• Anxiety or avoidance of eye contact		⸺	⸺

Exercise 7A.2.	**Sexual desire**	**Maladaptive**	**Adaptive**
	• Deeply satisfying sharing	⸺	⸺
	• Does not enhance closeness	⸺	⸺
	• Addictive encounters	⸺	⸺
	• Enhances closeness	⸺	⸺
	• Lust that objectifies partner	⸺	⸺
	• Paired with love and care	⸺	⸺

Exercise 7A.3.	**Pain**	**Maladaptive**	**Adaptive**
	• Signal of emotional harm	⸺	⸺
	• Leads to adaptive avoidance	⸺	⸺
	• Leads to depression/melancholia	⸺	⸺
	• Chronic harm turned on self	⸺	⸺
	• Feels unavoidable; "stuck" in it	⸺	⸺
	• Leads to grieving for a loss	⸺	⸺

Exercise 7A.4.	**Enjoyment/joy**	**Maladaptive**	**Adaptive**
	• Ignores the pain of others	⸺	⸺
	• Vanishes quickly with loss of external stimulus	⸺	⸺
	• Calming, soothing, quiet	⸺	⸺
	• Excessive urgency for it	⸺	⸺
	• Lasting pleasure	⸺	⸺
	• Experienced deeply within	⸺	⸺

Exercise 7A.5.	**Shame/guilt**	**Maladaptive**	**Adaptive**
	• Leads to self-recrimination	⸺	⸺
	• Leads to genuine regret, remorse	⸺	⸺

Exercise 7A.6.	**Interest/excitement**	**Maladaptive**	**Adaptive**
	• Compulsive attraction	⸺	⸺
	• Deeply satisfying; care for subject	⸺	⸺
	• Intense and driven involvement	⸺	⸺

* Relaxed but deep attention   ____   ____
* Excessive/manic energy   ____   ____
* Hope, optimism, looking forward to   ____   ____

Exercise 7A.7.   **Grief/sorrow**   **Maladaptive**   **Adaptive**

* Compassion for self   ____   ____
* Crying that leads to feeling worse   ____   ____
* Tears shed with memories of loss, painful   ____   ____
  but relieving
* Self-blame, self-attack   ____   ____
* Tears that cover up anger   ____   ____

Exercise 7A.8.   **Anger**   **Maladaptive**   **Adaptive**

* Conscious guiding of feelings   ____   ____
* Unreflective venting of feeling   ____   ____
* Planning best course of action   ____   ____
* Little forethought of action   ____   ____
* Loud swearing, yelling   ____   ____
* Clear statement of wishes   ____   ____
* Frustration, hopelessness   ____   ____
* Rush of energy to limbs, but well controlled   ____   ____

Exercise 7A.9.   **Fear**   **Maladaptive**   **Adaptive**

* Actions to protect self   ____   ____
* Attacking, thwarting self   ____   ____
* Paralyzed action, unable to cry out   ____   ____
* Able to run, scream, freeze as needed   ____   ____

EXERCISE 7B: WHAT'S THE ACTIVATING OR INHIBITORY FEELING UNDER THE DEFENSE?

Qualifier: There are no definite answers to these patient responses. There are only possibilities that need to be checked out with the patient. The answers that are given are ones commonly encountered in our clinical work. But patients often have idiosyncratic responses, so be open to variations from what is given below.

Directions: In the examples that follow, suggest one or more underlying affects from the following list that the patient might be experiencing. Again, of course, the answer will vary according to the context; this exercise is intended only to get you thinking. Also, any supposition by a therapist will need to be confirmed by a patient.

Anger	Excitement	Anxiety
Sadness	Enjoyment	Shame
Tenderness	Sexual Desire	Guilt
Fear (flight)	Pain/anguish	Contempt/disgust
Positive feelings toward the self		

Exercise 7B.1.   Patient says, "I feel butterflies in my stomach."

Possible underlying affect(s): _____

Exercise 7B.2.   Patient crosses legs and folds arms.

Possible underlying affect(s): _____

Exercise 7B.3.   Patient sighs deeply.

Possible underlying affect(s): _____

Exercise 7B.4.   Patient makes a fist.

Possible underlying affect(s): _____

Exercise 7B.5.   Patient slowly and repeatedly strokes fingers through hair.

Possible underlying affect(s): _____

Exercise 7B.6.   During difficult discussion, patient suddenly feels back pain.

Possible underlying affect(s): _____

Exercise 7B.7.   Patient covers eyes.

Possible underlying affect(s): _____

EXERCISE 7C: EXPOSURE—EXPERIENCING AFFECT ON THREE LEVELS

Directions: By using the three-level process taught in Section II of this chapter, try to create therapist responses that would facilitate exposure to affect. We will provide a clue by telling you the Affect Phobia that is present. For each of the patients described below, indicate what the therapist might say to help the patient do the following:

1. Label the affect.
2. Identify the physical feelings of affect in the body.
3. Imagine desired action in fantasy.

In the example's answers, we also provide hypothetical patient responses to follow each of the possible therapist interventions.

Example: **The Troubled Widow**

PATIENT: Since my husband died, I still can't get over the fact that he refused to take better care of himself so he could be here with me. [Affect Phobia: Phobia of anger]

Answers: **What therapist might say to label feeling ("Label" hereafter):** There's a lot of emotion in your voice as you describe this. What do you feel about the fact that he didn't take better care of himself?

PATIENT: I hate to say it, but it makes me angry.

What therapist might say to elicit physiological experience ("Physiological signs" hereafter): Where do you experience that anger in your body?

PATIENT: It's a rush of energy in my torso and arms!

What therapist might say to elicit imagined actions ("Imagined actions" hereafter): If you allowed yourself to experience all of that anger toward him that you've been holding back, what would you want to say and do?

PATIENT: I can feel the energy in my legs. I'd want to lunge at him and shake him hard, for not taking better care of himself! It's hard to say, but it's true.

THERAPIST: It is not uncommon to have such feelings, you know.

Exercise 7C.1. **The Ungrateful Neighbor**

PATIENT: Last week I was so sick with the flu that I couldn't get out of bed. My neighbor brought me over a pot of chicken soup, and it really helped. But I hardly even thanked her. I don't know why. [Affect Phobia: Phobia of closeness]

Label: _____

_____

Physiological signs: _____

_____

Imagined actions: _____

_____

Exercise 7C.2.   **The Unhappy Painter**

PATIENT: I was really getting this rush from painting again, and then something happened. I just couldn't let myself have it. [Affect Phobia: Phobia of excitement]

Label: _____

_____

Physiological signs: _____

_____

Imagined actions: _____

_____

Exercise 7C.3.   **The Stressed Husband**

PATIENT: My wife knew how stressed I had been and she had drawn a bath for me and cooked me this fabulous meal with all of my favorite foods. But I got in a bad mood and I just couldn't enjoy it. [Affect Phobia: Phobia of joy or closeness]

Label: _____

_____

Physiological signs: _____

_____

Imagined actions: _____

_____

Exercise 7C.4.   **The Distressed Man Working Late**

PATIENT: I've been working late with my boss. She didn't do anything inappropriate, but I'm starting to feel really weird around her. What kind of a pervert am I, anyway? I mean, my wife and I have some problems and all, but I'm pretty happily married—or so I thought. [Affect Phobia: Phobia of sexual feelings]

Label: _____

_____

Physiological signs: _____

_____

Imagined actions: _____

_____

EXERCISE 7D: HOW TO DEEPEN THE EXPERIENCE OF THE AFFECT

Directions: Identify which of the following therapist responses would be most likely to deepen the patient's affect. Once again, there are many possible responses to the following situations. These exercises are meant only to prompt your thinking about how your responses may move patients toward greater or lesser experience of feeling.

Example: PATIENT: My father was always shaming me in front of my brothers and sisters. It was such a part of my childhood.

Answer: **What therapist response would deepen the anger?**

   ✓   A. Can you think of a specific time that happened and tell me about it?

          B. Would he shame your other brothers the same way?

          C. You seem to have come through it well.

          D. He was probably projecting his own shame onto you.

Explanation: The most appropriate answer here is **A**, because specific memories tend to lead to elicit more affect than generalizations about an event that "always happened." B is gathering more history. C is intended as a supportive comment, but could be interpreted as minimizing. D is an analysis of the father's behavior, not the patient's feeling.

Exercise 7D.1. THERAPIST: How do you experience that sadness right now?

PATIENT: There's this queasy feeling in my stomach. And my throat is tight.

THERAPIST: Is that sadness?

PATIENT: No, I guess that's me trying to control the sadness.

What therapist response would deepen the sadness?

          A. I wonder if you could just try to let yourself cry?

          B. Just let yourself relax and focus on your breathing. See what comes up.

          C. What would happen if you tried loosening your throat and didn't fight it so hard?

          D. Can you tell me what words or images come with the sad feelings?

Exercise 7D.2. PATIENT: I know it's over with my boyfriend, and that he ultimately wasn't good for me, but I still think about him all the time. I came from a very cold family where no one touched each other. He was the first one I kissed and the first one I made love to. (*Looking sad*) The sex wasn't good at all, so I don't know why I made so much of it.

What therapist response would deepen the longing for closeness?

          A. You must have longed so much to be held and touched. Can you tell me about a specific time when you were being held by him that you keep thinking about?

          B. Since your family was so cold, it is understandable that you would have been vulnerable to the holding and touching that you that you didn't get from them.

_____ C. There'll be others for you. You need to let him go.

_____ D. If you learn to love yourself, you won't need to look for others to fill that capacity.

Exercise 7D.3.

PATIENT: [Toward the end of a session] I won't call again this week, I promise. I'm fine.

THERAPIST: You said it was very helpful to reach out and call last week. We agreed that you would call if things became very difficult, so you did. You've also been reaching out to other people and letting them help you through this struggle. We know you give to other people all the time. But it's important to allow yourself to receive. This can begin here with me, and then extend to your friends and family.

PATIENT: Well, you're a therapist. So I guess you're just doing your job.

THERAPIST: That sounds pretty clinical. Is there something I've been doing that would make me come across as emotionally detached?

PATIENT: Well, no, you seemed really concerned when I called.

What therapist response would deepen the feeling of care from another?

_____ A. So, by thinking of me in this impersonal way, do you think you might be putting up a barrier with me—as you do with others?

_____ B. Of course, I think many people would feel concern under such circumstances.

_____ C. Yes, I was very concerned about you and glad that you called. How does it feel to hear me say that?

_____ D. So you shouldn't hesitate to call if you need to. I'll see you next week.

Exercise 7D.4.

PATIENT: (_Tearfully_) I don't want to cry here in front of you.

What therapist response would deepen the sadness?

_____ A. It would be good if you could just let go. Isn't this the place to do it?

_____ B. Could you tell me what specific thoughts or memories are making you feel so sad?

_____ C. What's the hardest part about crying in front of me?

_____ D. You don't need to right now, if you don't want to. We can get back to this on another day.

Exercise 7D.5.

PATIENT: (_Shaking his fist_) What can I do? My father just wants me to live his life.

What therapist response would deepen the anger/assertion?

_____ A. When you say "live his life," what do you mean by that?

_____ B. Do you notice you are shaking your fist? How does your body feel right now?

_____ C. It must really be frustrating to feel like you're always in his shadow.

_____ D. He probably never was able to have the freedoms you have, so he resents it.

Exercise 7D.6.   PATIENT: My wife is so supportive of me with everything else, but she's really frustrated with our sex life. Whenever we try to make love, I get really turned on at first but as time goes by I feel more and more ashamed of myself for wanting it.

What therapist response would deepen the affect?

_____ A. What is it about wanting it that's the most shameful?

_____ B. We've seen a number of times that it can be difficult for you to ask for things you want. Is there anything you could say to your wife so that you would feel less pressure?

_____ C. How sad that you can't let yourself enjoy one of the deepest and most pleasurable parts of your relationship!

_____ D. To help your relationship, it seems like it'll be important for you to be comfortable with your sexual feelings. This may be hard to talk about, but what things turn you on the most as you get started?

EXERCISE 7E: HOW TO REGULATE ANXIETIES ABOUT FEELING

Directions: In the following examples what might the therapist say to decrease the inhibitory affect (A on the Triangle of Conflict—anxiety, shame, guilt, or emotional pain) that is preventing the patient from experiencing the adaptive affect (F). Remember that there are a number of ways to reduce inhibitory affects, including providing support/reassurance/information, using humor, and using the basic cognitive intervention (i.e., "What's the hardest [scariest, most painful] part of _____?").

Example: PATIENT: I don't want to break down in front of you [the therapist].

Answer: **What the therapist might say:** What's the most difficult thing about letting your feelings out here with me?

Exercise 7E.1.   PATIENT: I can't bear to feel this angry at my mother.

What the therapist might say: _____

_____

Exercise 7E.2.   PATIENT: (*Looking ashamed*) I feel so guilty about having these sexual fantasies. I must be such a pervert.

What the therapist might say: _____

_____

Exercise 7E.3.   PATIENT: [After first session] It feels a little indulgent coming here and talking about nothing but me for an entire hour.

What the therapist might say: _____

_____

Exercise 7E.4.   PATIENT: [After being questioned by therapist about missed sessions] Even though I need to talk about my brother's death, I guess I've been dreading coming here because I'm afraid even to start feeling my grief, because I might never stop crying.

What the therapist might say: _____

_____

Exercise 7E.5.   PATIENT: (_Looking uncomfortable_) When you praised me just then, I really wanted to dismiss it.

What the therapist might say: _____

_____

EXERCISE 7F: SYSTEMATIC DESENSITIZATION—RESPONSE PREVENTION AND EXPOSURE

Directions: For each of the following first hypothesize what affect is the focus of the patient's Affect Phobia. Then indicate what the therapist might say to achieve these two aims:

- Block or circumvent defenses (response prevention).
- Expose patient to the phobic affect.

This exercise is challenging, because you need to determine the affect focus. So if you are having difficulty with one item, read the answer (see the Appendix) and then try to do the next one.

Example: PATIENT: I felt really tense when she complimented me. I couldn't take it in.

Answer: **Phobic Affect:** Feelings of pride in self.

What the therapist might say: How would it feel if you relaxed for a moment [response prevention] and let yourself feel some pleasure from that compliment [exposure]?

Exercise 7F.1.   PATIENT: When she tries to talk about our relationship, I get so tense that I want to just hide behind the newspaper.

Phobic affect: _____

What the therapist might say: _____

_____

Exercise 7F.2.

PATIENT: I don't think I've ever even cried during that whole time after Mom died. I held it together for everyone else in the family; I was the strong one.

Phobic affect: _____

What the therapist might say: _____

_____

Exercise 7F.3.

PATIENT: When you ask me how I feel about my promotion, I find my mind just going elsewhere, or thinking about things I've got to do.

Phobic affect: _____

What the therapist might say: _____

_____

Exercise 7F.4.

PATIENT: A job opened up at work that I really want, but I've been pretending to the people in my department that it's no big deal. I can't stand to ask for things I want, so I go out of my way to avoid it.

Phobic affect: _____

What the therapist might say: _____

_____

Exercise 7F.5.

PATIENT: I was starting to get really excited about my writing again, and then I heard my father's voice warning me not to "get too big for my britches." Since then I haven't written a thing.

Phobic affect: _____

What the therapist might say: _____

_____

CHAPTER 8

Affect Restructuring, Section 2: Affect Expression

Chapter Objective   To demonstrate how to help patients integrate and express feelings adaptively (i.e., without Affect Phobias) in all their relationships.

Therapist Stance   Serving as teacher, guide, and collaborator.

Anxiety Regulation   Helping patients manage the fears, shame, and pain involved in giving up long-held Affect Phobias, and helping them anticipate and plan for new and changed relationships.

Topics Covered

I.   Overview of Affect Expression

II.   Building Expressive and Receptive Capacities

III.   Bearing Interpersonal Conflict

IV.   Integrating Feelings

V.   Role Playing of Difficult Interactions

VI.   Providing Information to Aid Expression

VII.   Identifying Pitfalls in Affect Expression

VIII.   Repeating Practice Until Affect Expression Flows Naturally

Indications for a Focus on Affect Expression

• A patient's Affect Phobias have been sufficiently desensitized in fantasy that the patient's feelings can be experienced without significant conflict.

• Practice or skill building is needed in the interpersonal expression of affects.

I. OVERVIEW OF AFFECT EXPRESSION

Affect Expression as the Ultimate Goal of Treatment

In Defense Restructuring, patients learn to identify and give up their maladaptive response patterns. In Affect Experiencing, they learn to experience emotions that were previously unbearable due to excessive inhibitory affects. But the pure experience of feeling—Affect Experiencing—is not the ultimate goal of treatment. That goal is Affect Expression—the ability to experience and communicate the fullness of affect in an adaptive manner that not only furthers the patient's goals, but also generally benefits those around him or her. Often patients say things like this:

PATIENT: I can't get over it. . . . Since I managed to tell my mother how mad I was at her and how hard it's been for me, our relationship is better than ever. And to think how hard I worked not to tell her that!

Affect Expression is a direct measure of therapy progress; you and the patient can assess the results of your work in the form of improved relationships and improved functioning.

Affect Expression Is Not Venting

It is important for therapists and patients to remember that Affect Expression is not venting, explosive acting out, or regressive discharge, but a well-guided expression of wants and needs:

- Assertion rather than aggression.
- Crying fully over losses.
- Expressing tenderness openly and without shame.
- Pursuing interests enthusiastically.
- Giving and receiving sexual pleasure freely.
- Laughing or feeling at peace when experiencing joy.

These capacities are the basis of self-soothing, self-protection, and mature, healthy functioning.

Some Important Components of Affect Expression

Achieving well-guided expression of wants and needs means working with the patient on three overlapping areas of Affect Expression:

1. **Building expressive and receptive capacities,** so that the patient is able to express affects to others and respond to the affects others express.

2. **Bearing interpersonal conflict,** so that the patient is able to face and tolerate conflict, use it productively, and stay positively connected.

3. **Integrating feelings,** so that the patient is able to blend and balance affects in a mature way.

These are important areas of functioning to note carefully throughout treatment. However, during Affect Expression, these capabilities move to the forefront.

Key Interventions for Affect Expression	The key interventions for strengthening Affect Expression include **providing information and skills training** as needed in such areas as communication, social skills, and assertiveness; **role playing** for skills practice and anxiety regulation; and *in vivo* **desensitization**—the patient's real-life exercise of Affect Expression with people who are important to him or her.

In Vivo or Real-Life Desensitization

Patients with Affect Phobias have spent years or decades avoiding their feelings rather than expressing them—and have had this behavior reinforced by the relief that avoidance brings. Even after extensive work on Affect Experiencing (Chapter 7), it is possible that long-established behavior patterns will not be easily changed.

Affect Expression requires *in vivo* or real-life desensitization to help patients reconnect with and reattach to others. Thus patients will need to practice expressing their feelings when they are face to face with important people in their lives—dozens or even hundreds of times. While some patients are able to do this on their own as soon as they have gone through Affect Experiencing, most will require at least some instruction or practice with a therapist on this focus. Such work may involve the process of integrating affects, teaching and providing information, and role playing.

Integrating Affects for Optimal Forms of Affect Expression

As patients work toward optimal ways of expressing their inner feelings, they learn that specific affects (such as anger) must now develop into more sophisticated blends of affects (e.g., assertion mixed with care for others). This process of integrating affects is central for patients to learn mature, adaptive, cognitively guided expression of feeling. Achieving an open but well-guided blend of feeling means that a patient has "succeeded" in developing an optimal form of Affect Expression: balancing shame with mature pride, fear of rejection with love, tempering anger with compassion, and so on.

Teaching and Providing Information

Although cognitive, interpersonal, and behavioral therapists have routinely incorporated skills training into their treatment repertoire, psychodynamic therapists have been reluctant to do so. Providing information with encouragement and coaching is a fundamental method of learning and should not be forbidden in Short-Term Dynamic Psychotherapy (STDP)—just applied intelligently. Here are a few guidelines:

1. Work on resolving defenses and conflicted feelings first.
2. Teach what the patient does not already know.
3. Allow dependence, while at the same time always supporting and planning for the patient's eventual autonomy and greater independence.

When to Focus on Affect Expression

Many forms of therapy use Affect Expression as their starting point. For example, cognitive, interpersonal, and behavioral therapies often begin with social skills training or assertiveness training, which are ways to teach patients how to interact with others and express wants and needs appropriately. In contrast, in STDP, Affect Expression becomes the focus only **after** the underlying defensive patterns have been given up (response prevention) and **after** the exploration of the conflicts has freed up affective responding (exposure until desensitization occurs).

Affect Expression Follows Defense Restructuring and Affect Experiencing

There are several reasons why it is important to work in this order. Consider, for example, patients with conflicts or phobias over anger. If they try to learn assertiveness skills without resolving the Affect Phobia, their avoidance of anything associated with anger may lead to a number of problems:

1. Anxiety may make it difficult for them to learn the skills even on a theoretical level.
2. They may learn the theory, but have great difficulty acquiring the skills with the therapist.
3. They may acquire the skills with the therapist, but be unwilling or unable to put them into practice.
4. They may put the skills into practice and behave assertively, but be "white-knuckling" (i.e., doing so only at the cost of great internal distress).

For these reasons, achieving optimal forms of Affect Expression—expressing positive and negative affects in an integrated, balanced, adaptive manner in all aspects of life—is the endpoint rather than the starting point of this therapy.

Character Change

As Harville Hendrix (1992) supports the belief that no matter how much work is done in therapy, significant character changes are made in sustained, loving relationships in the real world. The practice is in each day-to-day relationship. The implicit goal of treatment is not to provide the ultimate relationship, but to help the patient be able to find, maintain, and grow in loving relationships outside of therapy. Affect Expression allows the patient to consolidate and continue the work he or she has begun with the therapist. By the time patients are ready to move from Affect Experiencing to Affect Expression, they may well be starting to make significant changes in the areas of expression and reception of feelings, integration of feelings, and bearing conflict. For that reason, this transition is a good time to reassess a patient's interpersonal affective functioning. Are the patient's relationships significantly improved, or improving? Therapists can start to explore this quite straightforwardly with open-ended questions, such as "How are you doing with your boss [or your husband/wife, or your friend]?"

The three areas of Affect Expression (expression/receptivity, bearing conflict, and integrating feelings) are addressed later in this chapter, with other questions that can help in assessment. After that, we turn to the particular treatment techniques of role playing and providing information.

Therapist Stance: Serving as Educator, Coach, and Collaborator

Helping patients find optimal responses to problematic situations requires careful judgment and active engagement on the part of the therapist. "Neutrality" is likely to lead to collusion with patients' defenses, perpetuating their long-standing maladaptive behavior patterns.

Therapist as Educator and Coach

During Affect Expression work, the therapist educates and coaches the patient in order to move from newly freed feelings toward authentic functioning and relating. Teaching is often essential, but it must not be condescending, pedantic, or overly authoritative. Such interventions as guidance, advice, providing information, instruction, role playing, and modeling—which might have been less helpful when Affect Phobias were present—can now be used more fruitfully. Standard educational techniques, such as encouragement, support, and praise, are also useful.

Therapist as Collaborator

Although the therapist will and should have opinions about what might or might not be helpful in the patient's relationships, these opinions should be offered in a collaborative, exploratory spirit rather than an authoritative one, as in all the other treatment objectives.

Discovering Values and "Ideal Self"

Because Affect Expression involves the patient's actions in the world, not just in the therapist's office, finding optimal responses necessitates clarifying the patient's values and ideals. Some questions that may be helpful in determining optimal responses include the following:

- What would be an optimal adaptive response to the presenting problems?
- What kind of person does the patient wish to be in relation to others?
- Who might provide a model of exemplary behavior? Does the patient have heroes or heroines who represent ideals toward which to aspire?
- What is the patient's "ideal sense of self"?

Often a patient must build an image of an ideal self if there is not one already—with the therapist's help. Therapists must pay particular attention to patients' values and beliefs, as these may differ from their own. Cultural differences among the therapist, the patient, and the surrounding environment also need careful scrutiny.

When the patient's ideal self is not in agreement with conventional wisdom in mental health, the therapist should talk this over with the patient and collaboratively decide what ways of optimal responding make the patient feel most comfortable.

THERAPIST: Well, here's one way you might go about this. It's a way that lots of people have found helpful, but that doesn't necessarily mean you will. So I'd like you to tell me what you think about it and how it fits with your own style. If my suggestion doesn't feel right to you, we should explore some other possibilities.

With their therapists acting as collaborators, patients gain a new type of relationship and an opportunity to build a greater awareness of the regard they should be given. When psychodynamic conflict—and therefore "resistance"—have been reduced, patients often welcome encouragement and guidance when it is given respectfully, because these are responses that have often been missing in their experience.

Collaborating to Find an Optimal Form of Expression

PATIENT: I don't date much, because I feel like I have to marry the woman if I go out with her once.

THERAPIST: That seems like an exaggerated level of obligation!

PATIENT: But I feel noble being this way. Women get so hurt.

THERAPIST: I wonder if you would consider your "noble behavior" from another perspective? To be so concerned about hurting women could be seen as patronizing or even infantilizing. In some ways it might be another way of creating distance [D]. Instead of a caretaking relationship where your needs are buried, wouldn't you prefer a more adult, give-and-take relationship?

PATIENT: Well, huh . . . I see what you mean. When you look at it that way, maybe it's not all that noble.

Anxiety Regulation: Anticipating Other People's Reactions

Supporting the Patient to "Reconnect" with Others

In Affect Expression, patients need to apply behaviors learned in therapy to relationships in the outside world. Although the imaginal exposure of Affect Experiencing (Chapter 7) should have reduced the Affect Phobia so that this work will be possible, a patient still may feel significant anxiety about expressing these affects to others. Even though positive change gives a feeling of mastery, it can provoke anxiety. The therapist needs to support the patient in "reconnecting" with others in new ways.

Anticipating Difficulties in Relationships

Anxiety can be regulated by anticipating the patient's fears and preparing the patient for others' reactions.

THERAPIST: It seems like you want to speak strongly [F—anger/assertion] to your mother about her criticizing you all the time. Let's imagine how she might respond if you said something. [Anticipation of reaction—either negative or positive]

PATIENT: Oh, she would blow up. I've never said a word in opposition to her.

THERAPIST: Then we might expect that she would be upset at first. [Teaching and exposure to the feared response]

PATIENT: Yes! It terrifies me to even think about it [A].

THERAPIST: What's so terrifying [A]? Let's try to imagine how you can handle a range of responses so that it is not so difficult. [Exposure]

This could be followed by role-playing the interaction with the mother to prepare the patient in advance for what might happen. (For more on role playing, see Section V below.) Arranging for significant others to come to a therapy session and become acquainted with the change process can also be helpful.

II. BUILDING EXPRESSIVE AND RECEPTIVE CAPACITIES

Assessing Expressive and Receptive Capacities

Healthy interpersonal affective functioning requires not only that patients be able to express affect to others adaptively, but that they be able to take in or resonate to affect that is expressed to them and respond adaptively. Therapists need to assess whether their patients are comfortable with the expression of feelings in their real-life relationships, as well as whether they are receptive to others' communications. Here are some questions a therapist should consider in evaluating this, along with questions the therapist might ask to elicit information:

1. Is the patient able to express emotions adaptively?

   THERAPIST 1: When you were missing your mother so much, were you able to tell your husband about it?

   THERAPIST 2: When you got so mad at John, what did you do? Were you able to get him to stop?

2. Is the patient able to receive emotions adaptively?

   THERAPIST 1: When he complimented you, how did it feel? Were you able to savor that?

   THERAPIST 2: When your daughter was so sad, were you able to share her grief?

   THERAPIST 3: When your boss told you to get off the phone, how did you react?

3. Is there remaining anxiety, guilt, or shame about the expression or reception of feeling that has not been sufficiently addressed?

   THERAPIST: Do you feel more able to tell your wife when you're angry at her, and to hear her when she's angry at you—or are you still feeling somewhat uncomfortable with conflict?

4. Is there secondary gain that still lingers, so that the patient does not have the motivation to respond differently?

> THERAPIST: Does it still feel rewarding to hold back?

5. Is there insufficient knowledge or skills to allow for ease of expression?

> THERAPIST 1: Do you know what to do when you start to feel sad?
>
> THERAPIST 2: Do you know how to tell the difference between grief and depression [as discussed in Chapters 1 and 2]?

Assessing Expression of Specific Affects

Here are some examples of how to assess whether conflicts centering around specific feelings have been adequately desensitized:

Anger

Does the patient feel able to stand up and fully assert wants, needs, likes, and dislikes? Is assertion comfortably experienced without fear or shame?

> PATIENT: I can see myself walking into the boss's office right now and saying, that we have to have a talk! My body feels pumped up and good. I don't feel scared at all! I can't wait.

Grief

Though a significant loss will always be sad, the memories should not carry a "sting" or a gut-wrenching pain after the grieving process. The patient should be able to feel and put in perspective both positive and negative feelings about the loss; he or she should also feel able to continue life functioning, and feel hope about replacing the loss (to the extent possible).

> PATIENT 1: I miss her so much! We used to have such fun just reading the paper to each other. But I also have to admit it—her cancer was so devastating to watch, and so painful for her, that I feel a deep sense of relief that she's finally gone and no longer suffering.
>
> PATIENT 2: When I think of my husband now, I can do it without feeling so angry. Sometimes I get a burst of irritation when I remember him smoking, and still wish he had taken better care of himself so he could be here with me. But I'm more at peace with that now. I know he loved me, and he will always be in my heart. That makes me able to carry on.

Closeness

Can the patient bear to be open and vulnerable with significant others? Can tenderness be expressed in a heartfelt manner? Can the patient feel care and gratitude deeply? Can he or she make eye contact when doing so? Is the patient comfortable about confiding in trusted people and being confided in?

> PATIENT 1: I told her that I have never felt closer to anyone in my life, and

that she had treated me better than I have ever been treated. I held her tight, and I really let her know how deeply I felt that.

PATIENT 2: Now I don't feel so blocked in feeling warmth. Recently I let myself feel touched by someone's kindness, and I really liked the openness of that feeling.

Self-Care or Compassion

Does the patient take good care of him- or herself? Is there compassion for his or her own mistakes, as well as an ability to roll with the punches?

PATIENT: Well, I didn't do a good job of that interview, but I'll practice my interviewing skills and do better next time. I don't always have to be perfect!

Other Positive Feelings

Can the patient give him- or herself over to the joy, excitement, or pride from a positive experience? Are positive feelings allowed to permeate the body?

PATIENT 1: [Joy] At times now, I find myself just sitting quietly and feeling quite peaceful. It's a whole new world, and it's just wonderful.

PATIENT 2: [Pride] You know, I've stopped criticizing my every move and started to let myself feel really good inside about the work I have done!

PATIENT 3: [Sexual feelings] The old anxiety is gone, and I am feeling freer and freer just to let my body feel turned on—passionate, even! And (*laughing*) I don't even feel immoral!

PATIENT 4: [Interest/excitement] I suddenly noticed that I was immersed in what I was doing—and not on guard every minute. I was excited about what I was making, and letting myself feel it.

If these capacities continue to be blocked, or if Affect Expression generates self-attacking remarks, consider more work on Self- and Other-Restructuring. (For more work on building the foundations necessary for expressive and receptive capacities, see Chapters 9 and 10 of this book, as well as CC, pp. 291–296 and 315–337.)

III. BEARING INTERPERSONAL CONFLICT

Making Conflict Productive

It is not possible to have a good relationship without conflict. The ability to bear conflict and use it productively (to "fight fair") is in some ways a specialized form of expressive and receptive capacities, but it is so important that it is worth singling out. The therapist may benefit from considering the following questions.

1. Does the patient communicate in a mature way?—not blaming or criticizing, but honest and decent?

   PATIENT: I'm not happy with the fact that you were late today.

2. Does the patient blend positive and negative feelings in what he or she says?

   PATIENT: I really care about you, so I'm going to tell you something you did that upset me, in the hope that it will make us closer.

3. Does the patient communicate in "I" statements rather than "you" statements? That is, does he or she say, "When you do X, I feel Y," rather than "You're a jerk for doing X" or "You're immature to do X"?

4. Are requests made in a manner that optimizes the likelihood of positive response—for example, "It would mean a lot to me if you would stop doing that," rather than "Stop doing that"?

As described above, communication should be handled so that both parties benefit. This is the goal of "fair fighting" overall—to turn the "zero-sum game" (or actually negative-sum game) of destructive conflict into the "positive-sum game" of productive conflict.

IV. INTEGRATING FEELINGS

People Are "Mixed Bags"

Feelings don't happen in a vacuum. People are "mixed bags," and life is a "mixed bag." There will inevitably be a mix of emotional reactions to any given person or situation.

Putting Feelings in Perspective

Mature socialization and wise relating—the ideals of empathy and compassion—mean taking a range of emotions into consideration at the same time. The therapist must strive to help patients put feelings "in perspective" by combining cognitive guidance with awareness of feelings.

Enough tenderness needs to be integrated with anger that anger doesn't get punitive. Sufficient assertion (anger) and limit setting need to be integrated with the longing for closeness that people are not taken advantage of or abused. Sadness needs to be tempered by joy, and losses need to be replaced (to the extent possible). This process can be called **playing feelings in concert** or **emotional integration.** Sometimes the mixture of emotions comes naturally, but more often work needs to be done to strive to invoke positive feelings when feelings are negative, or vice versa.

Helping Patients Integrate Feelings

When patients have trouble integrating feelings, the therapist must help them do so by focusing on the full range of feelings, and identifying the ones that are out of balance.

For example, does the patient have problems with the following:

1. Such strong feelings of anger that the patient cannot take into consideration the tenderness in the relationship?

2. Such excessive gratitude or need that the insensitivities or abuses of others are ignored?

3. Such excessive grief that finding new ways to meet needs is not possible?

Guided imagery can be used to integrate affective experience, just as it has been used to focus on single affects (Chapter 7). All feelings need to be modulated by considering the feelings of others. Here are some examples of how therapists might work to help patients integrate opposing feelings:

Integration of Opposing Feeling

THERAPIST 1: You seem much more comfortable with tender feelings now. But are there conflicts in the relationship that need to be dealt with as well?

THERAPIST 2: You seem almost too grateful that your husband brought you gifts, but you seemed not to react or have feelings about his yelling at you.

THERAPIST 3: You gave yourself over to the joy of snowboarding so completely that you didn't see the rock in the middle of the trail. Maybe you needed to blend in a certain amount of fear to keep you vigilant and safe.

When a patient has difficulty mastering these capacities, it suggests a need to look for work that remains to be done. Are there defenses that need to be restructured, Affect Phobias that need to be desensitized, or issues of self or others that are blocking integration? (For more on integrating feelings and putting feelings in perspective, also see CC, pp. 288–290)

V. ROLE PLAYING OF DIFFICULT INTERACTIONS

Improving Affect Expression through Role Play

Role playing is common in our daily lives. Examples include talking over a problem with a friend or playing out interactions in one's imagination to determine a helpful proper course of action. Role playing—both during and outside therapy sessions—can be a helpful way for patients to practice and improve their interpersonal communication. From the standpoint of psychotherapy, there are several ways to think of role playing. In the cognitive-behavioral framework, it represents skills training and practicing. From a psychodynamic perspective, it can be seen as a therapist-assisted enactment of the mature defense of **anticipation,** in which problems that may occur in the future are anticipated and prepared for in advance.

From the perspective of Affect Phobia, role playing can be thought of as exposure treatment for the anxieties centering around Affect Expression. For that reason, it can be helpful to regulate the anxiety centering around role playing.

Role Play with Anxiety Regulation

PATIENT: I am much more open than I used to be with my friends, but sometimes I still don't quite know how to say what I want to say.

THERAPIST: Well, how would it be to take a specific situation where you held back, and role-play what you would have wanted to say?

PATIENT: I don't know where to begin.

THERAPIST: Why don't you go back to the moment when you felt stuck and start there? You may not have anything on the tip of your tongue, but take a moment and see what comes up.

PATIENT: Well, with my roommate, I want to ask her to do her share of cleaning up the apartment.

THERAPIST: How might you ask her?

PATIENT: Um . . . Mary, I've been wanting to ask you to take the garbage out when it's your turn. . . .

THERAPIST: (*Role-playing Mary*) Oh, I just forget. Why is it such a big deal?

PATIENT: Well . . . I guess . . . because it smells bad in the kitchen for days.

THERAPIST: (*Role-playing Mary*) OK, OK! I'll try to do it.

PATIENT: Thanks, that would be great.—Gee this is hard to do!

THERAPIST: What was the hardest part of imagining saying those things to Mary? [Anxiety regulation]

Of course, role plays in therapy sessions may be quite a bit longer than this. It can also be helpful to role-play various possible scenarios: for example, the therapist above might suggest a role play in which the roommate is less easily convinced. It may also be helpful for the therapist to model adaptive behavior by playing the patient, particularly initially. (To learn more about regulating anxiety over expressing affect, and about role playing, see CC, pp. 286–287 and 301–304.)

VI. PROVIDING INFORMATION TO AID EXPRESSION

Sometimes patients lack basic information that would help them better guide their actions. When this is the case, the therapist may need to teach or inform the patient, to fill in real gaps in knowledge. As discussed in Section I, teaching is an important component of Affect Expression.

Offering Suggestions or Direct Advice

When you think a patient doesn't know something and could benefit from being told, it can sometimes be helpful to offer direct advice or suggestions, always being careful to solicit the patient's response:

THERAPIST 1: If you have trouble getting out of bed, would it help to set your alarm one hour earlier? What do you think?

THERAPIST 2: If you do this, you will likely avoid a great deal of suffering in your life. Do you see it that way?

THERAPIST 3: I think it would be helpful for you to practice relaxation three times this week. Do you?

Of course, if advice or assignments are given, there are many therapeutic opportunities in the follow-up. If the advice was followed, how did it feel to the patient? Was it relatively easy to follow, or was the behavior still accompanied by significant anxiety (which might signal the need for more Defense Restructuring and/or Affect Experiencing)?

If the advice was not followed, it is important to explore the reasons, in the same nonjudgmental way you would explore anything else. Noncompliance could result from any number of reasons, including good judgment, competing demands, or residual conflict. It may take some perseverance to reach a conclusion:

THERAPIST: I know exactly what you mean about it being a busy week, but I wonder if it's possible that some of that same old guilt might have held you back from doing what you needed to do?

PATIENT: Yeah, I suppose that's right, because when I think about it now, I do start to freeze up a little bit.

Thus, even when the therapist is being "directive," it is always in the spirit of collaboration. (For more on therapist stance, also see CC, pp. 283–286.)

Pitfalls of Teaching

It can be difficult to distinguish a patient's true need for advice from a passive, dependent defense. In such cases, try Socratic questioning:

THERAPIST: You tell me you have no idea what to do. Have you ever seen anyone handle a similar situation in a way that you admired or thought was effective?

If patients are not comfortable with underlying feelings, they will just be "going through the motions" when following your teaching. (For more on teaching and sometimes why not to teach, also see CC, pp. 298–301.)

THERAPIST: You want me to tell you what to do, but I would do you no service if I didn't explore all the issues around your request. Can we first see if you are comfortable with the anger necessary for assertion?

Some Distinctions in Communication

Basic information on communication has helped many patients improve their relationships. This section covers a number of distinctions in interpersonal communication that many patients simply don't know. Often they are able to put the information to good use once they are aware of it.

Passive (Inhibited), Assertive (Adaptive), and Aggressive (Disinhibited) Expressions of Affects

There are a number of ways anger can be expressed—keeping silent (passive), or speaking up (assertive), or losing one's temper (aggressive).

Passive: Patient says very little and smiles compliantly, but is upset inside.

Assertive: "I don't like it when you're late. I'd like you to let me know when you're not going to be on time."

Aggressive: "You #&$#!!! You don't give a ##$$% about me or my time!"

Similar distinctions can be made for the expression of all the affects. However, such affects as grief, it makes more sense to speak of expression as inhibited (rather than passive), adaptive (rather than assertive), or disinhibited (rather than aggressive). Of course, deciding which category a particular piece of behavior falls into requires judgment and will depend on an individual's cultural background and milieu.

Appropriate Suppression of Emotion

In addition to the distinction between appropriately expressed emotion (assertive/adaptive) and inappropriately expressed emotion (passive/inhibited and aggressive/disinhibited), emotion can also be "appropriately suppressed." Appropriate suppression does **not** mean never speaking up (i.e., it is **not** passive). It means consciously choosing to hold back until an appropriate time, using the mature defense of suppression (e.g., keeping a stiff upper lip, holding one's tongue, or counting to 10—but eventually expressing what is felt in an appropriate way).

Acting out: Patient throws coffee cup across room and storms off.

Appropriate expression: "I really want this to stop. Why are you doing this? Can we talk about this?"

Appropriate suppression: Patient waits until she and her spouse get home before confronting him about his behavior at the party.

Suggestions for Self-Help Books

Not all information needs to be provided by the therapist. Some of the better self-help books can provide helpful guidance for developing more adaptive behaviors. Here are some books that many patients have found helpful, which deal with specific affects or related topics:

- *The Dance of Anger* (Lerner, 1985): Anger/assertion
- *Coping with Difficult People* (Bramson, 1981): Anger/assertion
- *Toxic Parents* (Forward with Buck, 1989): Abusive parents
- *Necessary Losses* (Viorst, 1986): Grief
- *The Drama of the Gifted Child and the Search for the True Self* (Miller, 1990): Building self-compassion
- *Getting the Love You Want* (Hendrix, 1988): Closeness
- *Don't Say Yes When You Want to Say No* (Fensterheim & Baer, 1975): Assertion
- *The Two-Step: The Dance toward Intimacy* (McCann, 1985): Closeness

VII. PITFALLS IN AFFECT EXPRESSION

Affect Expression has a number of possible pitfalls, which therapists should be aware of. This section focuses on the following:

- Expressing emotions before experiencing them (superficial responding).
- Compliance.

Expressing Emotions before Experiencing Them (Superficial Responding)

It is tempting in active STDP to encourage patients toward "adaptive" behavior before they have made sufficient progress in resolving their internal Affect Phobias—in other words, to work on Affect Expression before Affect Experiencing. As discussed in Section I, there is the potential when this is done for patients to respond by rote (superficially), rather than authentically from their own feelings.

Even patients who have done a significant amount of work on Affect Experiencing can respond superficially. The important point is that when a patient gives an example of Affect Expression—outside or during a session—the therapist should assess the patient's internal experience to see whether it is one of continued conflict (anxiety, shame, etc.) or of relative ease or relief in the expression.

If there is continuing inhibition (nervousness, discomfort) about expression of feelings, this means that the Affect Phobia is still present to some degree. Then the focus of therapy can return if necessary to Defense Restructuring (Chapters 5 and 6), Affect Experiencing Anxiety Regulation (Chapter 7), and/or Self- and Other-Restructuring (Chapters 9 and 10), as indicated.

Example

PATIENT: (*Somewhat tensely*) I've been thinking over what we've been talking about—how I let things bother me and I don't speak up—and I realized that there was something bothering me here that I should talk to you about.

THERAPIST: What's that?

PATIENT: That time when you called the night before and canceled the session, I realized that that bothered me. I mean, I'm supposed to give you 24 hours' notice if I cancel, but you just called up the night before. It didn't feel fair somehow.

THERAPIST: You know, I'm really glad that you felt like you could bring this up with me. And if you'd come in and asked me how I thought you should do it, I don't think I could have suggested anything better. [Reinforcement of assertive behavior] I want to respond to what you said, and I will, but first I just wanted to check in and see how it felt to tell me that. [Note that the therapist provokes some anxiety—though in a supportive way—by not responding immediately to the patient's complaint.]

PATIENT: (*Relaxing*) Horrible. Like I'm doing something really wrong. Like I'm really being a jerk.

THERAPIST: So you're doing great on the outside, in terms of behavior, but we've really got to work on freeing you up on the inside. I don't think it's a lot of fun for anyone to tell people that they upset you, but we need to get you to the point that when you do it, it feels like a relief rather than feeling horrible. [The therapist is suggesting a need for more work on anxiety regulation to reduce inhibition about speaking up.]

The therapist should then return to dealing with the concerns the patient brought up. (For more on superficial responding, also see CC, pp. 304–306.)

Compliance: Living from the Outside In

When patients are overly compliant, it often means that they are living "from the outside in" rather than "from the inside out." As with compliance in Defense Recognition (Chapter 5), therapists need to assess whether patients are living in reaction to someone else's wants or needs. Here are some questions to consider in relation to this:

- Are patients able to respond to their own feelings, or only to what others appear to want of them?
- Are patients more able to stand their ground in the face of opposition?
- Have patients stood their ground with their therapists or "just gone along"?

PATIENT 1: I watch him like a hawk, but I can't tell what he wants of me. I don't know what to do.

THERAPIST 1: Have you ever thought about what **you** want to do?

THERAPIST 2: I may be right, or I may be wrong . . . but this is the way I am seeing it. Do you see it differently? Does this fit your experience?

PATIENT 2: Well (*pausing*), I guess it does.

THERAPIST 2: (*Listening carefully for compliance*) You sound somewhat hesitant. I wonder if you have some other thoughts about what has been happening, but that it's hard for you to share them with me.

PATIENT 2: I guess you're right. I kind of do the same thing with you that I do with my mother—just kind of going along with her, even when I have some reservations but I don't tell her.

VIII. REPEATING PRACTICE UNTIL AFFECT EXPRESSION FLOWS NATURALLY

Patients need repeated practice to replace dysfunctional ways of relating with more effective ways. Encourage patients to practice—in and outside of therapy—until their inhibitions are reduced. The more work that is done between sessions, the faster change will take place.

If the patient's fears remain and Affect Expression is inhibited, then patient and therapist may need to return to Defense, Affect, and/or Self- and Other-Restructuring as needed, in order to resolve any remaining conflicts.

When to Consider Termination

However, it is important to keep in mind that not all the work of change has to be done while a person is in therapy. Therapy that is short-term strives to "get the change process started" and provide patients with the tools to continue growing and changing after treatment ends. If patients' adaptive emotional responses are becoming easier and more natural with each repetition, this suggests that enough work may have been done in therapy, and that the patients will be able to continue the process on their own. If so, it may be time to consider termination (see Chapter 12 for how to handle the process of termination).

Summary of Affect Expression Steps

The basic steps of Affect Expression are summarized in Table 8.1.

Table 8.1. Steps in Affect Expression

- Encourage *in vivo* desensitization (i.e., real-life practice).
- Help patient build expressive and receptive capacities.
- Coach patients in bearing interpersonal conflict.
- Help patient integrate affects for optimal expression.
- Provide skills training as needed.
    Give direct advice if patient can utilize it.
    Teach skills where there are deficits.
    Provide assertiveness training.
    Role-play difficult interactions.
- Repeat practice.

CHAPTER 8 • EXERCISES

EXERCISE 8A: IDENTIFY INHIBITED, ADAPTIVE, AND DISINHIBITED RESPONSES

Directions: Indicate whether each of the following patient expressions of the given affect is **inhibited**, **adaptive**, or **disinhibited**. Remember that in the case of anger/assertion, these three options correspond to **passive**, **assertive**, and **aggressive** responses. Put the correct description on the line following the example.

Example: **Anger: Inhibited, adaptive, or disinhibited?**

A patient's friend is talking incessantly, and the patient is not able to get off the phone. The patient:

Answers:

A. Interrupts gently, saying, "Sue, I've enjoyed talking with you, but I really need to get going now. I'm sorry to be so abrupt—let's talk again soon." _Adaptive_

B. Sighs loudly, and says with much annoyance, "I've got to get going." Then hangs up abruptly. _Disinhibited_

C. Listens cordially, and acts interested while feeling bored and irritated. _Inhibited_

Explanation: The answers above are given with respect to the dominant middle-class European American culture that we authors (and most therapists) come from. The answers may need to be modified to be more appropriate to you, your patient, and/or the cultural milieu you both find yourselves in.

A. **Adaptive** (Appropriately assertive). Note that the comment begins and ends with something positive (this is called a "positive sandwich").

B. **Disinhibited** (aggressive).

C. **Inhibited** (passive).

Exercise 8A.1. **Excitement: Inhibited, adaptive, or disinhibited?**

Your patient just received a large promotion and is at a restaurant with friends. She does the following:

A. Worries that her friends will feel outdone and so remains silent.

_____

B. Insists on buying dinner for everyone, even though some people clearly want to leave. _____

C. Says, "Hey, I got some really great news today!" _____

Exercise 8A.2. **Anger/assertion: Inhibited, adaptive, or disinhibited?**

Your patient's coworker has just taken credit for an idea of hers, and she finds herself alone with the man in a private office. She says:

A. "I didn't like what you said in the meeting this morning, and I want to talk to you about it." _____

B. "You bastard, I'm going to get you for what you did today!" _____

C. "I thought you did a really nice job in the meeting today." _____

Exercise 8A.3.

Joy: Inhibited, adaptive, or disinhibited?

Your patient just had a moving spiritual experience. He conveys it to his friends as follows:

A. He says, "I had a really moving experience this morning." _____

B. He remains silent, not wanting to offend. _____

C. He strongly urges his friends to come to his meditation group, saying, "Anyone who misses out on this doesn't have a clue about spiritual things." _____

Exercise 8A.4.

Sexual excitement: Inhibited, adaptive, or disinhibited?

Your patient is saying good night to his or her date. They clearly find each other attractive. Your patient does the following:

A. Pushes the date against the wall and starts kissing. _____

B. Looks at the ground and hopes that the date will kiss him or her. _____

C. Makes eye contact, moves closer, and watches for the date's signals. _____

Exercise 8A.5.

Grief: Inhibited, adaptive, or disinhibited?

Two years after the death of his wife, a man is having lunch in a restaurant with some close friends. One of his friends reminisces about the man's deceased spouse. The man responds as follows:

A. Keeps his face impassive and focuses straight ahead. _____

B. Tears up, and says that she would like being remembered this way. _____

C. Breaks out in uncontrollable sobs and cannot speak. After a while, friends help him out of the restaurant. _____

Exercise 8A.6.

Anger/assertion: Inhibited, adaptive, or disinhibited?

A neighbor asks your patient for honest feedback about whether he has been inconsiderate in letting his dog out on garbage day. Your patient responds:

A. "Oh, no. It's no problem." (Her stomach churns and chest tightens.) _____

B. "Yes, thanks for asking. It has been an annoyance to me, and I would like something to be done. I appreciate your concern." _____

C. "Yes, I wondered how long it would take you to figure that out," or (sarcastically), "Oh, no, why would I mind garbage all over my lawn every week?" _____

EXERCISE 8B: HELP INTEGRATE FEELINGS AND FIND THE MISSING AFFECT

Directions: In order to integrate feelings for appropriate expression, it is often necessary to determine whether an affect is "missing" that would provide balance. For each of the following patient statements, first form a hypothesis about which affect the patient needs to experience and express in order to achieve balance or integration. Then make up a therapist response that might elicit the missing affect from the patient (we have provided suggestions in the examples that follow.)

Example: PATIENT: I just feel so miserable since my father died. I know he did all those terrible things to me, but I can think only of how much I love him and miss him. Isn't that strange?

Answer 1:   **What affect is needed to balance the sadness?** _Anger_

Explanation: Feeling angry, of course, is the normal, adaptive response when someone does "terrible things" to you. Here the patient is able to acknowledge longing and sadness, but seems to know there's something missing. Indeed, the patient's use of "miserable" suggests that there may be self-attack caused by unconscious feelings of anger, and that integrating all the feelings toward the father may help resolve complicated mourning.

Answer 2:   **What might the therapist say to help elicit the affect?** (Here are two possibilities):

> Well, there are always mixed feelings for people close to us and that may be what is bothering you. Can you imagine feeling angry at him? What is the most difficult part about feeling angry?

> It does seem a little strange that there wouldn't be other feelings mixed in with your sadness and longing. If there were another feeling there, what do you think it would be?

Explanation: In the first response, the therapist suggests the affect directly, does some exposure ("Can you imagine feeling angry . . . "), and then introduces anxiety regulation ("What is the most difficult part . . . "). Of course, these interventions don't need to be combined into a single speaking turn, but could be presented one by one. The second response encourages the patient to identify the affect.

Exercise 8B.1.   PATIENT: I know my boss's mother is in the hospital, but you wouldn't believe how much she loused up my schedule! I mean, she's still my boss. I think she should suck it up and get on with her job.

What affect is needed to balance the anger? _____

What might the therapist say to help elicit the affect? _____

_____

Exercise 8B.2.

PATIENT: It's a relief that my father's dead. He was terrible to me—the only feeling I have toward him is fury. [For months after her father's death, patient has expressed nothing but her rage toward him, despite clear instances of her father's caring for her and sorrow about how he had treated her.]

What affect is needed to balance the anger? _____

What might the therapist say to help elicit the affect? _____

_____

Exercise 8B.3.

PATIENT: It's just so wonderful to be with her! She's so understanding that I can tell her anything. So how can I get upset when she is in a bad mood and loses her temper? I just put up with it.

What affect is needed to balance the closeness? _____

What might the therapist say to help elicit the affect? _____

_____

Exercise 8B.4.

PATIENT: My husband says he hardly recognizes me now that I stand up for myself. I asked him if he missed the "old me," and he said no, he really can see that the changes I've made are helping me—and even though it's tough on him, they're helping our relationship, too. But he jokes about how now that I'm so tough I won't just cuddle up with him, and I worry that it's not just a joke.

What affect is needed to balance the anger/assertion? _____

What might the therapist say to help elicit the affect? _____

_____

EXERCISE 8C: HELP THE PATIENT WITH INTERPERSONAL EXPRESSION

Directions: In each of the following exercises, choose the aspect of Affect Expression that is likely to be **what the patient needs most help with**. Then think of a statement the therapist might make in using this intervention (again, we have provided two in the example that follows). For the example and each of the six exercises, **only one of the interventions from the following list** is to be chosen (each is used once only):

> A. Addressing secondary gain.
> B. Mature expression of anger.
> C. Receptive capacity for praise (positive feelings toward the self).
> D. Information: The difference between grief and depression.
> E. Conflict over assertion.
> F. Conflict over closeness.
> G. Blending of positive and negative feelings.

Example:

THERAPIST: When your boss told you that you'd done such a good job on your presentation, how did you feel? What did you say to her?

PATIENT: I was embarrassed; it was in front of all those people. I just said that everyone else had basically done all the work, even though that's totally not true.

Answers:

What does the patient need help with? C. Receptive capacity for praise (positive feelings toward the self).

What might the therapist say? (Here are two possibilities):

It seems that it's really hard for you to take a compliment. Can you imagine something else you might have said that would have been fairer to yourself? [Guided fantasy]

What was the hardest part about hearing her say what a good job you'd done? [Anxiety regulation]

Exercise 8C.1.

PATIENT: I've really been working on setting limits with my wife, and it's helping. She thinks it's helping, too.

THERAPIST: I'm really glad to hear that. You know, you came in talking about how lonely you felt, and we were able to discover that part of the problem was that she was doing lots of things that made you angry, but you felt powerless to stop her and so you just pulled back. Now that you aren't doing that as much, I wonder if you are feeling less lonely?

PATIENT: Well, I guess maybe a little. I mean, I don't feel as beaten down as I used to feel—but other than that, I don't think things between us have changed that much.

What does the patient need help with? _____

What might the therapist say to help elicit the affect? _____

_____

Exercise 8C.2.

PATIENT: I told my boss that I appreciated his confidence in me, that I was glad he valued my work so much, but that if he wasn't able to pay me more I would start looking for a new job.

THERAPIST: Good for you! We've been working on this for a long time, so I know that wasn't easy for you. Tell me, how did it feel to do that?

PATIENT: I was glad I said it, but I felt bad afterwards. It felt disloyal to say that to someone whom I've been working with for years.

What does the patient need help with? _____

What might the therapist say to help elicit the affect? _____

_____

Exercise 8C.3.

PATIENT: So finally I'd just had it up to here with my boss, and I said, "I'm sick to death of your bullshit!"

What does the patient need help with? _____

What might the therapist say to help elicit the affect? _____

_____

Exercise 8C.4.

PATIENT: After we talked about my mom's death last session, I was just feeling really down, and I was scared the depression was coming back. I would start to cry, and I wouldn't know whether to fight it or to really let myself go.

What does the patient need help with? _____

What might the therapist say to help elicit the affect? _____

_____

Exercise 8C.5.

PATIENT: Well, I made another angry scene—but the whole time I was doing it, I was thinking to myself, "Why are you doing this? You don't really need to, but there is some real delight in blasting him." And, as usual, my husband was extra sweet to me afterwards.

What does the patient need help with? _____

What might the therapist say to help elicit the affect? _____

_____

Exercise 8C.6.

PATIENT: Although I told her I was really stressed from work and needed some quiet time to recuperate, my wife just kept talking on and on over dinner. So I finally said to her, "I really need some peace and quiet. Please be quiet!" I asked for what I wanted, and I wasn't nasty, but she'd made a really nice dinner for me, and I guess I spoiled it. She was pretty upset.

What does the patient need help with? _____

What might the therapist say to help elicit the affect? _____

_____

PART III | SELF- AND OTHER-RESTRUCTURING

Introduction to Part III

An Overview of Self- and Other-Restructuring

In *Changing Character*, Self-Restructuring and Other-Restructuring were treated together in a single chapter. For this book, we have chosen to discuss them in two separate chapters. We have done this to highlight basic differences between the two objectives, as well as to clarify interventions specific to each. Nevertheless, issues of self and other are intertwined in Short-Term Dynamic Psychotherapy (STDP); the difference lies primarily in whose perspective is being emphasized.

Chapter 9: Self-Restructuring

In Chapter 9, the focus is on **the inner image of the self and the receptivity to one's own feelings.** This chapter illustrates how to work toward a more accurate and compassionate view of the self to foster greater self-care and autonomy. Patients who need this kind of work might say:

PATIENT 1: It just doesn't seem that important to care for myself.

PATIENT 2: I don't deserve to ask for anything.

PATIENT 3: I never feel proud of myself.

PATIENT 4: I spend a lot of time figuring out what other people want, but I don't really know what I want.

Chapter 10: Other-Restructuring

Chapter 10 focuses on **the inner images of others and the receptivity to others' feelings.** This chapter addresses how to modify the inner-held view of others and how responsivity to others' feelings can foster healthy connection and interdependence of the self with others. Patients who need this kind of work might say:

PATIENT 1: When anybody says they care for me, I never let myself believe it.

PATIENT 2: He offered to help me, but I felt too guilty and told him not to bother.

PATIENT 3: (*To therapist*) I'm just another clinical case to you.

PATIENT 4: I don't trust anybody very much. And it takes me a while to trust you again when we miss a session.

Defense and Affect Work Can Come First When Self is Strong

Although the restructuring of defenses and affects inevitably has some impact on the inner images of self and others, higher-functioning patients suited for STDP (Global Assessment of Functioning [GAF] scores over 60, good impulse control, etc.) tend to need relatively little self- and other-work. Thus treatment can begin (as we have begun in Part II of the book) with rapid restructuring of defenses and Affect Phobias.

Other patients with moderate impairment (GAF scores of 51–60) may have pockets of difficulties with relationship to self and others, and thus may need varying degrees of remedial self/other work during the short-term work.

Self- and Other-Work Comes First When Self Is Impaired

Patients with significant impairment (e.g., GAF scores under 50) may need a sole focus on Self- and Other-Restructuring before Defense and Affect Restructuring can begin. Otherwise, attempts to restructure Affect Phobias can elicit self-attack or become blocked.

Prerequisites for Short-Term Treatment

Thus relatively adaptive senses of self and others can be thought of as prerequisites for rapid Defense and Affect Restructuring. When these capacities are lacking, the therapist must build them, before or along with work on other core conflicts. In actual practice, therapy is likely to alternate between focusing on images of self and others, and work focusing on defenses and affects; the relative emphasis on these two aspects of therapy will depend on the patient's overall level of functioning, including the patient's level of functioning.

Why Does Self- and Other-Restructuring Follow Defense and Affect Restructuring in This Book?

It may be confusing that the coverage of Self- and Other-Restructuring in Part III comes **after** that of Defense and Affect Restructuring in Part II, since Self- and Other-Restructuring must at times come first in treatment. There are two main reasons:

1. Typical STDP begins with restructuring defenses and affects.
2. The need for extensive work on self-image and image of others suggests a somewhat different form of treatment with a more impaired patient, and sometimes is not "short-term" at all.

Therapy Takes Longer When the Self Is Impaired

Significant impairments in self-image or relationships to others tend to make therapy a longer process; sometimes 50–100 sessions or even more can be necessary. Nevertheless, the therapist's attitude should always be one of making treatment as efficient as possible, given the level of the patient's difficulties.

Summary

Self- and Other-Restructuring is designed to shine a spotlight on an extremely important area for healing and ultimately for character change. As noted in Chapter 1, this model sees optimal relatedness as the well-integrated balance of autonomy and healthy interdependence, expressiveness, and receptivity. Together, Chapters 9 and 10 propose a vision of an esteemed self that has well-defined boundaries, but is still flexible and responsive to a give-and-take with others.

A positive self-image and adaptive connections to others constitute the foundation on which mental health is built. To lay this foundation, the therapist must pay particular attention to the defenses and affects associated with the self and with others.

Self-Restructuring: Building Compassion and Care for Self

Chapter Objectives	To demonstrate how to restructure the sense of self, through desensitization of Affect Phobias about positive feelings toward the self. Showing how to help patients (1) view the self with compassion (both strengths and vulnerabilities); (2) respond to needs for autonomy as well as interdependence; (3) become their own "good parents."
Therapist Stance	Using a caring therapist–patient relationship to expose the patient to a positive and compassionate view of self.
Anxiety Regulation	Regulation of guilt and shame associated with self-perception, self-care, and self-compassion.
Topics Covered	I. Overview: Restructuring for a Positive Sense of Self II. Building Receptive Capacity to One's Own Feelings III. Changing Perspectives on the Self: Encouraging Patients to Imagine How Others See Them IV. Finding and Encouraging the Lost Voice V. Encouraging "Parenting" of the Self VI. Reducing the Externalization of Needs VII. Repeating Interventions until Phobias about Self-Feelings Are Desensitized and Self-Worth Improves
Indication for a Focus on Self-Restructuring	• The patient's Global Assessment of Functioning (GAF) score is below 50 (serious symptoms, or serious impairment in functioning). • Problems occur with self-care, self-esteem, self-confidence, or the like. • Problems occur with impulse control (acting out, angry outbursts, substance misuse, eating disorders, etc.).

- Defense or Affect Restructuring becomes blocked due to excessive self-attack or negative sense of self.

I. OVERVIEW: RESTRUCTURING FOR A POSITIVE SENSE OF SELF

A positive self-image is the foundation on which mental health is built. In this chapter, we look at ways to build or strengthen that foundation.

Desensitizing Affect Phobias about Positive Self-Feelings

Previous chapters have shown how to treat phobias connected to specific affects. Self-Restructuring focuses on treating Affect Phobias specifically related to the following:

- Positive self-image (self-perception, self-esteem, sense of self, etc.).
- Self-compassion; responsivity to self-feelings and needs (care for the self).

In other words, Self-Restructuring means desensitizing Affect Phobias about positive feelings toward the self. Adaptive functioning requires an ability to know and care about oneself and one's wants and needs. This chapter highlights some specific methods for building positive feelings toward the self. The interventions are designed to help the patient develop a healthy autonomy and sense of self, while at the same time maintaining a balance between independence and interpersonal connection, as taught in the next chapter.

Lack of Receptivity to Self-Needs

Many patients who need Self-Restructuring work are unaware of their own inner signals, neglect them, or don't feel entitled to respond to them or to voice their own needs. Generally, they were taught as children to adapt to situations by denying parts of themselves. Many patients were taught to be very receptive to other people's needs, but not receptive to their own needs. When this lack of "receptive capacity" to one's own wants and needs continues in adulthood, it can create a constant state of self-inflicted deprivation:

PATIENT 1: I feel selfish when I indulge myself the least bit.

PATIENT 2: I don't feel like I ever deserve special treatment.

Lack of Receptive Capacity Means Longer-Term Treatment

The ability to respond to internal signals is basic, and is often a prerequisite for the affect work that we have described in previous chapters. For example, therapists cannot help patients become more assertive about their needs if they are simply not aware of what those needs are. The more these capacities are lacking, the more emphasis needs to be placed on Self-Restructuring, and—in general—the longer therapy will take. In such cases, there is less rapid uncovering of conflicts, and more emphasis on supportive and ego-building methods. We have chosen to cover these deviations from "pure" Short-Term Dynamic Psychotherapy (STDP) here in this chapter and the one that follows.

Steps for Self-Work

When lack of self-esteem or self-care is evident, and patients need Self-Restructuring, therapists will need to:

- Ask directly whether patients can recognize their needs.
- Identify when patients are neglectful or self-abusive, rather than caring for the self.
- Desensitize Affect Phobias centering around self-image and self-care, to help patients (1) view themselves with compassion (both strengths and weaknesses); (2) meet their own needs for both autonomy and interdependence; and (3) learn to act as their own "good parents."

In the remainder of this section, we discuss how to desensitize and restructure Affect Phobias about self-image and self-care, followed by discussions of the therapist stance and anxiety regulation in Self-Restructuring. In Section II, we discuss receptivity to self-needs and present an overview of the main areas of self-functioning.

Restructuring Conflicts about the Self: Desensitizing Affect Phobias of Self-Feeling

Types of Affect Phobias about Positive Self-Feelings

Conflicts or Affect Phobias related to self-responding are very common. For example, people are often horrified at the thought of feeling proud:

THERAPIST: You must be proud of that promotion. You worked so hard for it.

PATIENT: Feel proud? I guess I should, but it feels self-centered to celebrate the promotion, or make a big deal out of it.

THERAPIST: It's unfortunate that you never were allowed to pat yourself on the back.

Similarly, many patients cannot bear to be indulgent of themselves:

THERAPIST: If your neck and shoulders are in knots from bending over the computer, I wonder if you ever consider getting a massage.

PATIENT: Never! That would be much too self-indulgent. I'd feel too guilty.

THERAPIST: How sad that you are so neglectful of yourself.

Systematic Desensitization for Self-Restructuring

Positive feelings about the self form the basis of healthy autonomy, so that when conflicts about self-feelings are present, the therapist needs to desensitize them—just as we have seen earlier with Affect Phobias in general. The principles for desensitization of Affect Phobias related to self-feeling are the same as previously described: exposure to compassionate feelings for self, with response prevention and anxiety regulation as needed, repeated again and again.

As discussed in Section III of Chapter 1, self-feelings do not represent a single category of affect, but rather a blend of Tomkins's interest/excitement and enjoyment/joy directed toward the self. In clinical work, we typically group all of these under "positive feelings toward the self" on the adaptive Feeling Pole (F) of Malan's Triangle of Conflict. Some examples of self-feeling include **self-esteem, self-interest, self-respect, self-confidence, self-compassion, and self-care** (see Figure 9.1). These positive self-feelings are inhibited by anxiety, guilt, shame, pain, or contempt/disgust on the Anxiety Pole (A), and result in behaviors on the Defensive Pole (D) such as self-attack, self-neglect, or self-hate, which block or avoid the self-nurturant or self-supportive behaviors that we will detail below (see Section II) in our discussion of areas of self-functioning.

Exposure and response prevention with anxiety regulation will help decrease the phobic avoidance of these adaptive responses. Consider this example:

THERAPIST: If you put aside your self-deprecation [D] for a moment [response prevention], what would it feel like to just let yourself feel proud [F] of what you did [exposure]?

If the patient resists:

THERAPIST: What's the hardest part about just letting yourself feel proud? [Anxiety regulation]

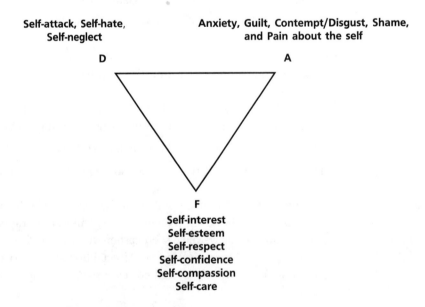

FIGURE 9.1. Self-feelings on the Triangle of Conflict.

Therapist Stance: Encouragement and Shared Affect

The Caring Relationship Is the Intervention

When there has been a significant impairment in self-image, the relationship with the therapist will be a crucial first step toward self-acceptance. The therapist then must become a model of caring, acknowledging the patient's positive qualities and showing compassion and understanding for limitations.

Using Socratic Questions to Elicit Feelings

For impaired self-functioning, the therapist's own emotional response is the most important part of the intervention. But it is important that the therapist's feelings **not be directly stated** at first, because statements like "I feel sad for you" are too easily defended against and dismissed. Instead, the therapist's feelings should be elicited socratically **from the patient**, via such questions as "What do **you** imagine that I might feel for you?"

This Socratic approach often needs much focus and repetition, but over time it helps build within the patient the capacity to resonate to the therapist's feelings, and ultimately the feelings of other significant people.

THERAPIST: What can you sense that I feel right now when you say that?

PATIENT: I don't know.

THERAPIST: Take a moment and see if you can imagine what I might feel.

PATIENT: Gee, this is really hard.

THERAPIST: How would you feel if someone told **you** the story you have told me? [As noted above, it is important that the therapist does not tell the patient what the therapist is feeling, but tries to elicit that perception in the patient—in this case by changing perspectives, as will be covered in Section III.]

PATIENT: I guess I would feel really sad. Maybe you do feel a little sad?

THERAPIST: Yes, I do. Maybe more than a little.

Therapist Acknowledgment of Feelings

Once an awareness of the therapist's feelings has been elicited from the patient, these feelings may be acknowledged by the therapist. It is important, though, that the therapist acknowledge only honest feelings. Sometimes the therapist feels strongly, and sometimes not; nothing should be faked. But it is rare that a therapist has no concern whatsoever. Therapists are in the business of healing, so the simple wish that the patient resolve problems and build a better life can be Socratically elicited and then acknowledged.

THERAPIST: What do you think I feel?

PATIENT: I guess you are concerned about me, and want the best for me.

THERAPIST: Yes, of course I do.

When the Therapist's Concern Seems Greater Than the Patient's

Sometimes the therapist may seem more concerned about the problem than the patient does. Here is one way to deal with this:

THERAPIST: Do you notice that I seem to feel more compassion for you than you do for yourself. Isn't that sad? How does that sit with you?

PATIENT: I don't know. [Often the therapist will not get an immediate response to this intervention, but if it is gently repeated over several sessions, it can eventually make an impact.]

PATIENT (*Weeks later*) I suddenly thought, "You care more about me than I care about myself . . . and that's not right!!" [This is the patient's first small indicator of self-compassion.]

Therapists' Dislike of Patients

A therapist needs to realize that feelings of irritation toward or lack of care for the patient are signs of potential defensiveness—in either the patient or the therapist. Sometimes, if a patient uses defenses that are irritating or antagonistic (passive aggression, sarcasm, devaluation, etc.), it can be very helpful to convey this in a compassionate way to the patient. (Also see CC, pp. 173–175, 319–321, and 333–337.)

PATIENT: I think you are irritated with me. You seem irritated.

THERAPIST: Yes, I think I do feel somewhat irritated. And I tell you this not to be critical, but to explore what is going on. This reaction may reflect my own issues—but it also may tell us about ways you interact with others. What do you think?

Anxiety Regulation: Decreasing Anxieties about Adaptive Self-Feelings

Desensitization of conflict about adaptive self-feelings requires anxiety regulation, just as desensitization of conflict about other feelings does. A patient needs to be exposed to successive degrees of positive feelings about the self—from the therapist, from others, or from memories of past figures—until the anxiety subsides (see also CC, pp. 337–338).

THERAPIST 1: What's the worst thing about feeling good about yourself?

THERAPIST 2: What would be the guilt about indulging yourself this way?

THERAPIST 3: You say you can't think of anyone who cared for you, but what about your grandfather? What is the most difficult thing about acknowledging that he was really proud of your accomplishments?

We now discuss some of the most common anxieties about positive feelings toward the self.

Self-Care Feels Like Selfishness

Many patients argue that care for self excludes care for others. They fear that developing pride, self-esteem, or genuine self-interest will make them selfish or arrogant. Here are some possible ways to teach patients about adaptive self-care.

Suggested Responses   THERAPIST 1: Caring for yourself does not have to compete with caring for others. When people neglect their own feelings, their caring for others can easily become resentful, obligatory, and draining. The more you can meet your own needs, the more you should feel able to be genuinely giving—and truly charitable toward others. What do you think?

THERAPIST 2: Having self-esteem does not mean holding yourself out as superior to others. People who are arrogant or insulting to others are more likely to have low self-esteem that they are covering with grandiosity. Do you know anyone like that?

THERAPIST 3: Can you think of someone with genuine self-confidence, who does not have to act in a way to make others feel inferior?

Too Much Pain to Bear (Grief That Blocks Change)   Another common reason why patients find it hard to accept positive changes in their self-image is that change—no matter how positive—can be very painful. **Each opening to tender feelings brings grief, because experiencing something wonderful for the first time carries the realization of all that was missed, as well as the fear that it may be lost in the future.** In other words, beginning to experience joy or closeness for the first time brings tremendous sadness about living so long without these emotions. Many patients' defenses against grief keep them stuck in joyless, loveless patterns—for fear of the pain that comes with tenderness.

PATIENT: All these years I didn't feel lovable. It's so sad that I have neglected myself for so long that it's almost unbearable to face.

THERAPIST: Have you been able to cry in your lover's arms and let him [or her] know how deeply you are feeling?

Helping Patients Bear the Pain   It is the therapist's task to help patients bear the pain and grief involved in opening to positive feelings about the self, so that patients can experience more of the full range of self-feeling.

Example 1   PATIENT: You know, it's really weird—all that time I was married, I wanted my wife to do things like give me backrubs, and she wouldn't. Now I have this wonderful relationship with someone who would love to give me backrubs, and I can't let her do it. I just choke up, and I have to make her stop.

THERAPIST: Why do you "have to make her stop"?

PATIENT: Well, I can't just burst into tears every time she gives me a backrub.

THERAPIST: What would happen if you did burst into tears a few times? [Anxiety regulation]

PATIENT: It's embarrassing. I should just be able to enjoy it after all this time, but I haven't been able to.

THERAPIST: You know, this is a pretty common reaction when people finally start to get some of the things they longed for. It really brings home the amount of deprivation you lived through, and it's very common for grief to come up like this. How do you imagine she would feel if you really started to cry when she was giving you a backrub?

PATIENT: Now that you have me think about it, I bet she'd be fine. She'd be understanding. I guess I have been tensing up and not enjoying what she is giving me, because I am so afraid of looking like a fool if I cried. And I've been missing out on a lot by not showing who I really am.

Example 2

PATIENT: I've been in a lot of relationships that I ended because I thought the person just wasn't right for me. Now I'm in a relationship that's really good and that I really want to last, and I find myself picking little fights over nothing.

THERAPIST: What do you make of that?

PATIENT: Well, I've been trying to watch when I do it, and it seems like it happens when I'm afraid that he's going to wind up not wanting me.

THERAPIST: So I wonder if you are creating a self-fulfilling prophecy. You feel afraid he might not want you, and then you do something that might in fact cause you to appear less loveable.

PATIENT: Oh, I really am, aren't I?

THERAPIST: Yes, but I bet there's a good reason. Can you imagine feeling that you are really valuable and loveable to this person?

PATIENT: Terrifying! I couldn't bear it if he left me.

Loss of Identity Can Be Terrifying

Because giving up old ways of being can be very frightening, **it is important to help patients build new supports before they give up the old ones.** As noted throughout this manual, to get patients to relinquish maladaptive behavior patterns, more adaptive ways of responding must be developed to replace the maladaptive ones. Building new supports is particularly crucial for helping patients restructure their self-image. Patients cannot uncover and give up unconscious defenses if they are shoring up a fragile sense of self. A therapist must help a patient build a stronger sense of self to replace the maladaptive one.

Ways to Build New Supports

Some ways the therapist can help build new supports to replace maladaptive defenses include the following:

1. Teaching new behaviors (e.g., the distinction among passive, assertive and aggressive behaviors that we have discussed in Chapter 8).

2. Supporting and encouraging the patient's struggle for change.

THERAPIST: It's hard to give up old habits that are perhaps the only way you have known. It will take time and effort, but gradually you can learn to set limits with people and not have that guilty feeling.

3. Helping the patient take small steps that he or she can tolerate.

THERAPIST: You don't have to change the way you assert yourself with people all at once. We can work on doing this a little bit at a time, as it feels right to you.

4. Helping the patient imagine an ideal self who could cope with the problems in a different way.

THERAPIST: Could you imagine how you would ideally like to respond in these difficult situations, and begin to build a new image of yourself?

5. Identifying people that the patient sees as heroic or as possible role models.

THERAPIST: Do you know of anyone who has handled situations like yours in a way that you admired?

II. BUILDING RECEPTIVE CAPACITY TO ONE'S OWN FEELINGS

Resonance to Inner Signals

One of the main healing mechanisms in Self-Restructuring is the improvement of patients' receptive capacity. **Receptive capacity** means patients' ability to "take in," "receive," or resonate to their own internal signals of wants, needs, and self-value. The receptive capacity is a missing capability regarding the self that must be built. Receptivity includes the ability to do the following:

1. Accept and understand one's own value.
2. Accept one's strengths and limitations.
3. Perceive and respond to bodily signals and nurture the self.
4. Feel entitled to pursue one's own wants and needs.

Healthy Autonomy Is Built upon a Reservoir of Care

When a patient has mastered these capacities, a healthy autonomy will result. **Autonomy** is generally defined as independence or freedom. **Autonomy of the self** is the capacity to govern oneself, control oneself, have authority over oneself—in short, to stand on one's own when necessary. It means being centered or in touch with one's own feelings and being able to meet most of one's basic needs. Autonomy has often been mistaken to mean never needing others, but in STDP autonomy is seen as a result of healthy connection. Care from others helps to build care for self; concern for self is learned from others, held within, and drawn upon as needed. This **reservoir** of closeness, tenderness, and positive feelings originates from others (especially from caretakers in early life) and needs to be replenished from time to time. The reservoir is critical for autonomy, because optimally it should be made up of sufficient positive feeling to sustain the self when others are absent, hurtful, or disappointing. Contrast these two patient–therapist exchanges:

PATIENT 1: I feel so miserable when I am alone, I can hardly bear it.

THERAPIST 1: Are you ever able to remember the love of your family in such times?

PATIENT 1: I know my family loves me, but I don't let that comfort me.

THERAPIST 2: With all that you've been through, how do you manage to sustain yourself?

PATIENT 2: I am comforted by knowing that my friends and family wholeheartedly support me.

Teaching, guidance, and encouragement are helpful to get patients to attend to inner signals (of distress, fatigue, need, anger, hunger, isolation, lack of meaning in life), as we have discussed in regard to building supports in Section I (anxiety regulation).

Lack of Receptivity Prevents Change

Lack of receptivity is a defensive stance and one of the biggest obstacles to character change. When patients are unable to be receptive or responsive to their own feelings (or the feelings of others—see Chapter 10), their maladaptive assumptions from the past cannot be corrected by new experiences. Then old deprivations continue, and old behavior patterns are carried into the future. Even when nurturing people or situations are available, patients often feel undeserving or unworthy and refuse to savor such care. In such cases, the patients' receptive capacity **must** be built before character change can occur.

Receptive Capacity Is Often Overlooked

Despite the importance of receptivity for change, this capacity is typically not addressed in treatment.

- More emphasis has been placed on **therapist interventions** than on **patient responses** to therapist interventions. Yet empathy, concern, or compassion from therapists will be devalued or dismissed by patients if they are not able to be receptive to such feeling.
- More emphasis has been placed on the **expression of feeling** (discussed in Chapter 8) than on **receptivity to feeling**. Yet the two are equally important, and being receptive to what one feels or what others are feeling is often a prerequisite for appropriate self-expression.

(For more information on the receptive capacity, also see CC, pp. 293–297, 315–319, and 354.)

Areas of Self-Functioning

Deficiencies in receptivity to one's own needs can be subtle and thus not immediately evident. This section alerts therapists to areas of impairment in self-functioning that are often overlooked:

- Biological needs
- Psychological/emotional needs
- Sexual needs
- Social needs
- Spiritual needs

For each of the five areas of self-functioning listed above, we supply sample questions that a therapist might use for assessment. However, there is no expectation that a therapist will need to use all of these questions.

Biological Needs

Although rarely addressed directly in therapy, biological signals and needs (fatigue, hunger, pain, elimination, physical comfort, etc.) are basic and need to be responded to adaptively. Therapy work will be impaired if a patient is chronically overtired, overstressed, undernourished, or not meeting other basic physical needs. Here are some questions a therapist might ask:

- "Are you receptive and responsive to the signals your body is sending you?"
- "Do you eat healthily when hungry? Do you sleep regularly and well?"
- "Do you respond in a timely fashion to bladder and bowel functions?"
- "Do you feel worthy of eating well [or dressing warmly, being relieved, etc.]?"
- "Do you feel like you are entitled to be cared for in these very basic ways?"
- "Do you care for your medical and dental needs?"

For example:

PATIENT: I'm exhausted from overwork.

THERAPIST: Are you ignoring your body's signals to rest?

PATIENT: I don't pay attention to those kinds of things.

THERAPIST: Remember, you deserve to respond to your physical needs. You seem to push your limits too far.

Psychological Needs

Meeting one's own psychological needs represents Affect Restructuring applied to the self, with a special emphasis on self-perception or self-image, and on one's own feelings.

First, can patients feel joy (healthy pride) in themselves or their accomplishments without shame or guilt? Do patients value and accept themselves? Here are questions a therapist might ask:

- "What parts of yourself do you respect the most?"
- "Do you feel you are a person of worth, equal to others?"
- "What are you most proud of about yourself?"

Second, can patients feel interested or excited about various aspects of themselves? A therapist might ask these questions:

- "Do you have hobbies or interests that you feel excited by?"
- "Do you have interest in some aspects of your work?"
- "Do you feel interested in yourself—your goals, plans, hopes, or dreams?"

Third, can patients feel sadness or grief on their own behalf when losses occur? Here are some questions a therapist might ask:

- "When you feel sad, do you respond to yourself with self-compassion or self-contempt?"
- "Do you feel entitled to grieve?"

Fourth, can patients feel fear on their own behalf when they are doing something dangerous, or when they are vulnerable to loss of control in some destructive way? Some questions a therapist might ask are as follows:

- "Are you able to recognize when you are in a dangerous situation?"
- "Are you able to protect or remove yourself if you are in danger?"

Fifth, can patients feel shame or anger for their **actions** rather than for the **self** as a whole when they hurt another? Can they simultaneously feel grief for the other's pain and compassion for their own failings, so the action is not repeated? Here are some questions the therapist might ask:

- "When you do something that hurts someone, are you able to empathize with that person's feelings, yet without attacking yourself mercilessly?"
- "Are you able to feel genuine remorse, and the desire to make amends, when you hurt someone?"

Finally, can patients feel tenderness and compassion for themselves on an equal basis with others? The therapist might ask these questions:

- "Do you feel as entitled as other people to be cared for?"
- "Do you respond to yourself with self-acceptance or self-denial?"

Sexual Needs

It's surprising how frequently sexual topics are avoided in therapy. These are difficult questions for the therapist to ask, yet they are crucial ones in many cases. Therapists may need help to become more familiar and comfortable with exploring sexual feelings. Are sexual needs being responded to? Are these needs handled in a constructive way? Questions the therapist might ask include these:

- "How do you respond to your sexual needs?"
- "Do you let yourself have a full, enjoyable sexual experience?"
- "Are you able to ask your partner for things you'd like?"
- "Do you enjoy giving your partner pleasure?"
- "Are you able to masturbate?"
- "What are the masturbatory fantasies that bring you to orgasm or that make you the most aroused?" (These can signal some of the deepest conflicts in the individual's life and can help identify sexual orientation.)

Social Needs

Closeness to others is discussed in detail in the following chapter, so we will just note it briefly here. Are social needs being attended to? Is too much isolation or alienation tolerated? Are friends sought out for shared activities or to confide in? Here are some questions the therapist might ask:

- "Do you have people whom you trust and who support you?"
- "Do you have friends to do things with in your free time?"
- "Do you have people close to you in whom you can confide?"

Spiritual Needs

Spiritual needs often go unmet in our patients' lives and unattended to in therapy. However, many patients find that a nurturant, sustaining, and inspiring world view is essential for emotional well-being. The therapist needs to explore whether the patient has a sense of purpose and meaning in life—and, if not, why not? The therapist also needs to inquire about the patient's spiritual or religious life, as well as the patient's beliefs (or lack thereof) about living and dying. The therapist might ask these questions:

- "Do you have a religious or spiritual side? Is this something you would want to develop?"
- "How do you feel toward life in general? What makes life worthwhile for you?"
- "Do you have conflicts or fears about death?"
- "Do you feel satisfied with your life?"
- "Do you have a peacefulness or acceptance of life that is soothing? If not, do you ever let yourself feel at peace?"
- "Do you feel you have a relationship with God or a higher power? What is that relationship like? Is this experience nurturing or sustaining for you?"
- "Do you have an active spiritual or religious life—or do you have spiritual needs that are going unmet? Is there a religious or spiritual community that you are part of, or feel drawn to, or long for?"

Exposure, to Enhance Receptive Capacity

Desensitizing Conflict That Has to Do with Receptive Capacity

Receptivity can be avoided via many defenses—externalization of needs (see Section VI), feelings of emptiness, devaluation of others' feelings, or numbing of feeling, to name just a few. Therapists need to help patients prevent those defensive responses and expose patients to their feelings about the self, using the same techniques discussed throughout this book. Exposure to their feelings will improve both the patients' receptivity to the feelings of others, and ultimately their own self-worth.

Use of Imagery

As with the desensitization of other Affect Phobias, it is important to focus a patient's attention on inner experience, including bodily sensations. Generally, guided imagery is used to encourage the patient to recognize, acknowledge, or respond to his or her own and others' feelings. This attention includes both negative and positive feelings, as well as a particular focus on the relationship with the therapist, to illustrate the here-and-now experience of feeling.

THERAPIST: We've talked about how hard it is for you to let yourself slow down. Is there something that you'd like to do to take care of yourself, but you never seem to do?

PATIENT: It's embarrassing [A], but I always dream about giving myself a nice hot bubble bath.

THERAPIST: Why don't you take a minute now to imagine what it would be like at the end of a long hard day to tell yourself that you've worked hard enough, and you deserve a long relaxing bubble bath? Imagine just letting yourself sink into the steaming water. (*Therapist pauses, then notices a change in patient's expression.*) What are you feeling in your body right now?

PATIENT: It feels relaxed, and there's a lightness in my chest.

Although it is difficult to face negative feelings, it is often even more difficult to accept care from one's self because of the painful contrast to all that has been lacking, as noted above in regard to anxiety regulation (see Section I). Therapists must repeatedly expose patients to positive feelings for the self in guided imagery.

THERAPIST: You've told me a lot of things that suggest that you have had a hard time being gentle with yourself in these situations. I wonder how it would be for you to respond to yourself in a more generous and soothing manner.

III. CHANGING PERSPECTIVES ON THE SELF: ENCOURAGING PATIENTS TO IMAGINE HOW OTHERS SEE THEM

Self-image can be strengthened and made more resilient by helping patients view themselves differently—either by viewing themselves directly, or by imagining how others might view them in a more compassionate light. Interventions in this section lead patients to new perspectives on themselves. We focus on positive feelings, but it is also important to be able to bear negative feelings, such as remorse.

Changing Perspectives Builds Self-Compassion

Changing the perspective on the self is a simple and powerful intervention. The point is to encourage patients to **stand outside themselves** to get a different, gentler, and more forgiving view of themselves. This can be seen as a method for developing a more compassionate "observing ego." In Section III of Chapter 10, we turn to this technique again to help patients change maladaptive views of others. Here, the emphasis is on enhancing patients' self-feelings.

Asking Patients about Therapists' Feelings for Them

As we have illustrated in the section on therapist stance, a valuable technique is to ask the patient to imagine how the therapist feels about him or her.

THERAPIST: How do you think I feel toward you hearing this story?

PATIENT: If I think about it, I guess you're concerned about me.

Sometimes one presentation of this technique is sufficient to help the patient begin to view the self more positively. At other times, extensive exploration and repetition of the Socratic questions concerning the patient–therapist relationship will be necessary before the patient can develop the inner capacity to genuinely feel the care and concern of the therapist—and others.

Patients' Resistance to Self-Acceptance

Of course, not all patients are so quickly amenable to this technique. More resistant patients often say things like these:

PATIENT 1: I'd find myself, or anyone who acted like me, disgusting.

PATIENT 2: You must find me disgusting.

Then the therapist has more work to do to reduce the enormous shame about the self:

THERAPIST: Do you see how harsh you are on yourself? Does anyone deserve this harsh a judgment?

There are a number of ways to dispute and reframe maladaptive cognitions, including humor and tenacious perseverance. A negative self-image often requires the therapist to be relentless and wrestle with the defenses. **Tenacity should be maintained until feelings of self-compassion are clearly beginning to develop.** Here are some examples of various ways this can be done:

• Patients can generate a new positive view of themselves.

THERAPIST: If you look at yourself from this perspective, can you feel a little better about yourself?

- Patients can imagine how they would react to others in similar circumstances.

    THERAPIST: If a stranger [or a friend] told you the same story you're telling me, how would you feel toward that person?

- Again, patients can imagine how their therapists might view them.

    THERAPIST: How do you think I might feel about you, given all the suffering you have been through?

- Patients can imagine how other people might view them compassionately.

    THERAPIST: Can you see how she might have been feeling very warmly toward you, but you couldn't let yourself see it?

- Patients can imagine how past figures might view them positively (including love that may have been unexpressed in conflicted relationships).

    THERAPIST: Even though he was too reserved to talk about it, what feelings do you think your father had in his heart for you?

Here is an extended example in which the therapist changes perspectives in several ways:

Example

THERAPIST: If a friend of yours devoted herself to caring for a dying mother, but insisted on beating herself up for not doing enough—just like you do—how would that make you feel?

PATIENT: That would be sad. I'd feel bad for her.

THERAPIST: What would you say to her?

PATIENT: I'd say, "You did the best you could. She had cancer, and there was nothing more you could do for her."

THERAPIST: So you would be very compassionate toward this woman.

PATIENT: Of course. So, in other words, why can't I be compassionate toward myself? I don't know; I just can't.

THERAPIST: You've just told me a heartbreaking story, but you say you feel nothing for yourself. How would you feel if you were in my place? What do you imagine **I** feel toward you?

PATIENT: I don't know, like—"Here's another patient; why can't she get it together?"

THERAPIST: Can you see how quickly you feel sad for your friend, but how much harder it is to imagine that **I** might feel sad for you?

PATIENT: Yes, it is easier to imagine feeling bad for someone else . . . but it's still hard to believe you would feel that way toward me.

THERAPIST: It seems like other people readily receive your care and concern, but you have a hard time believing in those feelings others have for you.

PATIENT: (Pausing) Yeah, it's sad that I don't—but it's so different from anything I'm used to.

THERAPIST: I wonder if this week you can begin to think about this differently—about my feelings and others' feelings for you. [Encouragement for between-session exposure to new feelings and self-perspective]

There are a number of variations on these techniques that can aid the change process.

Two-Chair Technique

A variation on the two-chair technique from Gestalt therapy—done in imagery—can be used to deepen the affect. Here is an example:

THERAPIST: Can you imagine someone sitting in that chair and telling you the story you have told me. How would you feel toward that person?

PATIENT: I'd say, "No wonder you are feeling so sad."

Role Playing

Role playing can be another powerful tool for changing perspectives. The therapist may take the role of the patient, and the patient can take the role of a friend, a family member, a coworker, or even the therapist.

PATIENT: I knew I needed to go to the gym because I would feel better. But I just let time go by, and then there was no time left. It wasn't that important.

THERAPIST: Let's try reversing roles. You play the therapist, and I'll play you telling the same story—and let's see if you have the same reaction.

Patients often need additional work and much repetition to reduce the inhibitions about change.

Patients Have Great Potential for Change

The underlying theme of all of these techniques is that most patients, once they have worked through fears of change, have a tremendous potential to reframe their own maladaptive patterns of thinking and feeling. The following sections offer some methods for developing autonomous functioning by helping patients begin to attend and care for their own needs (see also CC, pp. 321–323).

IV. FINDING AND ENCOURAGING THE LOST VOICE

When a child's voice has been silenced as a result of years of criticism or being ignored, it can be very difficult to revive. As an adult, a patient may have lost not only the capacity to **express** wants and needs, but even to be **aware** of what those needs might be. In cases where this is true, it is important to build the receptive capacity to patients' wants and needs by helping them find their "lost voice."

Expression of wants and needs (assertion) has been addressed extensively in previous chapters, particularly Chapter 8 (Affect Expression). Those techniques are most helpful for patients who are aware of wants and needs, but have phobias about expressing them.

PATIENT: I'd really like a raise, but I'm afraid my boss would think I'm greedy if I asked for one.

The Lost Voice: Unawareness of Wants and Needs

In contrast, there are patients who do not know that certain self-needs exist. For them, uncovering the wish or need—finding the lost voice—is a prerequisite to Affect Expression. When there is some evidence of unspoken wants or needs, it is important to build receptive capacity. Sometimes these omissions are not too difficult to spot:

THERAPIST: When your boss didn't give you the bonus he'd promised, but hired a new, expensive consultant, did you protest?

PATIENT: Oh, not at all. It would never occur to me to do that.

THERAPIST: What about your needs? Do you see how easily you let yourself be dismissed without protest [D]?

Blind Spots: Difficulty Finding the Lost Voice

At other times, the unvoiced needs are so deeply buried that neither the patient nor the therapist will be aware of them initially. Therapists need to remember that some needs may be entirely unconscious. It's important to listen carefully for discrepancies that could give clues. The list of self-needs presented in Section II can be helpful in assessing what might be missing.

Once the need is identified, then the patient needs encouragement to voice that need. Finding the lost voice can be thought of as the undoing of a defensive position (silence and repression) that not only blocks interpersonal expression, but also blocks the basic awareness of the patient's wants and needs.

PATIENT: We're going to the mountains—camping—again this summer.

THERAPIST: Hmm, don't I remember your saying you preferred the beach?

PATIENT: Yes, but my husband doesn't like the beach, so we never go.

THERAPIST: Do you ever tell him that you would like to go to the beach?

PATIENT: Oh, no! I've never even thought about asking him for that.

For this patient, and for many others like her, extensive work on interpersonal assertion (Affect Expression) will only be fruitful after her receptive capacity is improved and she is more aware of her own desires.

V. ENCOURAGING "PARENTING" OF THE SELF

Good Self-Parenting

Becoming a "good parent" to oneself can be a good metaphor for healing the self and achieving autonomous functioning. It can be an antidote for problems of externalization, feelings of emptiness, and the lost voice. Reparenting the self is accomplished by the patient's **no longer accepting the conditions of his or her childhood.** It is each person's responsibility **not** to maintain the neglectful or abusive conditions of the past. Patients need to learn to treat themselves as they ideally would treat their own children—with attention, care, and respect.

Examples of Building Self-Parenting

THERAPIST: 1: Your parents may have done the best they knew, but we have seen that many of your needs went unmet. And now you are the only one that can change this situation. It would be a tragedy to continue your suffering when you have the capacity to make things different. Now you must learn to treat yourself as your own "good parent"—caring for yourself, respecting yourself, attending to your own needs, and so forth.

THERAPIST: 2: It's common for people to respond the way they did as children—because it's so ingrained. But you have a great deal more power than you did as a child. As an adult, you have so many more skills and abilities—for instance, to think through a strategy of action and negotiate your needs. You no longer have to tolerate abuse or put up with indifference. You can have an impact on your world so that the same old patterns do not persist.

THERAPIST: 3: In many ways you have inadvertently been reacting to yourself as your caretakers did, harshly and critically—or neglectfully. Maybe it's time now for you to begin to react to yourself in the ways that you need. You cannot change how you were treated in the past, but you can change how you treat yourself now—and in the future. What do you think?

Weekly Plans to Restructure Self-Care

When patients are able to acknowledge the need for better self-care, therapists can help by collaborating on a plan for putting some of these self-supportive behaviors into action. First, specific self-care behaviors that the patients can focus on (e.g., leaving work at a decent hour, eating regularly, etc.) should be identified. It is important to choose behaviors that will feel genuinely nourishing to a particular patient, not like an added burden. Specific assignments will help to track how often those behaviors are accomplished—or avoided. These are small steps to expose the patient to better self-care.

Example 1

THERAPIST: You've told me it really helps you feel better to get some exercise [or take long baths, relaxed meals, forgive errors you made, call a friend, etc.]. What's a reasonable goal for you this week in terms of that?

PATIENT: I think I could work on doing that a couple of times this week.

THERAPIST: Good. Why not give that a try, and pay attention to what makes it hard to do? If you don't manage to do it, we'll work to see what's blocking you.

Example 2

THERAPIST: How would it be to spend 1 minute each day to see if you can feel compassionate toward yourself?

Therapist and patient can review the progress from week to week, to see whether the patient is blocked or phobic about self-care and how the patient can better respond to the self. It is important to have the patient note what thoughts or feelings block his or her receptivity to nourishing the self in these ways—so that these can be desensitized in therapy.

THERAPIST 1: I wonder if you feel as though your life doesn't deserve the same sort of interest and attention you devote to everyone else?

THERAPIST 2: It's sad to see you have such a negative view of yourself. Can we look at what might be keeping you feeling this way?

When patients do not "do the homework," it is important to regulate the shame about that:

THERAPIST 3: Remember, you are not here to perform for me. We can set up goals together for you to work on outside of therapy, and if you're unable to meet those goals, then you and I will work toward discovering what makes that hard for you. But it's for you, not for me.

VI. REDUCING THE EXTERNALIZATION OF NEEDS

Excessive Dependency versus Autonomous Capacity for Self-Soothing

As a part of assessing receptivity in an individual, the therapist must consider how much externalization is being used. **Externalization** means the degree to which the patient needs the "good feelings" of care or validation to come directly from others. In other words, is the patient addicted to the physical presence of people for reassurance and support (an excessive and maladaptive dependency), rather than being able to draw from his or her own reservoir of good feelings from time to time (healthy autonomy)?

THERAPIST 1: I asked him over and over to tell me if he thought I was an okay person. He said he did, but I don't know if he really meant it.

THERAPIST 2: Are you mad at me? Are you sure? Oh, it would be terrible if you were mad. Are you sure you're not mad?

Support, validation, and affirmation from others are needed throughout life. But all individuals need to be able to hold onto what is given and thus maintain their own reservoir of positive self-feelings to draw from when alone, or when others have been disappointing or let them down. Contrast these two statements:

THERAPIST 1: It was terrible when my boyfriend broke up with me, but I could comfort myself by thinking of the love of my friends and family.

THERAPIST 2: It was terrible when my boyfriend broke up with me—I hated myself, felt utterly worthless, and no one could console me.

Addiction to Others for Support Means Lack of Receptivity

People who lack receptive capacity never let their reservoir be filled; there is always a drought of self-soothing capacity. When there is an inability to rely on or trust positive emotional experiences, patients stay addicted to the actual physical presence of others for emotional sustenance (a defensive position). The patients then become addicted to the "externalized" affirmation and support from others, because they are not able to call upon and savor from within the memories of other nurturing figures.

Building Reservoirs of Positive Self-Feeling

Therapists can help patients build inner felt experience of positive self-feelings as a reservoir to draw upon. In the following example, the therapist directs the patient away (response prevention) from the defensive externalization of asking the therapist to boost her self-worth. The therapist then exposes her to the experience of feeling valued by the therapist.

PATIENT: I know you said you were proud of me, but I don't know if you really meant it. Do you really mean it? Will you tell me again?

THERAPIST: It doesn't seem like my telling you directly is getting through. Can you try to feel in yourself whether I meant what I said? (*Later:*) When you are at home alone and yearning to hear positive feelings from someone, can you take 5 minutes and try to remember those positive feelings within yourself that you have been given and may be pushing away? Can you try to remember them vividly—as though the person who cares about you is with you?

Problems with experiencing the positive feelings of others often have their roots in early childhood. Patients who weren't shown the pride or joy others took in them during their childhood may have difficulty recognizing and responding to these feelings in adulthood. As a result, some patients may seek excessive external validation from their therapists (as well as from others outside therapy), because they cannot hold positive feelings from others within themselves. Other patients may find positive feelings from others so uncomfortable or even painful—because they were so lacking for so long—that they close off by rejecting or devaluing such feelings.

Handling Feelings of Emptiness

Patients who are deprived of positive self-feelings come to feel so "starved" and "empty" that they do not believe they can ever be given enough. They often feel insatiable. However, the truth is that patients who have been deprived for so long will find that opening to others—even in small ways—can feel remarkably nourishing. Giving affirmation to such patients can often be like giving a Thanksgiving dinner to a starving person whose stomach has atrophied and can't handle it. One must "spoon-feed" the patients bit by bit while they develop the capacity to receive more. Patients who feel empty often need much practice and encouragement to hold onto caring feelings from others by remembering them and savoring them when alone. Doing so will help to build their receptive capacity, step by step.

VII. REPEATING INTERVENTIONS UNTIL PHOBIAS ABOUT SELF-FEELINGS ARE DESENSITIZED AND SELF-WORTH IMPROVES

Repeat These Interventions Over and Over Again

When a patient's self-image does not immediately improve, the therapist should not give in to discouragement, but resolve to persist. The therapist needs to return the focus repeatedly to improving the patient's sense of self. With each repetition, the therapist should be vigilant for small shifts in the patient's view of the self. Repeating your own adaptations of the examples in this chapter should help the patient begin to build new and more self-affirming inner images, and develop a more resilient and autonomous sense of self.

For many patients, restructuring the self-image will be sufficient to improve relationships with others as well. However, in the more resistant cases, distorted views of others remain a major obstacle in rebuilding the image of the self. The self-image will not be healed until an adaptive view of others is attained and the image of others will need to be healed in parallel. This process of restructuring the images of others is addressed in the following chapter.

Summary of Self-Restructuring Steps

Before we proceed, however, the basic steps of Self-Restructuring are summarized in Table 9.1.

TABLE 9.1. Steps in Self-Restructuring

- Defense Recognition for Phobias about Self Feeling
- Gently point out self-attack, self-hate, externalization of needs.
- Defense Relinquishing of Phobias about Self Feeling
- Point out costs of self-attack; help patient understand rewards (primary, secondary gain).
- Help patient build new supports to replace defenses.
- Conduct exposure to enhance receptive capacity in imagery.
    Assess self-needs that are not being met.
    Help patient verbalize positive self-feelings.
    Help patient identify bodily signals of positive self-feelings.
    Help patient imagine desired self-protective or self-nurturing action in fantasy.
    Help patient imagine how others see him or her.
    Use changing perspectives to elicit feeling.
    Encourage the receptive capacity of the patient.
- Engage in response prevention (D).
    Point out defense/avoidance.
    Encourage patient to stay with the feelings a little longer.
- Engage in anxiety regulation (A).
    Calm patient by offering support, reassurance.
    Explore the fears, shame, pain.
- Return to exposure as soon as anxiety is reduced.
- Return to Response Prevention if necessary.
- Return to Anxiety Regulation repeatedly.

CHAPTER 9 • EXERCISES

EXERCISE 9A: ASSESS EXTERNALIZATION OF NEEDS OR EXCESS DEPENDENCY ON OTHERS

Directions: Which of the following patients seem overly dependent on others in maintaining positive feelings about themselves? Circle the correct answer, and then explain why.

Example: PATIENT: It's hard to admit this, but women are really a way to keep my self-esteem afloat. When I'm in the "pursue and conquer" phase, I don't feel that emptiness. But once I know they are hooked, I get bored and need to look elsewhere.

Answer: **How externalized are this patient's needs (circle one)?**

~~Overly dependent~~ (circled)   Not overly dependent

Why? This patient externalizes his needs by using relationships in an addictive way in order to feel better about himself.

Exercise 9A.1.   PATIENT: I get a lot of fulfillment out of my job. It means a lot to me that my supervisor values the work that I do, and I enjoy the pat on the back. On the other hand, there's more to my life than this job.

How externalized are this patient's needs (circle one)?

Overly dependent   Not overly dependent

Why? _____

_____

Exercise 9A.2.   PATIENT: As a father and provider, I love the feeling of taking care of my wife and my kids. In fact, it gives me such a sense of satisfaction about myself that I sometimes feel lost without it. Like when my wife took the kids on vacation, I felt miserable—empty inside—and didn't know what to do with myself.

How externalized are this patient's needs (circle one)?

Overly dependent   Not overly dependent

Why? _____

_____

Exercise 9A.3.   PATIENT: During the last session, I was feeling really good about the decisions I'm making in my career. It was very reassuring to hear your perspective. But then, driving home, I started to have this anxiety. I wanted to call and ask you again.

How externalized are this patient's needs (circle one)?

Overly dependent   Not overly dependent

Why? _____

_____

Exercise 9A.4.   PATIENT: I got a master's degree, hoping that it would make me feel good about myself. But now I think I'm a failure unless I have a PhD. I hate that I'm that way, but I must admit I think about it a lot. It's the "nothing is ever good enough" syndrome.

How externalized are this patient's needs (circle one)?

Overly dependent   Not overly dependent

Why? _____

_____

Exercise 9A.5.

PATIENT: I really loved him, but we weren't right for each other. I'm sad, but I feel like it's for the best, and I am not agonizing about it.

How externalized are this patient's needs (circle one)?

Overly dependent   Not overly dependent

Why? _____

_____

EXERCISE 9B: HELP BUILD PATIENTS' RECEPTIVE CAPACITY

Directions: Would each of the following statements help a patient develop his or her receptive capacity? Please circle Yes or No.

Example: THERAPIST: I'm very touched by what you just said. (*Pausing a moment*) I wonder how it feels to you to have to tell me that?   (Yes)   No

Explanation: The therapist is modeling receptivity in the first sentence, and encouraging the patient to be receptive in the second sentence.

Exercise 9B.1. THERAPIST: How do you think your mother would be feeling about you in this situation?   Yes   No

Exercise 9B.2. THERAPIST: Do you notice how you're neglecting yourself today by missing a third of the session?   Yes   No

Exercise 9B.3. THERAPIST: I wonder if you can try to let yourself feel proud of yourself for what you did?   Yes   No

Exercise 9B.4. THERAPIST: What do you think I might be feeling toward you in this moment?   Yes   No

Exercise 9B.5. THERAPIST: What do you think your grandfather was feeling when he used to take you around to see his friends?   Yes   No

Exercise 9B.6. THERAPIST: What's most difficult for you about that party that was given for you?   Yes   No

EXERCISE 9C: HELP PATIENTS GRIEVE FOR WHAT WAS MISSING

Directions: For each of the following patient remarks, select the therapist response or responses that would most help the patient grieve for what he or she was missing. Place a check mark by your choice(s). There can be more than one.

Example: PATIENT: When you tell me that I'm working hard to make these changes with my family, I don't believe you—I just feel strangely sad. I think you must say that to everybody.

Answer: **Therapist response most likely to facilitate grieving:**

____ A. What's the hardest thing about believing me?

____ B. I don't usually praise people unless I mean it.

✓ C. When you hear my praise, it seems to bring up the pain of what you have always yearned for, but did not receive.

____ D. If a friend told you he or she had done all the things you just told me, how would you feel toward that friend?

Explanation: Response C directly addresses the deep longing that is only beginning to emerge. A is anxiety regulation to reduce the inhibition against being receptive to the therapist's praise. B is presenting reality, and also a therapist self-disclosure. D uses the technique of changing perspectives to heighten the ability to be receptive to praise.

Exercise 9C.1.   PATIENT: For the first time, I told my wife I needed to be held and she took me in her arms, but I couldn't relax. I was (*tearing up*) stiff as a board. I'm so frustrated with myself.

Therapist response most likely to facilitate grieving:

____ A. Don't be too hard on yourself. You have blocked your tears for many years, and it would be hard for you to let go and cry the first time.

____ B. Next time you're with your wife, imagine if your mother had responded that way just once—and how it would have felt.

____ C. See if you can stay with that feeling and imagine yourself relaxing into your wife's arms. Just see what comes up.

____ D. You really are learning to ask for what you need, aren't you?

Exercise 9C.2.   PATIENT: I can't imagine that anyone could understand me better than you do. (*Becoming tearful*) Oh, how I've longed to be understood.

Therapist response most likely to facilitate grieving:

____ A. You've so longed to be understood for all these years.

____ B. Your longing has gotten in the way of enjoying yourself

____ C. Understanding your longing is the first step.

____ D. Feeling worthy of appreciation allows you to take others in.

Exercise 9C.3.   PATIENT: My parents were such busy professionals that they never paid any attention to me. I spent a lot of time playing by myself.

Therapist response most likely to facilitate grieving:

____ A. Can you tell me about one of those times coming home to an empty house?

____ B. Not getting attention is really hard on a child.

____ C. That sounds like it would be so hard for you.

____ D. You must have felt so alone.

EXERCISE 9D: ADDRESS DOMAINS OF SELF-FUNCTIONING

Directions: In response to the following patient statements, try to formulate what a therapist might say that would address the domain of self-functioning that the person appears to need help with. Remember that these domains may include biological, social, psychological/emotional, sexual, or spiritual needs.

Example: PATIENT: Since my divorce 2 years ago I've dated several guys briefly, but they've been more like friendships. I didn't feel like sleeping with any of these guys, but I do miss just the physical release that sexuality brings. Sometimes I find myself eating late at night when I'm not even hungry, just trying to soothe myself.

Answer: **What the therapist might say:** It's such a difficult dilemma, isn't it? You haven't met the right person with whom you can be sexual, yet the natural biological need is there nonetheless. This is delicate, but I think it's vital to talk about. Are you able to masturbate and give yourself pleasure in this way?

Exercise 9D.1. PATIENT: I don't even have time for sleep any more. There's too much to be done at work and at home. And I don't see it changing.

What the therapist might say: _____

_____

Exercise 9D.2. PATIENT: I moved here about 3 years ago and have been pretty much on my own, with no real close connections. I'm on friendly terms with some people at work. But generally I'm pretty self-reliant.

What the therapist might say: _____

_____

Exercise 9D.3. PATIENT: It's all the same, day in, day out. I'm just so bored with myself.

What the therapist might say: _____

_____

Exercise 9D.4. PATIENT: I don't know why I'm doing what I do any more. I really don't think it's depression, but there **is** something missing. Since I turned 50, there just doesn't seem to be any purpose to life.

What the therapist might say: _____

_____

EXERCISE 9E: HELP BUILD PATIENTS' SELF-IMAGE BY "CHANGING PERSPECTIVES"

Directions: Imagine how you might respond to each of the following patient statements using the technique of "changing perspectives," in order to help the patient build a more compassionate and accepting sense of self. Then give a brief rationale for why that intervention might be helpful.

Example: PATIENT: What a jerk I've been! How could I fall for another guy who winds up treating me this way? I know better than this, yet I let my loneliness talk me into believing in him. I am such a fool.

Answers: **What the therapist might say:** Let me ask you. If a good friend of yours were telling you the story you've been telling me—of someone who really longed for a good relationship, but was let down by someone the way you were—what do you imagine you might be feeling toward that friend?

Possible rationale: There may be a need for the patient to reassess her choices and look at the underlying dynamics that drive them, but self-denigration will not be helpful. Changing perspectives may help increase her self-compassion by harnessing her compassion for others.

Exercise 9E.1. PATIENT: There are so many people with bigger problems than mine. Spending this hour each week in therapy just seems self-indulgent.

What the therapist might say: _____

_____

Possible rationale: _____

_____

Exercise 9E.2. PATIENT: Well, my grandmother was my real mother. My mother had no time for children. My grandmother was everything to me, and since she died 5 years ago, I just haven't taken very good care of myself.

What the therapist might say: _____

_____

Possible rationale: _____

_____

Exercise 9E.3. PATIENT: I can never relax and just **be** with someone. I'm always trying to think of what I can do for other people. I never know if I'm good enough.

What the therapist might say: _____

_____

Possible rationale: _____

_____

Other-Restructuring: Building Adaptive Inner Images of Others

Chapter Objectives	To demonstrate how to desensitize Affect Phobias about adaptive feelings in response to others. Show how to help patients (1) perceive others' strengths and vulnerabilities accurately and compassionately; (2) build receptivity to others' feelings while maintaining an adaptive balance between autonomy and interdependence.
Therapist Stance	Using a caring therapist–patient relationship to expose the patient to a more accurate and compassionate view of others.
Anxiety Regulation	Bringing anxiety, shame, and pain about closeness within adaptive limits through exposure in imagery to care and acceptance from others.

Topics Covered

   I.   Overview: Restructuring Affect Phobias about Relationships with Others

  II.   Building the Receptive Capacity to Others' Feelings

 III.   Changing Perspectives: Viewing Others Accurately and Compassionately

 IV.   Identifying and Restructuring Addictive Attachments

  V.   Recovering "Lost Loves": Caring Persons in the Past

 VI.   Repeating Interventions until Phobias about Relationships Are Desensitized

Indications for a Focus on Other-Restructuring

- The patient's Global Assessment of Functioning (GAF) score is below 50 (serious symptoms, or serious impairment in functioning).
- Relationships are seriously impaired (e.g., few or no friends, distrust, paranoia).
- Therapeutic alliance is poor.
- Defense or Affect Restructuring becomes blocked due to maladaptive images of others.

I. OVERVIEW: RESTRUCTURING AFFECT PHOBIAS ABOUT RELATIONSHIPS WITH OTHERS

Building Perspective on Relationships

The goal in restructuring patients' inner images of others is to help patients develop more adaptive and realistic perspectives on their relationships. The therapist can help patients toward this goal by examining their view of other people, as well as their view of the therapist with them.

Triangle of Person

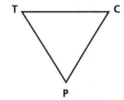

Evidence of the problems of intimacy and connection are everywhere in the world today, and of course such issues are central to the conflicts of many psychotherapy patients. As noted in Section VII of Chapter 1, the Short-Term Dynamic Psychotherapy (STDP) model is **not** based on a self that is separate from others. Individuals exist, grow, and develop in relation to others in dynamic interactions, and need both autonomy and deep connection. Adaptively perceiving and responding to others—both in the present (the Therapist Pole [T] and Current Persons Pole [C]) and in the past (the Past Person Pole [P]) on the Triangle of Person—are crucial parts of therapeutic change. (See Chapter 2, Figure 2.1, for the Triangle of Person.)

As discussed in Chapter 1, the STDP model works toward development of a mature and well-integrated self that can strike an adaptive balance between being autonomous (striving to meet own needs, expressing what's inside, setting limits, etc.) and being **inter**dependent with others (responding to the feelings and needs of others, being able to ask for what is wanted or needed).

Building Interdependence

Chapter 9 has focused on patients' inner images of the self, self-feelings, and building autonomy. In contrast, this chapter focuses on how patients view others and whether they can be open and receptive—with appropriate boundaries—to others' feelings, in both past and present relationships. Thus the interventions in this chapter are focused on building healthy interdependence and better interpersonal connections, while at the same time maintaining a balance with autonomy and support of self-needs. Building this balanced interdependence involves (1) accurate but compassionate perception of others (i.e., seeing and accepting the strengths as well as the limitations of other people); and (2) adaptive receptivity to others' feelings (ability to open up, but also to set limits as needed).

When a patient's sense of intimacy and connection is absent or impaired, it generally implies that there were not strong connections in the patient's early life. As a result, such a patient lacks positive (supportive, protective, etc.) inner images of others. Interactions to build openness and receptivity will help guide the patient toward more adaptive inner images of others and better interpersonal connection.

Therefore, to build connection and interdependence, the therapeutic work involves helping such patients become receptive to the positive qualities and care of others as well as understanding of the less than pleasant qualities of others—including therapists. It is also necessary to help patients feel compassionate toward others and respond constructively.

Healthy Interdependence Balances Self-Needs and Others' Needs

Being receptive to others does not mean agreeing with everything people say. Healthy interdependence is actually a balance between autonomy and connection. Maintaining such a balance depends on the ability to identify one's internal signals (both positive and negative) and articulate them to others, as well as being able to accurately identify and respond to signals of others. Openness and receptivity are not the only capacities needed; the full range of feelings is necessary for mature functioning. **Patients must be able to hold their own in relationships by setting limits and making requests; otherwise, opening to others can mean being easily taken advantage of or becoming a receptacle for others' needs.**

Unfortunately, some patients misperceive healthy interdependence as neediness, vulnerability, weakness, or immaturity; others misperceive it as excessively uninvolved, since healthy interdependence entails quite a bit of autonomy. So it is important for therapists to teach such patients to see the value in being open and close to others—as well as the value of saying no and setting limits when necessary. In other words, therapists must help patients maintain a balance between self-needs and the needs of others, between autonomy and connection.

Desensitization of Feelings in Relationships

Receptivity to others can be impaired by an Affect Phobia, when the affects associated with perception and acceptance of others are associated with excessive anxiety, guilt, shame, or pain. When this happens, the Affect Phobia needs to be desensitized through exposure to appropriate feelings in relationships (either positive or negative), prevention of defensive responses, and anxiety regulation.

Here are a few brief examples of interventions that can help patients not only to bear, but when appropriate to enjoy, shared feelings:

First, a therapist can focus on the inhibitory or self-attacking affects associated with others' positive feelings.

PATIENT: I can't help feeling that people are suckers if they are kind to me, like Joe . . .

THERAPIST: That's exactly the response that is so hurtful to you. What is the fear of letting in Joe's kindness?

We touch on this sort of anxiety regulation later in this section, and we focus on the receptive capacity to others' feelings in Section II.

Second, a therapist can help the patient be receptive to and put negative messages from others into perspective.

PATIENT: When he told me that my work could use improvement, I knew it was just because he had it in for me, so I just ignored it.

THERAPIST: Well, if you put yourself in his position, can you imagine any **other** reason why he might have said what he said?

The receptive capacity to others (Section II) includes the ability not just to take the positive from others, but to respond appropriately to negative messages. We have discussed the technique of changing perspectives in relation to Self-Restructuring in Section III of Chapter 9, but we return to it in relation to Other-Restructuring in Section III of this chapter.

Third, the therapist can help the patient change or let go of deep attachments to earlier, more destructive relationships—where the sense of self was created—to create emotional separation from maladaptive relationships.

THERAPIST: I wonder if letting yourself feel the sadness of all the things you didn't get from your parents might help free you from your pattern of choosing people who devalue you.

Detaching from maladaptive relationships is discussed in Section IV.

Finally, the therapist can help the patient build inner images of more affirming relationships—including with the therapist. The ability to internalize good people is crucial to this process.

THERAPIST: How was it when you sat next to your grandfather on the couch? What did he do that made it feel good to be next to him?

Techniques of this sort are discussed further in Section V.

Relationship of Other-Restructuring to Affect Expression

It is important to understand the relationship between Affect Expression and Other Restructuring. In Affect Expression (Chapter 8), one expresses one's own feelings, wants, and needs **to others**. In Other-Restructuring, the focus is on one's **perception of others** and one's **receptivity to how others feel.**

Without accurate perceptions of others, patients may not be able to use opportunities to correct misperceptions about other people. In other words, **Other-Restructuring can be seen as a prerequisite for Affect Expression—** just as Self-Restructuring is (see the Introductions to Parts II and III). When patients have a maladaptive sense of others, they may need work on Other-Restructuring before they are able to master Affect Expression. Before one can express feelings to others, there needs to be either trust in others, or a clear perception of the need to guard oneself. Therefore, patients need to become receptive to the positive qualities and care of others (building healthy interdependence) as well as able to pick up others' unpleasant or dishonest qualities (maintaining autonomy and protecting one's own boundaries).

Receptivity to Others Allows for Vulnerability and Change

Lack of receptivity to the feelings of others is a defensive stance that (along with lack of receptivity to self-needs) is one of the biggest obstacles to character change. When patients are unable to be receptive or responsive to the feelings of others, then the patients often feel uncomfortable or unworthy even when nurturing people or situations are available, and they refuse to savor such care. When this happens, their assumptions from the past cannot be corrected by new experiences. Then isolation and alienation from others continue, and old behavior patterns are carried into the future. In such cases, patients' receptive capacity must be increased before character change can occur.

Therapist Stance: Building Trust and Closeness

When close and trusting relationships have not been present in a patient's life, often the only way to teach these capacities is by building trust and closeness in the patient–therapist relationship. So the therapeutic relationship, which is so important in all phases of this therapy, is **even more crucial** in Other-Restructuring.

Trust in the Therapist Is Essential

It is important to remember that if a patient distrusts and fears others, the alliance with the therapist will probably be impaired. Little therapeutic work can be done until the patient can learn to trust and receive care, **while at the same time** remaining differentiated and autonomous with strong boundaries. The relationship with the therapist thus plays a central role in repairing a patient's sense of others and ability to respond to others' feelings.

As human beings, we learn to trust and set limits through relationships with people who are accepting of all parts of us. Therefore, the patient's relationship with the therapist will be a crucial first step toward building new inner images of others. The therapist must be an accepting figure—of both positive and negative messages coming from the patient.

Transference versus the Real Relationship

In psychoanalytic theory, exploring the patient–therapist relationship is often referred to as working "in the transference" (i.e., exploring the inner images that the patient holds about early-life caretakers, and that the patient may be "transferring" or projecting onto the therapist). Although a patient's transference is important to identify, in STDP the main focus is on the **real relationship** between patient and therapist, as well as on the **dis-**

tortions that the patient may be making and transferring onto the therapist. Consider this example;

PATIENT: You seem so cold and distant, just like my father! [An example of transference of the feelings toward the father onto the therapist]

THERAPIST: That sounds very uncomfortable. Can you tell me what it is that makes you feel that way?

PATIENT: You always ask about me, but you never talk about yourself.

THERAPIST: Yes, there's some truth to that. [Validation] But I wonder if you can think of any other reason why I might do that other than just being cold and distant? [First addressing the real relationship]

(See CC, pp. 85–89, for more discussion regarding the distinction of transference vs. the real relationship.)

Eliciting Patient's Ideas Before Sharing Therapist's Feelings

Note that the therapist elicits the patient's ideas about the therapist's feelings before stating them directly. As discussed in connection with Self-Restructuring (Chapter 9), this technique makes the sharing of the therapist's feelings much more powerful. Here is another example:

THERAPIST: What do you think I feel about your being mad at me?

PATIENT: You're probably thinking, "This guy is a real pain in the neck."

THERAPIST: Is there anything I have done to make you feel that way?

PATIENT: Actually, no. But I just worry that you might.

THERAPIST: I wonder if you can imagine any other way I might feel.

PATIENT: It seems hard to believe, but maybe you're understanding—and a little sorry.

THERAPIST: Yes, you bet I am.

Special Focus of Other-Restructuring

The example above is a form of Affect Expression (looking at the patient's expression of anger)—but it has a very specialized focus on how the patient perceives **another's feelings**. This focus is essential for restructuring how others are perceived, experienced, and reacted to. Note that the patient's initial perceptions are distorted and negative. The therapist gently leads the patient to a more adaptive, reality-based experience.

Difficulties with Sharing of Therapist Feelings

It is often a dilemma for therapists whether to respond openly or hold back. Many patients have not had exposure to others' positive feelings—or they have had too much exposure to negative feelings from others. The responses to these old patterns cannot be altered without a focus on how others feel, and often this process must begin with the therapist. It can be complex and challenging for therapists to share feelings and at the same time maintain professional boundaries, but it is an essential element of the therapeutic process.

Gratification versus Abstinence

The suggestion that therapists not immediately reveal their own feelings is one example of the long-standing debate over whether to **gratify** patients by answering their questions, self-disclosing about a similar problem, or offering reassurance or support—or whether to withhold such responses and remain silent or **abstinent**. These are difficult questions with no easy answers. The following discussion gives some examples and general guidelines.

A delicate balance needs to be maintained between gratification and abstinence. Gratification that is premature or excessive can cut off patients' opportunities for growth in self-soothing or autonomous functioning. Therapists need to think about whether gratifying communications stem from the therapists' own need to be seen as empathic—or even omnipotent. On the other hand, excessive abstinence by therapists can cut off opportunities for growth of closeness and can be equally undesirable.

Guidelines for Gratification

Skill is needed in the balancing of gratification and abstinence, and in understanding the patient's needs and boundaries. Some patients rely too heavily on praise from others because of an inability to resonate to positive feelings within themselves (externalization; see Section VI of Chapter 9). This is often caused by shame or a lack of healthy entitlement. Others reject praise for the same reasons.

In both of these cases, it can be helpful either to withhold praise until patients learn to access feelings within themselves, or to give praise and then address the patients' defensive dismissal. This parallels our discussion of therapists' feelings earlier in this section and in connection with therapist stance in Chapter 9: Therapists should first try to elicit the patients' feelings, but then acknowledge their own feelings.

Example: "Delay" of Gratification

THERAPIST: You told me about what happened at the award ceremony, but I wonder how you **felt** about winning the award?

PATIENT: Oh, I don't know; it doesn't seem like a big deal. What do you think?

THERAPIST: How would you feel about someone else winning this award? [The therapist delays immediately gratifying the patient by not answering the patient's question. Instead, the therapist tries to elicit the patient's receptive capacity to feel what the therapist is feeling by asking a probing question.]

PATIENT: Oh! I'd feel very happy for them. And proud for them.

THERAPIST: How sad that you can feel that for someone else, but not for yourself.

PATIENT: Yes, it is. But that is how I feel.

THERAPIST: Well, how do you **imagine** I feel about your winning this award?

PATIENT: Probably doesn't mean much to you either way.

THERAPIST: Why would you think that? Especially when you said how easily you would feel proud of someone in your place. Do I seem so unfeeling?

PATIENT: Well, no. You don't seem unfeeling . . .

THERAPIST: So what might I feel?

PATIENT: That's hard for me to think about.

THERAPIST: Sure, but I wonder if you could try not to avoid this right now [response prevention] and let yourself feel it [exposure].

PATIENT: I guess . . . oh, this is hard to say. I guess you'd be a little bit proud of me.

THERAPIST: Only a little bit? [The therapist says this because she in fact feels very proud of what the patient has accomplished—and the patient is diminishing the positive feelings.]

PATIENT: Well, I'll admit it—though I'm embarrassed to say so. I think you might be very proud of me.

THERAPIST: Of course I am! [At this point the therapist can reply to or "gratify" the patient's request, because the patient first has searched within himself, and developed a little more of the capacity to be receptive to the therapist's positive feeling.] Can you let yourself feel that on your behalf?

PATIENT: Maybe a little, and it feels good.

If the therapist had prematurely gratified the patient's request by saying, "Of course I am proud of you," the moment the patient had asked, then the patient would not have been given the opportunity to practice discovering the capacity to look within and feel the therapist's positive feeling.

Open Communication by Therapists

Clinical experience has shown that many patients are deeply touched—even brought to tears—by open communications by their therapists, because of the dramatic contrast to what they are accustomed to. Other patients devalue their therapists for such communications. Whether the patient responds positively or negatively to the therapist's open communications, either type of response is important information. It is grist for the therapeutic mill and needs to be explored. Contrast these two exchanges:

THERAPIST 1: You teared up when I complimented you. What do you make of that?

PATIENT 1: Just thinking how little I've had of that in my life. [Receptive response]

THERAPIST 2: You just rolled your eyes when I praised you. What caused that?

PATIENT 2: Well, honestly, it's too easy. Like I put one over on you. [Unreceptive response]

THERAPIST 2: How sad that you push away my positive feelings. I wonder if you do this with others as well?

Finally, gratification **in imagery** can provide a healing experience that is not possible in reality:

PATIENT 3: I wish I could put my head on your shoulder and cry.

THERAPIST 3: It's understandable that you would want that. We don't work in that way, but we can do something that may be even more helpful for you. Let's both imagine how it might be. Can you feel what it would be like if you imagined crying on my shoulder? (*Later:*) How do you think I'd be feeling toward you?

(For a more extensive discussion of when and how to gratify a patient, see CC, Ch. 10, pp. 325–330.)

Anxiety Regulation: Decreasing Fears of Closeness

Regulating Inhibitory Affects about Attachment

The function of anxiety regulation during Other-Restructuring is to decrease the inhibitory affects linked to relationships and others' feelings, so that the patient is able to bear care and acceptance from others as well as appropriate negative feelings. This means talking about the anxiety, guilt, shame, and pain associated with others' feelings until these inhibitions no longer thwart the feeling. For each of the following examples of working with patients' fears of experiencing others' feelings, we provide several possible therapist responses, depending on the direction in which the therapist wishes to move.

Examples

PATIENT: I don't dare believe that he cares for me. [Possible phobia about care from someone]

Possible Therapist Responses:

THERAPIST 1: What is so scary about imagining that he cares for you? [Anxiety regulation per se]

THERAPIST 2: Could you try to let yourself imagine that and see what fears come up? [Exposure to elicit and further understand the anxieties]

THERAPIST 3: See if you can allow yourself to feel being cared for by him, without fighting it so much [Exposure and response prevention to begin desensitization]

PATIENT: He has a lot of nerve telling me I let him down! [Possible phobia about anger from others]

Possible Therapist Responses:

THERAPIST 1: What is the most painful thing about hearing that you might have let him down? [Anxiety regulation per se]

THERAPIST 2: Can you try to imagine what he must be feeling—and see what hurts you the most? [Exposure to elicit anxieties]

THERAPIST 3: Can you put yourself in his shoes for a moment and try to understand his upset feelings? [Changing perspectives to begin exposure and desensitization of the conflict]

PATIENT: She started to cry, and I wanted to get out of there fast! [Possible phobia about sadness in others]

Possible Therapist Responses:

THERAPIST 1: What was the most difficult part of having her start crying? [Anxiety regulation]

THERAPIST 2: Can you imagine what it would have been like to stay there with her as she cried? [Exposure to elicit anxiety]

THERAPIST 3: Can you try to let yourself feel that? [Exposure to begin desensitizing]

II. BUILDING THE RECEPTIVE CAPACITY TO OTHERS' FEELINGS

Putting Others' Feelings in Perspective

Receptive capacity toward others is the ability to internalize or "take in" the positive messages from others, and to process and put in perspective the negative messages. This interpersonal receptive capacity includes the following:

1. The ability to discern one's own positive and negative feelings toward others,

2. The ability to accept and be nurtured by positive feelings from others.

3. The ability to acknowledge and deal with negative messages or behaviors from others.

Patients will need to enhance their receptive capacity toward others by opening themselves emotionally to nurturing human contact, while also maintaining the ability to defend themselves, set limits, and assert their needs.

As mentioned in Section I, receptive capacity can be thwarted by excessive inhibition—in other words, Affect Phobia. Building receptive capacity means breaking the conditioned association of inhibitory affects to adaptive feelings associated with attachment and interpersonal connection. The basic components of desensitization—exposure, response prevention, and anxiety regulation—are the same for Affect Phobias about relationships with others.

To reduce conflict about responding to others' feelings, patients need to be exposed to successive degrees of relatedness—to their therapists' feelings, to the feelings of current others, or to memories of loving past figures—with help in regulating the amount of inhibitory affect (anxiety, shame, etc.). This provides a systematic desensitization of the Affect Phobia of others' feelings. Most of the techniques described in this chapter represent forms of "affect exposure" that can be utilized in order to address maladaptive receptive capacities.

When exploring Affect Phobias about receptivity, the therapist should consider the following questions:

- What prevents the patient from resonating with others' emotional states?
- Is there anxiety (or other inhibitory affect) attached to a particular affect—in other words, an Affect Phobia?
- Is the patient overgeneralizing from past experiences?

Desensitizing Anger from Others

In the following example, the therapist works to build the patient's ability to bear anger from others.

PATIENT: When my girlfriend confronted me on what I was doing, I just wanted to hide [D]. I felt horrible [A—shame/pain].

THERAPIST: What was it that made you feel so bad? [Probing to understand what about experiencing the anger of others creates anxiety]

PATIENT: It wasn't the way she did it. She wasn't abusive or anything. She didn't even raise her voice. And I know she has a right to those feelings, but I just don't want to hear it.

THERAPIST: So you want to run from that? [Clarifying defensive behavior]

PATIENT: Absolutely. It reminds me of times that my father would get on me. [Discovering the source of the feeling's painfulness]

THERAPIST: So maybe you have a heightened sensitivity to people being mad at you because of your experiences with your father. And that could make you read more into her anger than is really there. [Interpretation that patient may be overgeneralizing]

PATIENT: Maybe so.

THERAPIST: Let's look at how you would react if you really paid attention to what she was saying.

In this example of exposure to the Affect Phobia centering around anger from his girlfriend, the therapist helps the patient begin to acknowledge and bear the girlfriend's anger by seeing that it is no longer the same degree of painfulness as when he was a boy with his father. The patient's receptivity is heightened by exposure to the girlfriend's angry feelings and by anxiety regulation (reduction of pain).

Empathy Involves Receptivity and Expressivity

Although this chapter has focused on receptive capacity, there is an aspect of **expressive capacity** that is particularly relevant to Other-Restructuring: the capacity for **empathic responding**. Empathy involves the ability first to be responsive to the feelings of others (receptive capacity), and then the ability to respond in an affectively attuned way (one sort of expressive capacity). Because the expressive capacity has been addressed extensively in Chapter 8, this chapter touches on the expressive capacity only briefly as it relates to Other-Restructuring.

In assessing a patient's capacity for empathy, look to see whether the patient can (1) resonate to the feelings of others; and (2) respond in a way that is affectively connected and mutually beneficial, rather than defensive, dismissive, or devaluing. For example, when someone is justifiably angry at the patient, can the patient say, "I think I'd be angry too, if I were in your shoes. I'm really sorry, and I'll do my best not to let this happen again"? In addition, it is important to remember that the receptive capacity can vary with different feelings. Some patients may respond empathically to anger but not to grief, for example. So the therapist should evaluate the receptive capacity across the range of basic affects.

When conflicts in empathic responding are identified, they should be explored and desensitized:

THERAPIST: What would have been the most difficult part about just letting her continue to cry on your shoulder? [Anxiety regulation about sadness]

(See CC, Ch. 8, pp. 294–296, for a review of how a patient can show receptivity in each major affect category.)

III. CHANGING PERSPECTIVES: VIEWING OTHERS ACCURATELY AND COMPASSIONATELY

In Section III of Chapter 9, we discussed the use of changing perspectives as a technique to open patients to more positive views of themselves. In this section, we focus on the use of changing perspectives as a way of building more adaptive views of others. As before, there are many ways that this can be done:

• The therapist can elicit new views from the patient.

THERAPIST: How do you feel about me, given that I was late this morning?

• Patients can generate more multifaceted views of others.

THERAPIST: When we discuss what your friend did from her perspective, can you feel a little better about her?

- Patients can imagine how they might more compassionately view others.

THERAPIST: Can you see how he might have meant something very different from what you thought? He might have been having a bad day rather than being angry at you.

- Patients can remember people who loved them in the past (whom they very often have forgotten).

THERAPIST 1: Maybe it was hard to remember how tender your grandmother was to you after she died, because it hurt too much. I wonder if you can begin to let yourself feel what your grandmother must have felt for you?

THERAPIST 2: You say you can't think of anyone who cared for you, but what about your uncle? What is the most difficult thing about acknowledging that he was really proud of your accomplishments?

- The therapist can use the two-chair technique (see Section III of Chapter 9) to change the patient's perspectives on others.

THERAPIST: Could you imagine your husband in that chair and have him talk to you?

- Patients can revise their assessments of conflicted past relationships, and the love that might have been unexpressed:

THERAPIST: If your mother were still alive, what would she feel toward you?

Changing Perspectives on Transference Distortion

Here is an example of the use of changing perspectives to attempt to prevent transference distortions (response prevention) and help the patient open up to compassionate feelings from the therapist (exposure to feelings from others):

THERAPIST: You suddenly got very quiet [D]. What's happening right now?

PATIENT: I'm just imagining what you must be thinking about me, after what I've told you [A—shame].

THERAPIST: What do you imagine I might be thinking? [Encouraging changing perspectives]

PATIENT: You must think I'm pretty horrible [A—shame].

THERAPIST: I wonder if you can consider my reaction to you from a different perspective? [Response prevention] When you look at me, does it seem like I think badly of you? [Encouraging patient to see whether this is a distortion]

PATIENT: (*Looking directly at therapist*) Well, I suppose not. No, it doesn't seem as though you're looking down at me.

THERAPIST: If you look at my face, what does it seem that I am feeling toward you? [More exposure to perspective of other]

PATIENT: (*Anxiously*) I have absolutely no idea.

THERAPIST: Well, stay with it for a minute [Keeping the focus]. If you allow your eyes to stay on my face for a moment . . . what can you sense from me at this moment?

PATIENT: You look concerned. Maybe a little sad. You're feeling sadness for me.

THERAPIST: Well, you've shared a sad story. Why wouldn't I look sad?

PATIENT: I see what you mean. It **is** a sad story. I guess I would feel the same way if someone told me that story.

In this case, the patient is able to see through the transference distortion to the feeling in the real relationship with the therapist. She then can build a more accurate view of the therapist and a more compassionate view of herself. After the patient is able to initiate this feeling on her own, the therapist may then confirm the patient's perception.

Resistance to Receptivity in a More Defensive Patient

Not all patients are so amenable to this technique:

THERAPIST: When you look at me, what do you sense from me?

PATIENT: I don't know. I'm not sure what you're thinking.

THERAPIST: Still, what do you imagine I might be thinking or feeling? [Encouraging exposure to receptivity in therapeutic relationship]

PATIENT: (*Angrily*) Beats me! What's the point? [Patients will often respond defensively when pushed for a shared experience of closeness.]

THERAPIST: What do you think you might be feeling if someone told **you** the story you have just told me? [Introducing another change in perspective]

PATIENT: Well, I would feel incredibly bad for them, of course. I suppose I would feel a lot of compassion.

THERAPIST: Isn't it remarkable that you can so easily have this feeling of compassion for another person, but you have such a hard time imagining that **I** might be feeling this way toward you? You are ready to provide this compassion for others, but you—with all of the painful memories you have shared—are unable to imagine receiving the same compassion from someone else. [Disputing logic of patient's resistance to receiving compassion from the therapist]

PATIENT: It makes no sense. But that's the way I feel.

THERAPIST: So we'll need to keep looking at this to see what makes you feel like you don't deserve other people's compassion.

It is often necessary to repeat these interventions and exposures numerous times in order to desensitize the phobia and build compassion. (Section V of this chapter, on recovering "lost loves," covers other interventions to help patients who have a lot of difficulty receiving care from others.)

Even More Resistance

In even more resistant cases, the patient may say something like this:

PATIENT: I wouldn't feel anything toward the person in my shoes. Or I would just think they were stupid or horrible.

THERAPIST: So there is a lack of compassion for yourself as well as others. We need to see why you have such a harsh view of humanity, because it makes life awfully difficult for you.

This degree of resistance indicates that much repetition of Self- and Other-Restructuring techniques will be needed to desensitize the Affect Phobias about positive feelings toward the self and others, along with continued exploration of the sources of this punishing and defensive world view.

IV. IDENTIFYING AND RESTRUCTURING ADDICTIVE ATTACHMENTS

The Repetition Compulsion and Addictive Attachment

There are many people who repeatedly choose unhealthy, destructive, or injurious relationships. In psychodynamic terminology, this phenomenon has been viewed as an example of the **repetition compulsion**—a term that refers to the symptom, not the etiology. It can also be looked at as **addictive attachment,** in which addiction is understood as "continued use despite negative consequences."

To understand why an abusive or neglectful partner would be so compelling, it is necessary to understand the nature of reinforcement. If a person is lonely and constantly deprived of human connection, even a little bit of love will take away the grinding pain for a moment. And that little bit of attention will then be much more rewarding than it would be for someone who has been well loved.

The Power of Intermittent Reinforcement

The power of addictive attachment is due to intermittent reinforcement—the most powerful form of reinforcement and the most difficult to change. In behavior modification research, if the number of bar presses needed to obtain food varies, a hungry pigeon will peck furiously and continuously—thousands of times if necessary—to get one single pellet. Likewise, we all have known people who will work feverishly to try to get a little crumb of attention, love, or acceptance from withholding or abusive others. A little bit of care can be tremendously rewarding in a life that is bereft of care, especially when pain of loneliness is relieved.

PATIENT: Oh, how I longed for her to love me. I did everything in my power to make it happen. And when she tossed me a crumb of attention, it would make my whole week!

Thus, addictive attachments can be viewed as conditioned reactions. Children are drawn to what is familiar. It is not reinforcing to be loved if this is an unfamiliar experience. The strong care and attention of love can feel quite unsettling or intrusive—at least at first. The normal caring of well-adjusted people can feel aversive. People who are loyal, true, or faithful can seem dull, stupid, or needy. Furthermore, a predatory lover's intense and well-honed charm can be highly alluring.

PATIENT 1: This new guy is so tender and sweet to me, in a real decent way. But I still can't help feeling disgusted. He makes my skin crawl.

PATIENT 2: When someone is chasing me, I couldn't be less interested. But the minute they begin to reject me, the relationship—for me—begins.

A caring person is often devalued as having bad judgment.

PATIENT 3: She must be pretty desperate to love me.

Such contemptuous feelings can defend against the pain of receiving tenderness. If steady care were "allowed in," it would elicit tremendous grief over what was missed.

PATIENT 4: He spoke so intimately to me that I suddenly had to leave. I was starting to cry and I had no idea why—but I didn't let him know. He's weird. I'm not going out with him any more!

The child who has been treated badly becomes addicted to the "tease" (intermittent reinforcement) of the maladaptive relationship, and to the longing for it to change. The addiction to hurtful relationships is a way of holding onto the old longing for past figures—hoping that the current figures will respond better or differently than the past ones did—without actually having to grieve. In contrast, the well-adjusted child is attracted as an adult to steady, loving relationships in which there is ongoing and unconditional love. Loving relationships of this sort are reinforcing, and partners who are difficult or abusive do not attract these people.

Letting Go of Addictive Attachments

Before addictive attachments can be let go, three capacities (which we have discussed above) need to be built:

1. **A receptivity to caring feelings from others,** beginning with the therapist. To do this, anxiety associated with being loved or connected must be decreased.

2. **A new sense of self as worthy and able to receive care** (i.e., less shame about the self). If the sense of self and others is compassionate, caring will be experienced as more rewarding than aversive.

3. **The ability to grieve for what has so long been missing.** If grief can be borne, then the tears that come with tenderness will be experienced as more relieving than punishing.

Love versus Need

One method to help a patient identify addictive relationships is to teach the distinction between love (cherishing or valuing) and need (addiction to the approval of others). The therapist needs to change the conditioning patterns by linking negative feelings to the abusive partner, and positive feelings to the self.

THERAPIST 1: Where is the anger at the abuse [or the demand for performance]?

THERAPIST 2: Where is the disgust at being treated so badly or abandoned so brutally?

THERAPIST 3: Where is the healthy pride [i.e., joy taken in oneself] to encourage an interest in finding someone who will treat you better?

Secondary Gain in Addictive Attachments

Working to free up the full range of affects associated with healthy attachments (especially in the relationship with the therapist) can begin to restructure the inner representations of self and others—and undo the imprisonment of addictive attachments. But when patients strongly resist the emotional separation from hurtful others, secondary gain is likely to be playing a major role. For example, the relationship may be providing the only "security" the patient has ever known, or the patient's identity may be defined by the relationship. In general, secondary gain will be given up **only** when something else equally valuable is available to replace it. (See Chapter 6 to review how to deal with secondary gain.)

V. RECOVERING "LOST LOVES": CARING PERSONS IN THE PAST

How Relationships Are Held in Memory

Restructuring painful past memories of others is a major part of restructuring the image of the self. The self-image develops and grows from interactions with others, and carries those impressions lifelong. The relationships with the early-life caretakers have shaped the patient's sense of self. Much of the time, the memories from these relationships guide feelings and behavior—but outside of conscious awareness. Therefore, the therapist must search for and excavate these old attachments, and tap into the reservoir of tender memories often hidden below defensive and painful ones. Therapists need to work with patients to help them remember who loved them, so they can cherish these memories and savor them from within.

Using Imaginal Exposure to Remember Past Loves

Losses of loved ones early in life can be intolerable, especially when there is no support for grieving. Therefore, some patients have had to do whatever necessary to keep from remembering what is too painful to bear.

PATIENT: After my grandmother died, my world was so cold that I just shut off all my feelings and wouldn't let myself think about her.

Exposure to the mix of tender and painful memories is needed until the grief process is desensitized, so that grieving can flow freely and the past can be remembered lovingly and without anguish.

Questions to Elicit Lost Loves

Some patients will spontaneously remember loving people from the past during treatment. But sometimes these memories do not emerge, and the therapist will need to inquire and help discover what relationships were nurturing. The following questions can be helpful in eliciting memories of forgotten loving people in the past:

"Who made you feel special?"

"Who did you idealize or look up to when you were growing up?"

"How did that person feel about you?"

"Who would smile and hold their arms wide open when you visited them?"

"Whose eyes would light up when you walked in the room?"

"Who carried you in their hearts? Whom do you carry in yours?"

Exposure to Warm Memories of a "Lost Love"

THERAPIST: Who were you special to when you were little?

PATIENT: I don't think there was anybody. At least, no one comes to mind.

THERAPIST: Well, take a few minutes and try to remember. Was there a family member, a teacher, a neighbor . . . ?

PATIENT: (*After a pause*) There was someone . . . our housekeeper, Minnie. She wasn't really a nanny, but she was really good to me. She'd hum me little songs and smile and wink. Oh, how I loved her!

THERAPIST: And it sounds like she loved you too.

PATIENT: (*Tearing up*) Yes, she did . . . she did. I haven't thought of her in years.

Being able to access and sustain loving memories from people in the past can have an enormous impact on how one feels about oneself. These positive feelings from others can make one more receptive to the love and care currently given by others. When patients can be reawakened to loving feelings that grief over deprivation has made unbearable to remember, there is often a profound and positive change in their inner images of self and others. Then they can allow the painful memories to be put in perspective and subsequently put to rest.

How Past Figures Would Feel Now

One very powerful intervention is to encourage the patient to imagine how past significant others would feel now. For example, when parents did not live long enough to know what their child accomplished, the patient can be encouraged to explore what the parents might have felt.

THERAPIST: If your parents knew how you had overcome your problems in school and become a successful professional, what would they be feeling?

PATIENT: (*Angrily*) You can't ever know that! They're dead!

THERAPIST: But you lived with them and experienced them for many years. What do your memories of them suggest that they might feel? What does your intuition tell you? What do you know of them in your heart?

PATIENT: They were always proud when I did well . . . so (*tearing up*) I guess they would be proud now. (*Pausing*) Yes, I know they would be. But it's so painful to think about it that I can hardly stand it. They'll never know.

The imagery should stay as close as possible to the specific behaviors of the person (or persons) being remembered, but often the patient will have to add to it with his or her intuition about what the relationship involved.

THERAPIST: Yes, that is painful. But try to stay with the positive feeling for a moment. How does their pride in you make you feel—in your body? [Acknowledging the grief, yet pushing for incorporation of positive feelings as well]

PATIENT: Warm and soft and sort of strong. It also makes me want to cry.

THERAPIST: Then can you let yourself cry with the tenderness of that memory? (*Later:*) Can you hold onto that feeling of their being proud of you, and cherish it?

When a patient can reexperience such affirming memories, the grief for what has been lost can be tremendously healing. Of course, the fact that the "lost love" may not be able to respond in the patient's current life will also need to be acknowledged and mourned, and eventually replaced by inner models of current nurturant figures.

Lack of Positive Memories

Some patients cannot bring up positive memories because they simply may not be there. Then it is important to face the truth of the situation, whatever that may be.

PATIENT: When I really let myself think about what my mother would feel about me now, I just can't come up with a positive response. I don't have any memory of her being critical or demeaning of me . . . so I don't think she'd respond that way. I just remember her not caring—or not paying attention. Like I didn't matter. The more I think about telling her about my accomplishments, the more it seems that it wouldn't matter that much to her.

THERAPIST: We'll have to go over this to make sure you're not missing some care that was there. But you have told me many instances of your mother's self-absorption. So if this is true, then it is important to face it—and grieve it. It will also be all the more important for you to find other supportive people in your life. We also should look at other members of your family back then, your friends now, and—importantly—your relationship with me. It will be important for you to be able to acknowledge and accept the care that you do have, as you face the truth of what your mother may not have been able to provide. [This is also a means of building supports before removing defenses to assist the patient in grieving a painful truth.]

Integration of Opposing Feelings

As in Affect Expression, it is important to integrate the patient's positive and negative feelings about significant others.

THERAPIST: Although your mother was often harsh, there seem to be a few good examples of her caring for you, too.

This needs to be carefully done so that it does not invalidate someone's experience of abuse from a parent. Although patients need to develop compassion for parents—even abusive parents—it is important that forgiveness be for the person and their human frailties, not for the abusive or hurtful behaviors.

THERAPIST: It has been really important for you to access the anger you have toward your father for his harshness and abandonment of you as a child. You just alluded again to there being very happy, warm times between you as well. It's important that we look at this side of the relationship, too. What memories of those times with your father touch you the most?

Historical Accuracy versus Efficacy

As with generating formulations (see Section VII of Chapter 4), we can never know for certain whether the memories that are reconstructed is historically accurate. The only test of their worth is whether the memories are sufficiently realistic or believable—and close to the known facts—to help patients feel better about themselves, and feel able to function better in their daily lives.

VI. REPEATING INTERVENTIONS UNTIL PHOBIAS ABOUT RELATIONSHIPS ARE DESENSITIZED

Persistence Is Key

Just as in Self-Restructuring (Chapter 9), a therapist should not succumb to discouragement if the patient's images of others do not immediately improve. In a case with continued resistance, the therapist will have to stay on this focus week after week, until the patient begins to see others in a more realistic light and to feel compassion for them.

The therapist will need to stay alert to subtle shifts in the patient's awareness of others, because building trust and understanding of others can be a slow, incremental process. But it is only with such trust and understanding that the patient can continue to gain autonomy and healthy interdependence after therapy is terminated. As we have noted repeatedly, optimal relatedness is the well-integrated balance of autonomy and interdependence, expressiveness and receptiveness. Therapy is successful when the patient's newly acquired "emotional intelligence" translates into adaptive interaction with others.

Summary of Other-Restructuring Steps

The basic steps of Other-Restructuring are summarized in Table 10.1.

TABLE 10.1. Steps in Other-Restructuring

- Defense Recognition—
- Gently point out defenses, externalization of needs.
- Defense Relinquishing—
- Point out costs; help patient understand rewards (primary, secondary gain).
- Help patient build new supports to replace defenses.
- Conduct exposure to enhance receptive capacity to others.
    Help patient perceive and be receptive to others' feelings.
    Help patient identify bodily signals of responses to others' feelings.
    Help patient imagine desired action in fantasy.
    Use changing perspectives to elicit feeling.
    Encourage the receptive capacity of the patient.
- Engage in response prevention (D).
    Point out defense/avoidance.
    Encourage patient to stay with the feelings a little longer.
- Engage in anxiety regulation (A).
    Calm patient by offering support, reassurance.
    Explore the fears, shame, pain.
- Return to exposure as soon as anxiety is reduced.
- Return to response prevention if necessary.
- Return to anxiety regulation repeatedly.

CHAPTER 10 • EXERCISES

EXERCISE 10A: EVALUATE PATIENTS' RECEPTIVE CAPACITY

Directions: For each of the following statements, **identify how the patient is responding to the needs of others.** Choose from the following list:

A. Insufficiently attentive/receptive.

B. Appropriately attentive/receptive.

C. Overly attentive/receptive.

Identify whether the needs are emotional, biological, or social needs. And also suggest what needs the patient might be avoiding, lacking, or not attending to.

Example: PATIENT: My secretary told me she needed this morning off for a routine doctor's appointment. I'm really worried about her, and I sent her home at lunchtime yesterday. She kept saying she's OK, but she looked a little pale to me. Of course, it happened at the worst possible time because of a big project we had due, so I wound up staying up all night typing it up. So that's why I'm a little tired today.

Answer: **Nature of patient's response:** C—overly attentive/receptive to secretary's biological needs; inattentive to his own needs.

Exercise 10A.1.   PATIENT: My secretary waited until the day before yesterday to tell me she needed this morning off for a doctor's appointment, when we've got this big project due. She's so inconsiderate! Of course I insisted that she reschedule. I could see she was just about to get an attitude, so I left. You just can't find people with a good work ethic these days.

Nature of patient's response: _____

_____

Exercise 10A.2.   PATIENT: My secretary told me a couple of days ago that she needed this morning off for a doctor's routine checkup. But we're in the middle of a big project, and we had a huge amount of work to finish. So I asked her if she could stay late yesterday evening. She wasn't thrilled about staying late, but I was glad we got the work done and she could keep her appointment.

Nature of patient's response: _____

_____

Exercise 10A.3.   PATIENT: My husband and I went shopping, and he got irritable because he was getting hungry. I asked him to get something to eat at the restaurant next door so I could keep shopping as the sale was just about to end.

Nature of patient's response: _____

_____

Exercise 10A.4.   PATIENT: I'd been looking forward to this sale for weeks, but then my husband got hungry—it was past his usual lunchtime—and so I went to get some lunch with him at the restaurant next door, and then the sale was over by the time we finished. I started to tell him to get something himself, but he just gets this look like a little puppy dog, and I can't stand to make him eat alone.

Nature of patient's response: _____

_____

Exercise 10A.5.

PATIENT: We were just about to leave the pet shop when a pet monkey was brought in. The kids were so thrilled! I kept asking them to leave, but they just wouldn't budge. I had to wait an hour before they would leave, and we wound up missing our train to my friend's.

Nature of patient's response: _____

_____

Exercise 10A.6.

PATIENT: We were just about to leave the pet shop when a pet monkey was brought in. The children really wanted to stay, but we were due at my friend's at 3 P.M., so I told them we simply had to leave immediately. Then, of course, my friend wasn't even home yet—she's always late.

Nature of patient's response: _____

_____

Exercise 10A.7.

PATIENT: My wife can be so overly emotional. I told you about her friend who has cancer. Well, she died last week, and my wife's just been crying and crying. I just don't get it. It's not like it was a surprise or anything.

Nature of patient's response: _____

_____

Exercise 10A.8.

PATIENT: My wife's been having a hard time. Her friend who had cancer died last week, and it's really hit her pretty hard. So I've been trying to just be extra nice to her and watch the kids more often. The other night we got a sitter so we could go to a movie, and we just wound up sitting in the park with me holding her while she cried.

Nature of patient's response: _____

_____

EXERCISE 10B: HELP PATIENTS CHANGE INNER IMAGES OF OTHERS

Directions:

Which of the following interventions do you think might be most likely to **help each patient change his or her inner image of others?** Many of these interventions might be helpful in different ways, but in this exercise we are focusing on the specific methods for restructuring the image of others. Place a check mark by your choice.

Exercise 10B.1.

PATIENT: I could never be angry with you. You've seen me through the hardest times of my life. So what if you didn't extend our time a little last week?

    A. We've seen many times how you hold in your anger in rather than express it.

    B. Sometimes people can have strong feelings of anger, even toward people they care about. So could we explore all the feelings you might have had toward me at that moment?

    C. It sounds like you didn't feel I was supportive to you.

    D. I know it's frustrating, but we need to recognize the time boundaries here.

Exercise 10B.2.

PATIENT: How do I know this guy isn't out to just use me like all the rest? Sure, he seems nice and all, but he's probably laughing behind my back.

    A. Was there anything he did, or a way he looked, that made you think he was laughing at you?

    B. Maybe you need to go slow and trust your instincts.

    C. Isn't being so cautious a way of protecting yourself that you've learned in order to survive?

    D. Maybe it scares you that he seems so normal. What do you think?

Exercise 10B.3.

PATIENT: My father was good to me, so good. He died when I was only 6. I remember feeling so abandoned by him. I know it makes no sense, but I always felt like there was something wrong with me because he left.

    A. Of course, your father didn't leave because you were bad. He had a disease, and he died because of it.

    B. If your father were here now, what do you think he would say to you?

    C. Often children feel that they caused a parent's death.

    D. How sad that you took it out on yourself.

Exercise 10B.4.

PATIENT: How must you think of me after what I've revealed? You must think I'm pretty low.

    A. You know, we all have feelings like that sometimes.

    B. I feel quite moved that you were able to trust me enough to say this.

    C. I think it might be you that's feeling critical of yourself, rather than me. What do you think?

    D. Does it really seem like I'm looking down at you? Have I done something that would make you feel that way?

EXERCISE 10C: IDENTIFY ADAPTIVE AND ADDICTIVE ATTACHMENTS

Directions: In the following exercise think about whether the statements below represent **adaptive or addictive attachments,** and give the appropriate response in each case. If the response is "Addictive" (remember that this can mean defensiveness or codependency), identify what the patient might be defending against. If the response is "Adaptive," note what affect is being accessed and used appropriately.

Example 1: PATIENT: He stood me up twice over the weekend, but that's the way Eric is— unreliable. But when I am with him, it's worth all the times that he lets me down.

Answer: **Adaptive or addictive? Why?** Addictive. Patient is too forgiving, and too willing to accept and make excuses for being treated with lack of consideration. She is also paying too high a price for the time she spends with Eric.

Example 2:   PATIENT: I feel like taking it slow with Phillip. I haven't been available for other people since Scott and I divorced, but I feel like I'm ready now. In my own time.

Answer: **Adaptive or addictive? Why?** Adaptive. Going at own pace, listening to own voice in process of getting to know someone new.

Exercise 10C.1.   PATIENT: We've been together every day and night ever since we met 3 months ago. He gets very jealous when I hang around with my friends, or particularly when I hang around guy friends at college. It makes me feel very safe that he's so protective of our relationship.

Adaptive or addictive? Why? _____

_____

Exercise 10C.2.   PATIENT: I adore my wife, but I keep thinking that there's someone out there who is better—someone who could make everything perfect.

Adaptive or addictive? Why? _____

_____

Exercise 10C.3.   PATIENT: It really doesn't mean that much that I get praise from you—you're easy to impress. What I crave is to get my boss to just once tell me I'm doing a good job.

Adaptive or addictive? Why? _____

_____

Exercise 10C.4.   PATIENT: I know I'm taking a lot of risks with this man, but there's this rush I get thinking that my husband might find out. It makes it all the more exciting.

Adaptive or addictive? Why? _____

_____

Exercise 10C.5.   PATIENT: I forgave her the first time she canceled meeting me for lunch at the last minute. But when she canceled a couple of other times—without much excuse—I became less interested in her, and I stopped calling.

Adaptive or addictive? Why? _____

_____

Exercise 10C.6.

PATIENT: There's a cute guy at work who has been flirting with me. Although it's nice to get the attention, and I find him very attractive, I'm not about to cheat on my fiancé. It's just nice to fantasize.

Adaptive or addictive? Why? _____

_____

PART IV

DIAGNOSTIC CONSIDERATIONS AND TERMINATION

CHAPTER 11 # Treating Specific Diagnoses: The Relationship between DSM Diagnoses and Affect Phobias

Chapter Objective	To clarify the relationship between Affect Phobias and specific *Diagnostic and Statistical Manual of Mental Disorders* (DSM) diagnoses.
Therapist Stance	Flexibility in making treatment patient-specific.
Anxiety Regulation	Varies with the diagnosis.
Topics Covered	I. How Affect Phobias Underlie Diagnoses and are Maintained by Primary and Secondary Gain
	II. Integrating Nature and Nurture: The Biopsychosocial Model
	III. Using Axis I Diagnoses to Inform Treatment of Affect Phobias
	IV. Using Axis II Diagnoses to Guide Treatment of Affect Phobias
	V. Conclusion: Focusing on Affect Phobias That Underlie Diagnoses

I. HOW AFFECT PHOBIAS UNDERLIE DIAGNOSES AND ARE MAINTAINED BY PRIMARY AND SECONDARY GAIN

Diagnoses Fall on the Defense Pole

The process of diagnosis categorizes disorders according to certain collections of **symptoms**. In contrast, the model of Short-Term Dynamic Psychotherapy (STDP) presented in this book views diagnostic disorders as a combination of underlying **Affect Phobias** and neurobiological vulnerabilities (see Section II). Thus STDP does not view individual diagnostic entities as the starting point of psychotherapy (as discussed in Section I of Chapter 2 and Section II of Chapter 3. Instead, many such entities are dealt with as Affect Phobias centering around feelings (the Feeling Pole [F] on the Triangle of Conflict) that need to be desensitized. The diagnostic collections of symptoms are seen, in part, as surface indicators or defenses (the Defense Pole [D]) against those Affect Phobias; for example, a patient's avoidant personality disorder might spring from an Affect Phobia over closeness. Thus STDP focuses on the underlying psychodynamic components of Affect Phobias as formulated in Chapter 4, rather than on diagnostic symptoms.

Primary and Secondary Gain Maintain Diagnostic Symptoms

Since symptoms and diagnostic criteria can often be viewed as defensive behaviors or inhibitory affects, it's worth recalling from Chapter 6 that defensive patterns are reinforced by (1) the immediate **primary gain** of avoiding the anxiety (or other inhibitory affect) of conflicted feelings, and (2) the **secondary gain** of subtle positive rewards earned through avoidance.

Treatment focuses on the **source of the symptoms**—the conflict or phobia of adaptive affects. The ability to experience these underlying warded-off affects without conflict can be seen as the **missing capability** that the patient can acquire through therapy.

PATIENT: My wife keeps trying to help me to be able to grieve for my father. I finally just got so sick of her bringing up the subject that I blew up, and she hasn't mentioned it since.

Deconstructing the Symptom in Terms of Primary and Secondary Gain

In the example above, the symptom of defensive anger could provide the patient with the primary gain of avoiding the emotional pain of feeling sad. The secondary gain may be that by yelling at his wife, the patient has made it less likely that she will confront him with the conflicted affect (sadness) again. The missing capability that the patient needs to acquire in treatment is the ability to tolerate his affect; this not only will allow him to grieve, but will ameliorate the conflict in his relationship with his wife. (For further discussion of symptoms vs. source of the disorder, see CC, pp. 396–399.)

II. INTEGRATING NATURE AND NURTURE: THE BIOPSYCHOSOCIAL MODEL

Integration of Many Factors

As discussed in Section II of Chapter 3, STDP views patients' problems as resulting from many factors, including biological/neurological, psychological, and interpersonal or environmental. DSM disorders are not only biologically predisposed; they also reflect what is conditioned through life experience. Thus Axis I and Axis II symptoms can simultaneously be viewed as biologically based disorders and as learned defensive response patterns. For example, learned helplessness that is conditioned through life experience can contribute to, and even elicit, a biological vulnerability to depression. As Kandel (1998) points out, what is learned or conditioned then becomes biology.

Nature *and* Nurture Combined

It bears repeating that the origin of our patients' problems is not a question of nature "versus" nurture, but represents a combination of both. Therefore, with problems such as depression, a number of interventions—medication, skills training, behavior therapy, and psychodynamic exploration—can all be useful.

Learned Behavior Can Be Unlearned

Because behavior that is learned can be "unlearned" and more adaptive behavior can be learned in its place, STDP focuses on the learned ("nurture") component of the problem. Even when patients have a biological predisposition to a certain Axis I or Axis II disorder, the new capabilities learned in therapy can be used to manage, moderate, or even prevent the emergence of genetically predisposed symptoms.

III. USING AXIS I DIAGNOSES TO INFORM TREATMENT OF AFFECT PHOBIAS

The bulk of this chapter is devoted to a review of the DSM-IV diagnostic groupings, with an eye to the implications for treatment in our Affect Phobia model. (For further discussion, see CC, Ch. 11.) This section explores Axis I disorders as representing defensive behavior patterns of Affect Phobias, which can help therapists to formulate a treatment focus and streamline the treatment process. Section IV of this chapter similarly explores Axis II disorders.

Mood Disorders

Major Depressive Disorder

Any Affect Phobia can give rise to depression. Consider the depressive effects that can result from impairment in the capacity for anger, grief, closeness, positive feelings about the self, sexual feelings, interest, or joy. Many STDP therapists report reduction or resolution of major depression as a result of exposure to conflicted feelings.

Primary gain: Can be the avoidance of the range of conflicted feelings (frequently grief, anger, and/or positive feelings about the self—but also sexual feelings, interest, or joy).

Secondary gain: Can be the freedom from responsibility of correcting situations, replacing losses, facing or testing oneself, interpersonal conflict, and so forth.

Missing capability: Can be assertion, grieving, self-care, enthusiasm, and/or mastery—a range of the activating affects that would replace the depressive stance.

Dysthymic Disorder

Dysthymia is a low-grade, chronic form of depression that many clinicians consider hard to treat if not unresolvable. However, clinical experience and preliminary research suggest that STDP, focusing on early-life neglect and loss, with emphasis on "reparenting of the self" and better connection to others (taught in Chapters 9 and 10), can significantly improve and sometimes eliminate lifelong dysthymia. The main Affect Phobia concerns positive feelings about the self in relation to early-life figures.

Primary gain: Can be the avoidance of the range of conflicted feelings, but often is the avoidance of pain of not feeling worthwhile or special.

Secondary gain: Can be the safety of avoiding risk of being rejected or unloved.

Missing capability: A positive sense of self in relation to others is often the affect most urgently needed. Healthy entitlement and feeling worthwhile then become the basis for other adaptive affects (such as assertion, grief, joy, etc.).

Bipolar I Disorder

Bipolar I disorder (with full-blown manic and depressive episodes) is generally less responsive to psychotherapy than it is to medication. Active mania is typically a contraindication to STDP, because of the difficulty with loss of impulse control when conflicted affects are elicited. However, patients with bipolar I disorder who are relatively stable may be responsive to STDP—particularly Self- and Other-Restructuring. If medication noncompliance is rooted in psychodynamic conflict, such therapy could improve the course of the disorder.

Primary gain: Can be the avoidance of the range of conflicted feelings by manic bursts or depression.

Secondary gain: Can be the distraction and gratification offered by the mania—the high and boundless sense of energy that accompanies a manic episode.

Missing capability: Can be assertion, grieving, self-care, enthusiasm, and/or mastery—any of the activating affects that would replace the manic or depressive stance.

Bipolar II Disorder

In contrast, some patients with bipolar II disorder (which involves hypomanic rather than full-blown manic episodes, and has fewer biological contributions than bipolar I disorder does) have been responsive to STDP where conflicted affects are desensitized. Clinical experience has found that many such patients have sustained multiple losses, and have an Affect Phobia concerning grief that is too painful to bear.

Primary gain: Can be the avoidance of the range of conflicted feelings by hypomanic bursts or depression – or the avoidance of grief in some cases.

Secondary gain: Can be the distraction and gratification offered by the hypomania.

Missing capability: Can be grieving, assertion, self-care, enthusiasm, and/or mastery—any of the activating affects that would replace the hypomanic or depressive stance.

Anxiety Disorders

Anxiety Disorders in General

Symptomatic behavior in many anxiety disorders (e.g., panic disorder, generalized anxiety disorder, specific phobias) can function as defensive behavior patterns that block more adaptive forms of responding. Symptomatic anxiety can indicate that the defenses are not working effectively enough. For some anxiety disorders (especially obsessive–compulsive disorder), it is important to consider other treatment modalities, such as cognitive-behavioral therapy or medication. Social phobia (particularly of the generalized type)—like avoidant personality disorder (see Section IV), to which it is closely related—often involves conflict over closeness or positive feelings toward the self.

Primary gain: The (partial) avoidance of the warded-off feeling. The conflicted feelings can be many, covering the full range of feeling.

Secondary gain: Can be the distraction from focusing on the issue at hand—freedom from responsibility of correcting situations, replacing losses, facing or testing oneself, and so forth.

Missing capability: The bearing of the warded-off feelings, as in depression.

Posttraumatic Stress Disorder

We do not view posttraumatic stress disorder (PTSD) as originally caused by an Affect Phobia. PTSD is caused by a traumatic experience that continues to be intensely relived, rather than by conflicts (anxiety, shame, pain) about underlying feelings. For example, a patient may have been traumatized in a multicar accident, and afterward police sirens (or memories of police sirens) cause the patient to "relive" the accident as though he or she were actually there. Such traumatic memories appear to be encoded in the brain differently from normal memories, and to bring forth the sights, sounds, smells, and other sensations of actually reliving the experience (as though the visceral experience might be being "recalled" from the hypothalamus rather than the cortex; see Stickgold, 2002).

Many of the typical defenses do not work to modulate or control the powerful surge of traumatic affect in PTSD, and many patients become flooded with traumatic feelings. Other patients with PTSD resort to more primitive defenses, such as dissociation or emotional numbing, to avoid the traumatic memory.

Exposure to traumatic memories, though effective in some cases, can retraumatize many patients. A promising treatment approach for PTSD is Eye Movement Desensitization and Reprocessing (EMDR; Shapiro, 1995), which uses bilateral alternating stimulation hypothesized to restructure the neurological underpinnings of the encoded memory. There is a growing body of empirical research demonstrating the effectiveness of EMDR for PTSD (see Shapiro, 2001).

Finally, **complex PTSD** is a form of PTSD that occurs in patients with repeated traumas and/or Axis II personality disorders. In such cases, treatment of Affect Phobias (used in conjunction with EMDR) may play an important role in restructuring warded-off feelings, and especially in restructuring the sense of self and relationships to others.

Primary gain: In general, the pain of a traumatic memory is relived, not blocked by defenses. When defenses are used, they generally take the form of numbing or dissociative symptoms, which help the patient avoid the intense and traumatizing anxiety and pain.

Secondary gain: As in primary gain, the traumatic experience generally is negative, comes unbidden, and is not blocked by defenses. However, when secondary gain occurs, it may be that the painful state or the feelings of helplessness become rewarded in some way (e.g., receiving more care from others, being allowed to stay home from work, disability compensation, etc.).

Missing capability: The emotional mastery of the traumatic reaction—that is, the ability to recall the traumatic incident with well-modulated emotions, but without unbearable pain, dissociative episodes, or numbing defenses. Although an Affect Phobia may not be the fundamental contributor to simple PTSD, fears of feelings may play a role in PTSD and especially in complex PTSD. In cases where Affect Phobias are involved, therapists who are trained in EMDR can combine EMDR with STDP, with potentially beneficial results (see McCullough, 2002,). From the standpoint of Affect Phobia, some aspects of PTSD could be helped by teaching assertion to replace feelings of "victimization," or building a positive sense of self that provides a sense of mastery and competence.

Selected Other Axis I Disorders

Somatoform Disorders

Somatization (physical symptoms without physical etiology) can be thought of as defensive displacement of some emotional pain or turmoil. There may be many Affect Phobias—or a phobia of feelings in general. In contrast to patients with obsessive–compulsive personality disorder (see Section IV), who avoid feelings by "going into their heads" (intellectualization, isolation of affect), patients with somatization disorder or other somatoform disorders may avoid experiencing emotions by "going into their bodies" (displacement of emotional pain into physical pain).

Primary gain: The avoidance of some warded-off feeling (typically anger/assertion, grief, or positive feelings about the self).

Secondary gain: May be the care or solace received from others for feeling physical pain as well as decreased responsibility.

Missing capability: The ability to express unexpressed wants and needs. Patients need to recognize that anger can make the stomach hurt or the head ache. Fear of grieving can lead to choking or chest pain. Loneliness can cause fatigue. Such patients need special attention to the recognition of their affects.

Sexual Disorders

Sexual disorders, as defined by DSM-IV, fall into two main categories: the **sexual dysfunctions** (disturbances in some phase of the sexual response cycle) and the **paraphilias** (sexual behaviors or fantasies involving unusual situations, activities, or objects). When physical causes are ruled out, some sexual dysfunctions (sexual desire disorders, sexual arousal disorders, orgasmic disorders, etc.) may be due to anxiety, guilt, shame, or pain, and thus may represent typical Affect Phobias about sexual feelings. Although other sexual disorders can be seen as defensive responses to anger (e.g., rape or sexual sadism, in which sex is used as a weapon), at base many if not most sexual disorders also involve phobias about closeness or tenderness. The more serious the sexual disorder (e.g., paraphilias such as pedophilia or voyeurism), the more likely it is that the Affect Phobia concerns grief and **the unmet longing for love** (again, phobias about closeness/tenderness/care). When relationships have been too filled with anguish and pain, some individuals turn to cross-dressing or fetishes as displacements for the loved one. Others resort to actions that cause harm (pedophilia, sadomasochism, etc.) as ways to meet the powerful longings for acceptance, love, or some form of connection. When sex is used defensively (even in behaviors that might be immoral or illegal), it most often arises from the tragic blockage of basic human wants and needs for love and care.

Primary gain: Often avoiding the pain of unmet longing for tenderness, closeness, or connection.

Secondary gain: In many paraphilias, the tremendous and addictive pleasure obtained from the alternative "love object"—which is powerful and hard to break.

Missing capability: Healthy human attachment—closeness/tenderness, care for self and others. (For an in-depth discussion of treatment of conflicted sexual feelings and paraphilias, see CC, pp. 258–267, 406.)

Substance Use Disorders, Eating Disorders, and Other Disturbances of Impulse Control

The Affect Phobias associated with substance use disorders, eating disorders, and other disturbances of impulse control can involve any of the basic feelings. The acting-out behaviors can be seen as defenses that help to avoid the pain or discomfort of those avoided feelings. Some patients may be biologically more prone to impulsive behaviors, putting them at greater risk for these disorders. Furthermore, a lack of environmental limit setting (or excessive limit setting, which can cause oppositional acting out) may further put such patients at risk.

Primary gain: Generally, the avoidance of some aversive affect state.

Secondary gain: The rewarding quality of giving in to the action or impulse: short-term comfort that results in long-term costs. In substance use disorders, the social network of other individuals who misuse substances can also be rewarding.

Missing capability: The ability to bear and control the full range of feelings. Rather than exposure treatment, such disorders need behavioral and cognitive treatments (and Twelve-Step programs, when possible) to help build capacities to control behavior. In mild forms of these disorders, therapists using STDP can ask acting-out patients to do two things: (1) try to wait 5 minutes as a means of building self-control before giving in to their impulsive behaviors (e.g., binge eating or drinking, or any restless, impulsive action); and (2) to observe what feelings emerge at that moment that they may be trying to avoid. However, as mentioned in Section IV of Chapter 3, Affect Restructuring is generally contraindicated in serious forms of these disorders. Self- and Other-Restructuring, and some aspects of Defense Restructuring, can help such patients to understand their self-destructiveness and build self-care mechanisms to help manage their impulses. When treatment proceeds to the point where impulse control has been good for 1–3 years, the more active techniques of Defense and Affect Restructuring may be appropriate.

Schizophrenia

Although historically many practitioners have attempted to treat schizophrenia with dynamic psychotherapy, we do not know of such cases successfully treated with STDP. Schizophrenia is largely rooted in biology, but research shows that nongenetic factors still account for over half the variance. Therefore, some form of psychotherapy (supportive, group, family therapy, etc.) may be useful to treat the learned or environmentally based component of the disorder. Although schizophrenic symptoms and behaviors are biologically predisposed, they are also influenced by the environment and can be used by a patient defensively. The Affect Phobias involved in such behaviors include terror of others and immense shame about the self. Because patients with schizophrenia often have great difficulty processing complex social stimulation, they act as though they are "allergic to people." In such situations they can be seen as reacting defensively, with schizophrenic symptoms, to create a safe distance.

Primary gain: Can be the avoidance of the anxiety—or terror—of relating.

Secondary gain: The (seemingly) safe cocoon of isolation or social distance the schizophrenic symptoms create.

Missing capability: To the extent that STDP may be helpful, the ability to bear human connection or the tolerance of relating to others is the suggested focus. When psychotherapy is attempted, the therapist must understand the tremendous fears (often about human interaction) that lead to decompensation. The therapist also needs to use supportive interventions, anxiety regulation, and very gentle attempts at exposure to closeness or connection that will not elicit the profound shame and terror about the self in relation to others. Obviously, provoking high levels of affect has a high risk of destabilizing schizophrenic patients. But a systematic desensitization of feelings of closeness (taking tiny exposures or steps toward adaptive interactions) may help such patients better tolerate social interaction.

IV. USING AXIS II DIAGNOSES TO GUIDE TREATMENT OF AFFECT PHOBIAS

Axis II personality disorders represent patients' typical, predictable, and pervasive character traits—their chronic, lifelong ways of responding. Axis II diagnostic criteria (symptoms) are viewed in STDP as—at least in part—defensive behaviors.

"Pure" Axis II Are Exceedingly Rare

It is important to remember that "pure" Axis II disorders are quite rare. Patients frequently meet criteria for several Axis II disorders, or have blends of symptoms across categories without necessarily meeting full criteria for any one Axis II disorder. In addition, there is usually overlap or comorbidity with Axis I symptoms.

Axis II Criteria Reflect Degree of Defensiveness

The more Axis II criteria that are present, the more we find the following:

- A greater probability of defensiveness.
- Greater impairment of the self and of relationships with others.
- A need for a longer course of therapy.
- A greater need to start treatment with Self- and Other-Restructuring and/or Defense Restructuring **before** Affect Restructuring.

Axis II criteria can be reported by the patient on a self-administered set of paper-and-pencil instruments, the Psychotherapy Assessment Checklist (PAC) Forms, and can then be easily and quickly counted by the therapist before treatment begins. (The PAC Forms and instructions can be obtained from our Web site: www.affectphobia.org.) Remember that most patients tend to overreport these diagnostic criteria by about 20% (or more in cases of obsessive–compulsive personality disorder; See the PAC Forms' instructions). Therefore, clinicians will need to assess whether the criteria that patients check off are actually met. Of course, a few patients underreport their symptoms, due to the nature of their defenses, their motivation for treatment, or their situation (e.g., alcohol or drug use, adolescence, mandated treatment). It's easy for the therapist to count the **total number of checked Axis II items** on the PAC Forms, which can give a quick "ballpark" estimate of the degree of impairment:

0–10 items: Normal range. (Everyone has some of these items.)

11–20 items: Mild defensiveness. (Such individuals are probably suitable for STDP interventions and may be able to work on Affect Restructuring fairly quickly.)

21–40 items: Moderate defensiveness. (Most of our STDP research subjects fell in this range and needed much work on Defense Restructuring, combined with varying levels of Self- and Other-Restructuring, before getting to Affect Restructuring.)

Over 40 items: Strong defensiveness and high probability of impairment in sense of self and relationships. (This range indicates the need for an initial and often extensive focus on Self- and Other-Restructuring before moving to Defense or Affect Restructuring. In general, a score of over 40 items on the Axis II scale is an indication for longer-term treatment.)

Axis II Clusters

The DSM-IV Axis II diagnoses are grouped into three clusters:

Cluster A: Odd, eccentric, or withdrawn behavior.

Cluster B: Acting-out or impulsive behavior.

Cluster C: Anxious or fearful behavior.

Cluster A Disorders: Odd, Eccentric, Withdrawn Behavior

Paranoid, Schizoid, and Schizotypal Personality Disorders

The primary Affect Phobia in the Cluster A disorders (paranoid, schizoid, and schizotypal personality disorders) is about closeness. Such individuals can be thought of as being frightened of, or "allergic to people." The typical defenses include projection, idealization, devaluation, and autistic fantasy. These defenses primarily avoid the **anxiety about interpersonal contact.** The following hold true for all three of the Cluster A disorders.

Primary gain: The avoidance of relationships that are too frightening, too close, or too stimulating for comfort.

Secondary gain: The omnipotent safety of being alone.

Missing capability: The ability to be able to find other people trustworthy, soothing, or comforting, beginning with the therapist. As with all systematic desensitization, it is important to begin at a safe distance, then move closer.

Cluster B Disorders: Acting-Out, Impulsive Behavior

Histrionic, Borderline, Narcissistic, and Antisocial Personality Disorders

The main Affect Phobia in the Cluster B disorders (histrionic, borderline, narcissistic, and antisocial personality disorders) is about positive feelings toward the self. The self is experienced—either consciously or not—as bad, inadequate, or shameful. Impulsive reactions (narcissistic rage at insults, borderline anguish over rejection, histrionic defensive emotionality, and antisocial need-driven tantrums) can all be seen as **defensive affects that result from the pain of unmet longings.**

Cluster B Needs Self- and Other-Restructuring

Much restructuring of the self and of relationships to others must be done before these defensive behaviors can be replaced. Patients with severe levels of these disorders typically are not responsive to STDP approaches and are better treated with long-term dynamic, cognitive, supportive, or skills-building models.

Borderline Personality Disorder

The primary Affect Phobia in borderline personality disorder involves a fragile self-structure and a lack of positive feelings about the self. A stable self-image cannot be sustained in situations of real or perceived rejection, insensitivity, or abandonment. Patients with borderline personality disorder can vary widely in their symptoms and degree of functioning. Less impaired patients may be well-disciplined and high-functioning individuals with good impulse control, yet may have some degree of identity disturbance (conflicts about positive sense of self, loss of sense of self in relation to others). More impaired patients may have more profound identity impairment, combined with a lack of impulse control (acting out, self-harm, etc.)

Primary gain: The avoidance of painful feelings of abandonment and the avoidance of the painful longing for closeness. Defensive behaviors include identity diffusion, feeling empty inside, temper outbursts, splitting, and self-abuse.

Secondary gain: To shore up an inadequate sense of self and/or to manipulate others. In contrast to patients with narcissistic personality disorder who gain a great deal from their defensive structure (and who have much to lose by giving it up), the acting out and self-abuse of patients with borderline personality disorder is not as desirable to these patients. Even so, loss of control and self-injurious behavior (e.g., self-cutting) sometimes can be the only way patients can distract themselves from their unbearable emotional pain of feeling unlovable, unworthy, or alone. In the most severe cases, the emotional pain is so great that only extreme physical pain can distract their attention from the emotional anguish, while obtaining the longed-for attention from others.

Missing capability: A strong sense of self in relation to others, and the ability to support and sustain a positive self image even when others are not doing so. This disorder requires long-term treatment and benefits from skill-building interventions (see, e.g., Linehan, 1993). In addition, STDP methods, especially Self- and Other-Restructuring, can be beneficial and reduce treatment length.

Narcissistic Personality Disorder

The primary Affect Phobia in narcissistic personality disorder involves intense shame due to a fragile self-structure and lack of positive feelings about the self.

Primary gain: Avoidance of the pain associated with longing for a sense of worth or value from others. Narcissistic defensive behaviors include the presentation of a false self, putting one's own needs above others', and seeking undue admiration.

Secondary gain: The safety, sense of power, stature, and control one achieves. If one never becomes close or becomes vulnerable to another, one is never devastated by the pain of abandonment or betrayal. Such defensive behaviors are highly reinforcing, provide a sense of power and stature, and are extremely resistant to change.

Missing capability: Authentic connection to others, to replace the safety of cool detachment. Genuine pride about self. The ability to **grieve** losses rather than to be so potentially devastated that one doesn't dare care.

Histrionic Personality Disorder

The primary Affect Phobias in histrionic personality disorder involve a lack of positive feelings about the self, and insecurity in relation to others. Patients with this disorder flirt or seek attention from others as an external way of shoring up the poor sense of self. When this does not work, intense emotional outbursts defend against the grief and pain of feeling unworthy. Patients with histrionic personality disorder and a Global Assessment of Functioning (GAF) score above 50 have been responsive to STDP.

Primary gain: From defensive emotionality, avoidance of more painful or vulnerable affects. From flirtation and manipulation, avoidance of anxieties around closeness to others and feelings about the self.

Secondary gain: The distraction and control that the defensive emotion provides, and the sense of worth that is achieved, if only temporarily.

Missing capability: Cognitive control of the defensive affects and ability to bear adaptive affects.

Antisocial Personality Disorder

The main Affect Phobias for patients with antisocial personality disorder involve feelings of closeness, care, compassion, tenderness, and empathy. Such patients have severe deficits in attachment.

Primary gain: Can be the avoidance of vulnerability in any form.

Secondary gain: Often the power and control one feels.

Missing capability: Closeness, attachment, tenderness, empathy. Indeed, for patients with antisocial personality disorder, "correct empathy" initially means **not** showing too much empathy; when such patients think they are dealing with a "sucker," it will be impossible to build a treatment alliance. Initially, "correct empathy" with such patients will be showing them that they cannot "put one over on" the therapist. Just as one must titrate closeness for patients with Cluster A personality disorders (i.e., present closeness in very small doses), one must titrate empathy for patients with antisocial personality disorder.

Cluster C Disorders: Anxious, Fearful Behavior

Avoidant, Dependent, and Obsessive–Compulsive Personality Disorders

The main Affect Phobias in the Cluster C disorders (avoidant, dependent, and obsessive–compulsive personality disorders) involve both conflicts about the sense of self, and conflicts about closeness or receptivity to others. The STDP model was initially tested on patients with Cluster C personality disorders and showed significant improvement. In such patients with GAF scores above 50, and without pronounced Cluster A or B pathology, therapists can begin pointing out defenses from the start and encouraging patients to give up the defenses as soon as possible.

Avoidant Personality Disorder

Defenses in avoidant personality disorder (rejection sensitivity; avoiding social situations, new things, or close involvement; etc.) ward off the adaptive affect of closeness because of fear of rejection, or shame about the sense of self.

Primary gain: The avoidance of the fear associated with feelings that arise in social interaction, and avoidance of the shame of feeling unworthy or unlikeable.

Secondary gain: The protection and comfort of isolation.

Missing capability: The ability to bear closeness and attachment to others with adaptive levels of inhibitory affects. The ability to feel self-worth and self- confidence when with others.

Dependent Personality Disorder

The primary Affect Phobias in patients with dependent personality disorder involve anger/assertion, and/or confidence in one's sense of self or sense of autonomy. Other people are needed to provide the missing capabilities (caretaking, decision making, initiative, etc.) that these individuals have not acquired for themselves. A person with dependent personality disorder becomes frantic when left alone with such responsibilities.

Primary gain: The avoidance of the inhibitory feelings (anxiety, guilt, shame, and/or pain) involved in autonomy, independence, or being alone. In such patients, defensive behaviors include seeking reassurance, indecisiveness, helplessness, or childlike behavior.

Secondary gain: The safety and comfort of relying on others, or the freedom from taking responsibility for one's own life. (Note that in CC, p. 417, the primary and secondary gains for this disorder were erroneously reversed.)

Missing capability: A sense of mastery and competence about the self, and having comfort rather than pain when alone. Feeling comfortable with autonomy.

Obsessive–Compulsive Personality Disorder

The main Affect Phobia in obsessive–compulsive personality disorder involves feelings in general. Emotions often can feel chaotic, so the symptoms of this disorder help to maintain control. If Cluster A responses indicate an "allergy to people," obsessive–compulsive personality disorder reflects an "allergy to feeling."

Primary gain: The avoidance of unpleasant feelings within oneself or in connection to others. Thus Affect Phobias can include any of the major affects: anger, grief, closeness, or sense of self. Defensive behaviors include being stubborn, rigid, having no time for fun, trouble throwing things out, isolation of affect, and intellectualization.

Secondary gain: Can be the quiet peacefulness of relative nonfeeling—the sense that things are in control.

Missing capability: To experience any feeling as comfortable instead of chaotic. Because such people are phobic about feelings in general, much anxiety regulation is needed. It is helpful to remember that **feeling is always present**—so the therapist should acknowledge whatever small amount of felt experience is available, then encourage and build on that.

Provisional Axis II Diagnoses in Cluster C

Two final disorders are not listed as formal diagnoses in DSM-IV or DSM-IV-TR, but are included in Appendix B ("Criteria Sets and Axes Provided for Further Study"). However, they represent problem areas often found in clinical work, and are included to help identify and treat such patients. These disorders should be grouped with the other Cluster C diagnoses.

Depressive Personality Disorder

Similar (though not identical) to an earlier diagnostic category called self-defeating personality disorder, depressive personality disorder may be the most straightforward of the Axis II behavior patterns to treat, and one of the most responsive to STDP. The main Affect Phobia involves positive feelings about the self, especially self-care. Defenses include feeling inadequate, having negative expectations, and excessive guilt or worry.

Primary gain: The avoidance of the range of conflicted feelings that might threaten attachment.

Secondary gain: The approval or care that is received from others because of the passive or submissive behavior, as well as the avoidance of interpersonal conflict.

Missing capability: Care for self that includes setting limits and asking for things (both aspects of assertion of basic needs), and greater receptivity to both positive and negative feelings from others, in order to be able to bear conflict in interpersonal relationships.

Passive–Aggressive Personality Disorder

Patients with passive–aggressive personality disorder (also known as negativistic personality disorder) are generally largely unconscious of what they are doing, so the disorder is difficult to identify and is frequently missed on self-report instruments. One indicator can be a patient's report of a pattern of inexplicable or apparently unjustified anger from a number of other people. The primary Affect Phobia in this category—as the name implies—probably involves a conflict over anger.

Primary gain: The avoidance of direct interpersonal conflict or expression of negative feeling (which such patients feel powerless to face).

Secondary gain: The compelling, and enormously reinforcing, pleasure of fighting back from a hidden position. It can be a powerful feeling to do something infuriating and get away with it by denying it. Before this long-standing pattern will be given up, the individual must not only develop the missing capabilities listed below, but also must see them as more valuable than the passive aggression.

Missing capability: (1) Safe ways to deal with conflict (i.e., assertion), or to become emotionally separate; and (2) valuing and enjoying closeness.

V. CONCLUSION: FOCUSING ON AFFECT PHOBIAS THAT UNDERLIE DIAGNOSES

In conclusion, we reiterate that STDP does not view diagnostic categories as the starting point of psychotherapy. Instead, many DSM-defined disorders can be seen as stemming from a combination of biological predispositions and the underlying psychodynamic components of Affect Phobias. The individual symptoms or DSM criteria represent either the defenses (D) that prevent the adaptive experience of feelings (F), or the anxieties (A) that result when those defenses fail. The focus of the therapy work is on the desensitization of the underlying specific Affect Phobias that have contributed to the patient's diagnostic symptomatology; this desensitization, when successful, has the potential to resolve diagnostic symptomatology.

CHAPTER 12   **Termination**

Chapter Objective	To demonstrate when and how to terminate treatment.
Therapist Stance	Serving as a partner in review of treatment and in celebration of change.
Anxiety Regulation	Anticipating and managing fears of setbacks, and encouraging patient to maintain gains on his or her own.

Topics Covered

   I.   Overview of Termination

   II.   Assessing What Changes Have Been Made

   III.   Assessing Why Changes Have Been Made

   IV.   Celebrating Progress and Acknowledging What Needs More Work

   V.   Exploring the Full Range of Feelings for the Therapist

   VI.   Replacing the Loss of Therapy

   VII.   Conclusion and Commencement

Indications for Considering Termination

- Much improvement is made in main problem areas.
- The main Affect Phobias are resolved, or improvement is ongoing.
- The patient has confidence in maintaining gains and keeping work going.

I. OVERVIEW OF TERMINATION

Termination for a focused course of Short-Term Dynamic Psychotherapy (STDP) can be considered when the following criteria are met:

- The main problem behaviors have significantly changed.
- The patient feels able to maintain and expand upon the changes.

Placing Tools in Patients' Hands

In STDP, problems do not have to be completely resolved before therapy ends. The STDP approach attempts to "jump-start" the healing process and place the tools of healing in patients' hands, so they can feel capable of con-

308

tinuing on their own as soon as possible. When, as often happens at termination, there are Affect Phobias (core conflicts) that are not fully resolved, patients need these things:

- Awareness of the defenses against the specific feelings.
- The tools to work on these defenses further.
- Confidence in their ability to proceed on their own.

PATIENT: I'm doing so much better at work now. I know how to handle my coworkers better, and things are going so smoothly!

THERAPIST: [After going over the positive changes and celebrating the work that was done] You know, you came to treatment for problems with assertiveness, and you've really improved. What are your feelings about stopping or cutting down on therapy?

This can elicit a range of responses, as follows:

PATIENT 1: I was thinking the same thing on the way here. I really don't need to come as much any more.

PATIENT 2: I think you're right. I don't need to come to therapy any more for assertiveness—I think I've got that problem pretty much under control. But it's funny: As things have been getting better at work, I've been feeling a lot of loneliness and realizing how much I'd like to be married. I was wondering if there are things I can do in therapy that would help me with my relationships.

PATIENT 3: I don't think I'm ready to stop therapy quite yet. I know I've made a lot of changes, but I still don't feel secure that I won't go back to the old ways.

Patients should feel comfortable about ending treatment, and confident that they can maintain the gains made and not get stuck again in old patterns. When patients are nervous or hesitant about termination, these feelings need to be explored. Sometimes this will be an indication of the need for continued therapeutic work; at other times, the process of talking through the fears about ending treatment will result in patients' deciding for themselves that it is an appropriate time to terminate.

Patient Satisfaction

Once the therapist and patient have agreed that therapy is to be terminated or phased out, they can begin a process of reviewing the changes that have happened for the patient. Simply put, the real test of treatment is this: **Has the patient received what he or she sought in coming for therapy?** Are the presenting problems resolved and stable, or at least well on the way to being resolved?

It is also important for patients to have some understanding of **why** the changes have occurred. The better patients are able to understand their patterns, the more able they will be to continue their progress in the future and prevent relapses to previous dysfunctional patterns.

Tapering Therapy Gradually

Termination does not have to be abrupt. Often the frequency of sessions is decreased to once every 2 or more weeks. This allows patients to consolidate the changes with decreasing help from their therapists. Patients learn to navigate on their own during this time, and take over the steering from their therapists. Even after regular sessions have ended, "booster sessions" scheduled on an as-needed basis may be helpful for a while in maintaining the gains of treatment. Behavioral research has provided abundant evidence of the value of booster sessions.

Extending Length of Time between Sessions

Ending therapy may be particularly difficult for people who have suffered painful loss or abandonment. In such cases it may help to taper therapy **very** gradually—first to every other week, then to once a month, then possibly to every 3 months until it is clear that the patients can maintain treatment gains on their own. Even if they never return for help, it helps patients to know that they can return to therapy if they need to.

Therapist Stance: Partner in Review of Treatment and in Celebration of Change

Termination, like every other phase of STDP, should be a collaborative process in which the therapist is an unceasing advocate for the patient's best interests. In the rest of this chapter, we discuss the therapist's role in reviewing and celebrating the changes the patient has made in therapy. In this discussion, we highlight only the therapist's role in introducing the termination process.

Suggesting That Therapy End

When the patient has made substantial progress with the presenting problems, the therapist stance is to encourage ending or cutting down the frequency of therapy as soon as the patient feels comfortable doing so. Of course, the therapist's belief that the patient may no longer need therapy or can begin thinking about termination can be tremendously affirming in itself. When Affect Phobias are well on the way to being resolved, the therapist should show faith and confidence in the patient's potential to guide him- or herself from this point on.

THERAPIST: You could be spending this money on a vacation [or on opera tickets, or on sports events]. Wouldn't you rather be doing that?

PATIENT: That never occurred to me.

THERAPIST: Well, think about it. When you came here, you were very discouraged, and you needed to be here. You wouldn't have been able to enjoy a vacation. But now you are enjoying life a great deal more. Think what you pay for therapy per month, and consider what enjoyment you could have in doing other things.

PATIENT: That's kind of fun to think about—I'd love to go to Ireland. But I'm not sure I'm ready to leave. Are you trying to get rid of me?

THERAPIST: Not at all. You may stay as long as you need. But the goal of therapy is not to **need** therapy any more, so I will be reminding you from time to time about what life holds for you when you are finished.

One important measure of the effectiveness of therapy is patients' increased ability to take joy in their own lives.

Anxiety Regulation: Anticipating and Planning for the Future

Needless to say, the prospect of termination provokes a significant amount of anxiety in most if not all patients. An essential part of the termination process is anticipating future difficulties so that the patient is more prepared to deal with them when they arise, and so that a patient's anxiety is lowered.

Maintaining Gains and Handling Setbacks

Change is not a linear process. There are steps forward, and then a falling-back and starting again. Patients need to understand that they will have setbacks, and they need to be prepared for them. The therapist can "inoculate" the patient by using the mature defense of anticipation, looking at potential future difficulties such as stressful periods, difficulties with relationships due to the changes made, and so forth.

Prepare for Future Difficulties

Maintaining the gains of therapy does not require that a patient stay in therapy. When patients understand why change happened, and know how to prevent or recover from relapses, they will be able to keep the changes growing and evolving outside of therapy. Research on STDP has shown continued improvement in the years following the end of treatment.

Consider the Family System

This process of anticipation should include an assessment of the impact of a patient's change on people around him or her. Often after significant character change has occurred, the patient's spouse/partner or another significant other can be brought into the therapy process to discuss how these changes have affected the relationship. No matter how much work has been accomplished in the therapeutic relationship, it is in loving relationships in the real world that character changes are nourished and sustained.

THERAPIST: Change doesn't just happen evenly and smoothly. You're bound to hit stressful periods and find old defensive patterns occurring.

PATIENT: Yeah, that's good to remember.

THERAPIST: And let's go over your main relationships, and try to imagine what problems might arise because of the different ways you are responding now.

PATIENT: That's a good idea. For example, I don't think my brother will be so pleased that I want to stop going to every one of the family reunions.

Follow-Up and "Booster" Sessions

As discussed previously, maintenance of changes in behavior can be monitored by follow-up sessions every 4, 6, or 8 weeks until patients feel able to sustain changes on their own. Even after treatment has been phased out slowly, booster sessions on a monthly or quarterly basis—or as needed—can be helpful in the first year after termination. Knowing that such sessions are scheduled or can be available can greatly reduce the anxiety of termination.

Booster sessions follow the same format as typical STDP sessions. The problem areas are reviewed, and defenses and affects are dealt with as needed. Patients have already had much practice on their core conflict issues, and should be able to face defenses and explore affects.

THERAPIST: OK, so it sounds like you're stuck in that old familiar pattern. We know you made a lot of progress there, but let's dig down deep into the feelings and see what conflicts are still lingering and giving you trouble.

Patients who undergo rapid and dramatic behavior change in lifelong patterns will usually require booster sessions. Relapse is not uncommon following rapid change, because new habits have not been sufficiently established to maintain the changes. The possibility of returning to therapy does **not** have to be ruled out, but therapists should encourage patient autonomy and limit booster sessions to as few as needed to achieve the treatment objectives.

Help Patients "Take Their Therapists with Them"

One of the most important interventions near the end of therapy is helping patients "take their therapists with them," as in this example:

PATIENT: I just don't know if I'd be able to make it on my own.

THERAPIST: Do you remember how you were having a hard time 2 weeks or so ago, and you said that you imagined what I would have said and it was just like having me there with you?

PATIENT: Yeah, I do.

THERAPIST: Well, as we get closer to termination, let's work toward taking what you have learned here with you. Then, even after we stop seeing each other every week, there's a sense in which you won't be doing it completely on your own.

Here is a more extended illustration:

THERAPIST: As therapy is coming to a close, are there any difficulties that you foresee?

PATIENT: Yes. I can't bear the thought of losing you in my life. Your support has meant so much. I don't know how I will manage, actually.

THERAPIST: I wonder if you can think about taking me with you? Do you know what I mean?

PATIENT: You mean like earlier in treatment, when you would ask me to think about what you felt about me during the week?

THERAPIST: Yes, that is exactly what I mean. Just because we won't see each other on a regular basis doesn't mean that we don't have feelings for each other. What do you think I'll be feeling toward you in the coming months?

PATIENT: Oh, I know you'll be wanting the best for me! (*Tearing up*) You'll be hoping I'm happy and doing well. I really feel that!

THERAPIST: Yes, I will. And can you hold onto that and let that comfort you?

PATIENT: I do that a little already. I'll try to keep it going.

THERAPIST: And do you think you are going to be able to remember the things you learned here and keep that going?

PATIENT: Oh, I'll never forget what I learned. I've changed so much, and even if I have some troubles, I'll never go back to the way I was.

THERAPIST: So I hope that can be the way you will be able to take this therapy with you—and to take me with you as well.

The usefulness of this intervention underscores a point we have tried to make repeatedly throughout this book: Therapeutic change depends at least as much on caring, authentic relationships as on specific "techniques" or "interventions."

II. ASSESSING WHAT CHANGES HAVE BEEN MADE

The following questions can be helpful in assessing the gains made at various stages of treatment, but are particularly important when considering termination. The main issue the therapist needs to consider is this: Have the goals of treatment been reached, or are there areas that still need to be addressed?

1. Can the patient experience nondefensive affect freely in the session? Can he or she be tender, cry, and get angry appropriately?

2. Is this affect expressed adaptively outside therapy? Are there repeated examples of the patient's being appropriately assertive, engaging in appropriate self-expression, feeling appropriately entitled to things, asking for things, crying with others, and feeling tender and connected?

3. How much defensiveness is remaining? How have defenses changed? Have they decreased in number, type, and intensity?

4. Is the patient able to engage in satisfying give-and-take relationships?

5. Is the patient involved in work that is productive and satisfying?

6. Is the core conflict formulation underlying the presenting problems (a) clearly seen, (b) no longer ego-syntonic, and (c) beginning to be replaced by more adaptive responses?

7. Is the patient's sense of self and sense of others more adaptive than maladaptive?

8. Is the patient able to express the wants and needs that were formerly blocked, and able to take in good things from those around him or her?

Assessing the Resolution of the Affect Phobias

To assess the extent to which core conflicts or Affect Phobias have been resolved, it helps to ask specific questions. Here are some examples of questions that may be useful.

Anger/Assertion

THERAPIST 1: How was it for you when I was late for the last session?

THERAPIST 2: So when your mother was going on about the things you didn't want to hear about, what did you say to her?

THERAPIST 3: When you first came in to therapy, I know that it was really hard for you to ask for help from coworkers. How is that for you now?

Grief

THERAPIST 1: I'm remembering back to when we first met, and it was very hard for you just to feel your sadness over your brother's death. Over the last few weeks, you've been able to cry quite freely about it, but I was wondering how that's felt to you?

THERAPIST 2: Just now it looked as though you were tearing up, and then you stopped. What were you feeling, and what got you to stop?

THERAPIST 3: When your brother called you on the anniversary of your father's death, what was your conversation like? I remember you said some time ago that you and he just never talked about that.

Closeness

THERAPIST 1: We're coming to the end of our therapy, and one of the things I'd like to know is this: How have you felt about me and our relationship over the months that we've been seeing each other?

THERAPIST 2: One of the main problems you came here to talk to me about was having a hard time feeling close to your boyfriend. I'm wondering: How does being with him feel now versus when you came in? Are you able to touch him more? Does that feel easier?

THERAPIST 3: You say that you're more able to talk to your friends now about what's going on in your life, and I remember that was hard for you when you first came here. Can you give me an example of a time recently when you were able to talk with a friend more freely?

Positive Feelings toward the Self

THERAPIST 1: You've given me some wonderful examples of times when you were able to set limits with people—something which was very difficult for you when you came into therapy. I'm wondering how it **feels** to you: Do you feel that you genuinely deserve to be treated well, or is this something you kind of have to force yourself to do?

THERAPIST 2: I have the sense that you're not as hard on yourself as you used to be. Is that true?

Using the PAC Forms to Assess Outcome

To assist with the final evaluation, the Psychotherapy Assessment Checklist (PAC) Forms (available from our Web site: www.affectphobia.org), can be readministered at or toward the end of treatment, so that changes can be noted. It may be most useful to readminister the PAC Forms a few sessions before actual termination, as the information they provide will be further evidence for gains made, while identifying any areas of difficulty that still need to be addressed.

For example, change can be seen if the presenting problems (rated on the 1–10 severity scale) were originally rated 8 or above (severe) and are now rated 3 or below (mild). What can the patient do to continue improvement? Are Axis I and Axis II symptoms still present? If so, are they significantly less severe than when treatment began? Is the patient satisfied with the treatment received? The Global Assessment of Functioning (GAF) score at termination can also be used as an indication of progress that the patient has made.

Example: Rating Problem Change

THERAPIST: Let's go over the main changes and see how you've done. There were three core issues we focused on: your inability to grieve your father's death, your shyness over public speaking, and your difficulty in trusting and opening to others. How do you think you're doing on each of these?

PATIENT: Well, I certainly did grieve my father's death, and I feel much better about that whole situation. I was in so much pain when I came, and now I feel much more at peace.

THERAPIST: How would you rate that problem now? On the 1–10 scale?

PATIENT: Oh, it's so hard to put numbers on things—but it's so much better.

THERAPIST: Yes, it is hard to put numbers on things, but could you take a moment and try. If 10 means that "it couldn't be worse," 1 means there is "no problem at all," and 5 means the problem is "moderately disturbing," where would that problem fall?

PATIENT: I guess it would be pretty low. I'm not even moderately upset about it any more. Maybe a 2 or 3.

THERAPIST: OK. You had rated that problem a 9 when you came in—so that's substantial change. Now let's look at the specifics of the change and how you think it came about.

III. ASSESSING WHY CHANGES HAVE BEEN MADE

The Reasons for Change

As treatment nears completion, therapists must help patients review not only **what** changes have occurred, but **why** those changes have occurred. Each change in behavior should, if possible, be made conscious. At this point a patient should be able to give specific examples of change, not vague descriptions. Ask the patient to try to say in his or her own words what led to the changes the patient feels therapy has made. Sometimes this takes 10–15 minutes or more of reviewing how the change came about until it becomes clear. This topic may need to be revisited over several weeks. Often the answer is slow in coming, and it may be entirely different from what is expected. The following patient–therapist exchange illustrates different types of patient statements about the reasons for change:

Responses like this first one suggest that restructuring defenses contributed to the change:

PATIENT: It's not easy to put my finger on it. . . . It seemed to make a difference when you pointed out to me how I was projecting onto people that they were criticizing me, even though they didn't give any real indication of that. When you showed me what I was doing, I thought it was silly of me to do that.

THERAPIST: So seeing that helped you want to give up that way of responding.

Responses like this second one indicate that desensitization of conflicted affects has been helpful in changing problem behaviors:

PATIENT: Yes, but that wasn't all of it. Because I couldn't just **think** my way out of it. What also helped was just getting more comfortable sharing my feelings with people. You helped me be more assertive, and helped me cry—and I didn't feel like such a freak. I was always so afraid that if I showed my feelings in front of people, they would think I was crazy.

Responses such as this last one suggest that Self- and Other-Restructuring has been an important factor in change:

THERAPIST: Is there anything else that you think helped?

PATIENT: I just got more confident about myself. I knew that I had told you all kind of embarrassing things about me, and you didn't think badly of me. In fact, you were always my advocate. So I figured I must not be as awful as I thought.

THERAPIST: That is certainly true. So feeling more comfortable in here helped you feel better in other relationships?

PATIENT: Yes, definitely.

Pinpointing Reasons for Change

The discovery of the reasons for change is often not as clear-cut and straightforward as in the examples above. It often can be very difficult or confusing for patients to describe the change process. An example follows:

PATIENT: You know, it's really hard to say. I remember my boyfriend being less critical with me after I told him that I was mad at him for something he did. It also had something to do with that session when you didn't get mad at me when I came at the wrong time and walked in on the other patient. I don't know why that would make a difference . . . but it did.

THERAPIST: Well, let's take some time and sort this out until it becomes clearer.

It is important that patients know why they changed, and what role they played in their changes. In periods of stress, people have a tendency to slip back to where they were before. Patients who understand the motivating factors behind their behaviors are more likely to be able to reverse a relapse into old patterns. As we shall see in the next section, it helps to discuss this explicitly with patients. (For a detailed case example of assessment of change, see CC, pp. 368–371.)

IV. CELEBRATING PROGRESS AND ACKNOWLEDGING WHAT NEEDS MORE WORK

Examine the Progress of Therapy in a Positive Light

As therapy comes to a close, it is important not only to measure and explain the changes that have occurred, but also to focus on positive feelings about those changes. Many patients are embarrassed by their pride in accomplishment or joy in succeeding. This stage in therapy is an opportunity for exposure to such feelings and a chance to desensitize remaining inhibition.

THERAPIST: It has been quite a journey we have been on together. How does it feel to you, looking back?

PATIENT: I guess I've done OK, haven't I?

THERAPIST: Do you feel just "OK" about all that you have accomplished, or are you holding back on stronger feelings?

PATIENT: Oh, I feel really proud of what I've done—and what we've done together. It's just still hard to let it show. But you've pointed this out to me a number of times, and I shouldn't restrain myself so much. In fact, I'm really, **really** proud of myself!

THERAPIST: And well you should be!

It is important for the therapist to join with the patient in not only noting but also celebrating the fruits of their labor together.

In addition to noting and celebrating the positive changes of therapy, it is important to note whether the patient can state disappointments as well as benefits of treatment fully and openly, since this is a good indicator of the patient's openness to a number of different affects.

THERAPIST: Since we're coming to the end of treatment, let's review the pluses and minuses. I'd like to know how you think therapy helped, but just as important, I'd like to hear what you wanted that you did not get.

PATIENT: Well, I got a lot of help with protecting myself and standing up for myself. That really is better now. But I don't think I have my relationship problems all worked out. I'm still too ready to distance myself from my friends and family [Defense Recognition]. And I don't want to keep doing this [Defense Relinquishing].

THERAPIST: I can hear that you catch yourself when you're distancing yourself, and that you don't want to do that any more. Do you feel able to do something about it in the moment and keep working on building more closeness with others?

PATIENT: Yeah. I've made some changes already . . . but I'm not completely sure I will do it right all the time. I still feel a little awkward with people.

THERAPIST: First of all, as we've talked about before, you won't need to do everything right all the time. You can try to stay more open, and if you find yourself backing off then just think about what was so hard for you, and try to do a little more the next time. [Therapist passes the tools of treatment to the patient.] If you feel stuck, you can always come back for a booster session.

V. EXPLORING THE FULL RANGE OF FEELINGS FOR THE THERAPIST

Expression of Feelings for the Therapist

In addition to celebrating progress and noting disappointments related to the **therapy**, it is important for the patient to be able to express a full range of feelings toward the **therapist**. Again, this is an important opportunity to use the therapeutic relationship to assess and make progress on any residual Affect Phobias about relationships. These feelings may include deeply felt grief about leaving the relationship, positive expressions of appreciation for the work that has been done, and feelings of disappointment about things the patient did not receive from the relationship.

Positive Feelings for the Therapist

It is important for the patient to be able to express positive feelings for the therapist. A way to assess the degree of tenderness the patient is comfortable with is to see how much is shown to the therapist at the end of treatment. Such feelings may have come up spontaneously during treatment, as the patient's life improved, but fond feelings are often expressed again at closure of therapy.

Just as the shared affect between patient and therapist is a vital ingredient throughout this therapy, it is also essential in the termination process for the therapist to be able to express heartfelt positive feelings about how he or she has been affected by working with this patient.

PATIENT: It's meant so much to me to have had your help. My life is so different now, and I couldn't have done it without you! I feel like you've given me an incredible gift and I'll always be grateful to you.

THERAPIST: Thank you. It means a lot to me that you feel this way. One of the real privileges of being a therapist is to be able to accompany people like you on their journey, and so I'm grateful to you, too.

Some patients have a hard time expressing these feelings. Termination can provide another opportunity for desensitization of conflicts about communicating tenderness. When such communications are absent from the last session or two, the therapist should encourage the patient to explore them. Often this is very hard for therapists to do, because it feels like "fishing for compliments." However, patients have a strong need to express positive feelings when treatment has been successful.

PATIENT: [*Blandly, quickly, and looking out the window*] Uh . . . it's been nice coming here.

THERAPIST: The way you say that makes me wonder if you have more feelings than you're letting yourself acknowledge. Let's take a little time to look at the whole range of things you might be feeling.

Often patients have a great deal that they want to say, but that they cannot bring themselves to say. If something is not said, it is often acted out—by giving gifts, or by calls after therapy is over.

THERAPIST: I wonder if you have any feelings toward me as we come to the end of treatment?

PATIENT: Oh, there's a lot I want to say, but it's hard for me to do it.

THERAPIST: What is difficult for you? [Even as therapy ends, anxiety regulation can assist a person's blocked feelings.]

PATIENT: I feel so shy! I don't know what you'd think if I said what I feel.

THERAPIST: I know you remember how often you have let this shyness keep you distant from people, but I've watched you become a lot more open. I wonder if you can push the hesitancy away like you've learned to do?

PATIENT: You're right. And I don't want to leave without telling you this. (*With tears in eyes*) You've saved my life, and I really love you for it.

THERAPIST: I'm really touched to hear that. Thank you so much.

When Does a Therapist Say, "I Love You," to a Patient?

Many patients and therapists have said that it means a huge amount if the therapist can say, "I love you, too," after similar feeling is expressed by the patient at termination. If done professionally and with clear boundaries, it can be very healing (assuming, of course, that it is a genuine expression of the therapist's feelings). There is no definite rule about this. Each therapist must decide what feels appropriate. However, a colleague described the following termination of her own therapy, which stayed with her and soothed her for decades:

PATIENT: (*Saying goodbye*) This is so hard for me to say, but you've meant so much to me and therapy has helped me turn my life around so much . . . that I just want to say, "I love you."

THERAPIST: And I love you, as well.

Negative Feelings toward the Therapist

In addition to being able to express positive feelings toward the therapist, it is very important that the patient be able to express negative feelings. In addition to patients' feelings of loss at the end of therapy—because every therapist at times makes mistakes, has empathic lapses, misses or has to shorten sessions, and so on—patients may also harbor disappointment in the therapist. Ideally, patients should feel safe enough to express these disappointments to the therapist, demonstrate that he or she can get angry with the therapist, be assertive, and openly voice criticisms—all in an adaptive way.

THERAPIST: No relationship is perfect, so I'm wondering: Are there some things you would like to say about how I didn't do all that you had wanted? Did you feel let down by me at any time? How I could have been more helpful?

PATIENT: Well, you know I really got a lot from therapy. But there are some things that bothered me, and I really would like to talk about them. I appreciate your bringing it up, because I might not have. I still carry some resentment about that session when you didn't show up. Although you apologized and I said I understood, I feel like in some way it changed the way I saw you.

THERAPIST: I'm glad you're able to tell me that. Were there things that you held back from saying at that time that might be important to say now?

It is important for the therapist to hear the patient's complaints and make a frank apology when indicated. However, if the anger or criticism is expressed in an explosive manner, it probably indicates a defensive response that should be explored, possibly covering a feeling of rejection or abandonment.

Patient's Need to Mourn the Loss of Therapy

Because of the collaborative nature of STDP and the tendency to phase out treatment gradually, the negative feelings about ending treatment are not usually as intense as they can be in more traditional forms of treatment. Nevertheless, there are still feelings of sadness and loss in separating from a close, supportive relationship, and these need to be addressed.

- Can patients state what they will most miss from the therapy relationship?
- Do they feel able to stand on their own and manage their own lives?
- Can they replace the therapy relationship with close, warm relationships in their lives (see Section VI)?
- Can they "take their therapists with them," so that the ending can be something nourishing rather than depriving (see Section I)?

VI. REPLACING THE LOSS OF THERAPY

Replacing the Therapy Relationship

In preparation for termination, patients need to have built a network of support, both because of its intrinsic value and so that they can continue to work through issues in their lives. The capacity to find and sustain other supportive relationships is at least as important as taking warm and supportive memories of their therapists with them—and probably more so. It is important for the therapist to work directly on building relationships with the patient, as in the following example:

Example: Finding New Supportive Relationships

THERAPIST: You've said that you feel very close to me. Who else is there in your life that you think feels similar to the relationship here?

PATIENT: Oh, I don't feel as close to anyone as I do to you.

THERAPIST: Well, I will do you no service if we create a situation here where you only feel close to **me**. The next step is to find relationships in your life that feel close like ours—or more so. Who in your life now comes closest?

PATIENT: There's no one. I don't trust anybody that much.

THERAPIST: We've worked on that issue a lot, and you do have trouble opening up to people. You know how you've isolated yourself.

PATIENT: Yes, I know I do. And it's not really true that there is no one. You helped me get closer to my neighbor—and she **is** a good friend. She's different from me, but she's nice.

THERAPIST: Then your assignment for the coming weeks, as therapy ends, is to continue building these kind of relationships. Look around you and see who else feels interesting and warm and caring, or who can offer you some good aspects of friendship—even if not a lot.

PATIENT: I think I can do that.

VII. CONCLUSION AND COMMENCEMENT

At the end of Section I, we have talked about the importance of patients' "taking their therapists with them." In a similar way, we hope that you—our readers—will take this therapy with **you.** Ideally, you have already learned skills from this book that will allow you to do more focused, powerful, and time-efficient psychotherapy. Wrestling with the exercises should have allowed you to begin the process of translating the theory we have described into the "hands-on" practice of doing the therapy.

We also hope that you are interested in building further skills and learning more about doing this or related forms of STDP. **On our Web site (www.affectphobia.org),** we discuss the benefits of videotaping your therapy sessions, and the further benefits of using a scale that we provide there to code those videotapes.

You may also want to join a group of therapists learning or practicing STDP, or attend some conferences where you can watch experienced therapists in this and related models of STDP. Our **Web site** provides further information and links to related **Web sites.**

Finally, we have tried to be as specific as we can in this book, giving examples of interventions that have proven effective over the years. However, craft or technique is only part of even the most powerful therapy. The rest is about heart, emotional attunement, clinical intuition, and the inexplicable magic of connection that happens between a therapist and a patient. We hope you will find, as we have, that there is ample room for improvisation and creativity within the structure provided by this model. We also hope that you will find ways to integrate this work into your own practice. Then let us know what you discover, as the work of making psychotherapy more powerful and effective is an ever-evolving science and art, in which we all play a part.

APPENDIX   Answers to Exercises

CHAPTER 1

EXERCISE 1A
Identifying Activating versus Inhibiting Affects

1A.1. Shame (Inhibiting). Causes a cessation of positive feeling. Leads to shutting down, closing off, feeling bad about the self.

1A.2. Grief (Activating). Promotes crying (tears flowing out of the body) and active processing of the loss (including positive tender memories, as well as the pain).

1A.3. Pride (Activating). Causes greater openness, self-confidence, and ability to act.

1A.4. Curiosity (Activating). Motivates exploratory activity, interest, and approach behaviors.

1A.5. Guilt (Inhibiting). Leads to cessation of certain actions that overstep cultural or social regulations/laws/mores.

1A.6. Self-Confidence (Activating). Promotes acting on one's own behalf.

1A.7. Anxiety (Inhibiting). Causes restraint, paralysis of action, doubt, worry. However, fear can also activate behavior, as when fleeing from danger.

1A.8. Justifiable Outrage (Activating). Promotes appropriate action taken to right a wrong. This refers to mature assertion, not the inappropriate acting out of regressive rage.

EXERCISE 1B
Identify the Affect

1B.1. *Pleased by finishing an assignment well.* **Positive feelings about the self (Activating).** These feelings include self-esteem, self-confidence, pride.

1B.2. *Almost crying about Bosnia.* **Grief (Activating).** Tearing up generally represents grief, but it can sometimes represent closeness or joy. Given this topic, our first guess would be grief.

1B.3. *Realizing he is working too hard, and going to bed.* **Positive feelings about the self/self-care (Activating).** Responding to fatigue by stopping what one is doing and going to sleep is caring for oneself.

1B.4. *Speaking up to tell someone to wait his turn.* **Anger/assertion (Activating).**

1B.5. *Felt bad and couldn't look at him.* **Guilt or shame (Inhibiting).** Though "bad" often refers to pain/anguish, the context here suggests that the reaction means guilt over transgressions in behavior, or shame relating to self-image.

EXERCISE 1C
Spot the Affect Phobia

Keep your mind open. These are just some of the possibilities; see if you can think of others. There can be many other possibilities

1C.1. *The concerned father.* **Blocked affect(s): Sexual desire** (he may feel shame about the arousal that touching his daughter may produce); **closeness/ tenderness** (it is possible that the inhibition is not necessarily about sexual feeling, but involves a discomfort with public displays of affection).

1C.2. *The teacher with migraines.* **Blocked affect(s): Anger/assertion** (it may be that he is afraid of asserting himself, and needs to develop the capacity to speak up and set limits); **positive feelings about the self** (often lurking underneath lack of anger/assertion are phobias about feeling entitled or worthy to one's wants or needs).

1C.3. *The married woman who cannot state her needs.* **Blocked affect(s): Anger/ assertion** (she needs to develop the capacity for healthy assertion of her wants and needs); **closeness/tenderness** (there may be lack of trust in other's acceptance of her, or fear of rejection); **positive feelings about the self** (again, lack of assertion or anger can be due to phobias about feeling entitled or worthy).

1C.4. *The young woman who feels like a fraud.* **Blocked affect(s): Positive feelings about the self** (she might feel so much shame associated with her sense of self that she feels unworthy of praise and thus unable to feel self-esteem or self-confidence); **trust in others** (she may also fear that others will attack her).

1C.5. *A young man who cannot have a girlfriend.* **Blocked affect(s): Grief** (it is possible that he cannot grieve because he cannot bear the pain of letting go and moving on, and so his persistent anger may be a way to avoid the grief—being angry and blaming his girlfriend may help avoid more painful feelings); **positive feelings about the self** (he may feel negative about himself—possibly unworthy or like a failure—and thus be unable to feel the self-esteem and self-confidence needed to seek a new girlfriend).

1C.6. *Anxious while sitting in her garden.* **Blocked affect(s): Enjoyment or joy** (people who have been highly defended for many years will often panic as they begin to relax their hypervigilant style, because they suddenly feel vulnerable—as though they will be attacked or something bad will happen; then relaxing and feeling joy is very difficult or impossible).

1C.7. *The man with panic about children.* **Blocked affect(s): Self-confidence** (he may be unable to feel self-confidence about his ability to be a good father); **closeness/tenderness** (he may be afraid of the intimacy, responsibility, or commitment of family life); **anger/assertion** (he may fear that he will not be able to negotiate successfully with her about important issues, such as when or when not to have children). (If he could do so, he would be much less likely to have a panic attack.)

Again, you may be able to think of possibilities other than the ones above. Remember that no hypothesis is valid until it rings true to the patient and fits with the historical data of the patient's life.

CHAPTER 2

EXERCISE 2A
Identify Poles on the Triangle of Conflict

2A.1. avoid my eyes (D). **2A.2.** guilty (A). **2A.3.** intellectualize (D). **2A.4.** nervous (A). **2A.5.** angry (F). **2A.6.** uncomfortable (A). **2A.7.** longing (F—closeness or grief, depending on the context). **2A.8.** grief (F).

EXERCISE 2B
Identify Poles on the Triangle of Person

2B.1. My sister (P—early-life family member). **2B.2.** In here (T—referring to therapy or the therapist). **2B.3.** Your father and grandfather (P and P). **2B.4.** My boss (C). **2B.5.** Your mother (P). **2B.6.** My wife (C). **2B.7.** Aunt Margaret (P). **2B.8.** To therapy (T). **2B.9.** Your brother (P—early-life family member). **2B.10.** My son (C).

EXERCISE 2C
Identify the Poles of the Two Triangles: D-A-F-T-C-P

2C.1. THERAPIST: It seems you get distant [D] and irritable [D—defensive feeling] whenever closeness [F] comes up between you and your wife [C], just like with your mother [P]. You seem to have some fear [A] that silences you [D] and makes you avoid [D] being close and loving [F]. Does this pattern I describe seem right to you?

2C.2. THERAPIST: I notice that you change the subject [D] with me [T] whenever you become sad [F] over your brother's [P] death. These feelings may be too painful to bear [A]—and have made you depressed [D] and numb [D] rather than able to grieve [F]. What do you think?

EXERCISE 2D
Identify the Poles of the Two Triangles: D-A-F-T-C-P

2D.1. THERAPIST: It's true, they really don't pay me anything like what other people get for what I do. The owner [C] told me they can't afford to pay me any more, but I notice he just built a huge new house. I shut down [D] when I get angry [F] at him [C]. I could send out my resumé [F—anger/assertion], but I would feel like such a traitor [A—shame/guilt/pain] to pursue another job [F—anger/assertion]. I just keep hoping that he'll figure out what I'm worth and give me a raise [D, rationalizing, passivity, denial].

2D.2. PATIENT: When my boyfriend [C] told me that he wanted to leave me for her [C], I just got so depressed [A—pain; D—passivity, helplessness] and so aggravated with myself [D—self-attack]. I've sacrificed everything to make him happy [D—masochism, martyrdom], and somehow I'm still not good enough [D—self-attack]. My friends tell me he's not good for me and I should leave him [F—assertion], but I just love him too much [D—rationalization and excessive longing, therefore defensive]—.

2D.3. PATIENT: I was stone-faced [D] at my husband's [C] funeral, and I really haven't cried [F] since. I look at my daughter [C] crying [F] uncontrollably, and it's just so embarrassing [A]. I can't stand it [A—expression of emotional pain].

EXERCISE 2E
What Does a Defensive Feeling Look Like?

2E.1. *Defensive Tenderness:* Behaviors 2 (exaggerated affection), 3 (calling spouse "sweetie" when angry), and 5 (sugary sweetness) can be forms of defensive tenderness. Behaviors 1 (ignoring presence of another) and 4 (negativity toward others) may be defenses **against** being tender (or other feelings).

2E.2. *Defensive Anger:* Behaviors 2 (violent reaction to minor incident), 3 (finger pointing), 5 (picking on someone), and 6 (tantrums) are ways that anger can be used in a defensive or maladaptive way. Behaviors 1 (biting humor), and 2 (saying nonsense) may be defensive ways to **avoid** expressing anger (or other feelings) directly.

2E.3. *Defensive Sadness:* Behaviors 2 (crying in the middle of an argument, to avoid anger) and 3 (pathological mourning that does not resolve, to block negative feelings about the loss) can both be examples of sadness used defensively. Behavior 1 (manic addiction to exercise or shopping) can be a defensive way to avoid sadness. Behavior 4 (being happy when the person one is jealous of loses out) presents a more complex picture. Taking pleasure in someone's pain (something everyone does from time to time) is a defense—a form of sadism, to a greater or lesser degree—that helps to avoid one's own sadness and pain over not having whatever is desired. Severe cases of sadism can also reflect a very fragile and tormented sense of self. Sadism is a defense against the positive feelings of self. It can also be a barrier to self-confidence that could lessen the jealousy or envy by helping the individual feel worthy or capable of attaining what is desired.

2E.4. *Defensive Excitement:* Behaviors 2 (frenzied planning of a wedding to an unfaithful lover), 3 (loud displays of "I'm thrilled!"), and 4 (frantic activity after a loss) can be examples of defensive excitement. Behavior 1 (lack of interest) can be boredom or depression—which can be a defense against any of the activating feelings.

2E.5. *Defensive Sexual Desire:* Behaviors 2 (initiating sex when an argument seems likely) and 3 (sex without intimacy) can be defensive uses of sexual desire. Behaviors 1 (frequent arguing before going to bed), 4 (excessive need for a platonic closeness), and 5 (the feeling of being ugly and unloved) can all be defensive ways to avoid sexual feelings (or other feelings).

CHAPTER 3

EXERCISE 3A
Match the Patient with a GAF Interval

3A.1. The Crying Daughter

Specific Areas of functioning: Psychological: 61–70. **Social:** 71–80 or above. **Occupational:** 71–80 or above.

Current GAF rating: 61–70. **GAF rating for the past year:** 81–90.

Explanation: Crying when one's mother has just died unexpectedly is healthy and normal. It is also within normal range in a grief process to regret things left unsaid. If this were the extent of her distress, she would receive a score of 71–80 for a "transient and expectable" reaction to the death of her mother. However, she appears to be feeling a lot of guilt and ruminating about this as well as losing sleep, which suggests "mild symptoms" in the 61–70 range. Her social and school functioning is otherwise good, given the circumstances.

Prior to her mother's death, she had good functioning in all areas and was generally satisfied with life—placing her at least in the lower end of the 81–90 category. For her to receive scores in the higher end of this category, more information would be needed about whether she was involved in a wide range of activities and was socially effective. To fall in the 91–100 category, she would need to describe situations where she was sought out by others.

3A.2. The Student with Suicidal Thoughts

Specific functioning: Psychological: 21–30. **Social:** 51–60. **Occupational:** 41–50.

Current GAF rating: 21–30. **GAF rating for the past year:** 51–60.

Explanation: His functioning is moderately impaired in two areas (social and occupational/schoolwork), with serious psychological symptoms (plans for suicide). His moderate impairment in social functioning is based on his feeling of alienation from most of his classmates and his inability to join groups or team sports. However, he does have a few friends, and this keeps him from being rated as seriously impaired socially (e.g., no friends; 41–50). His current GAF score is 21–30, reflecting his constant preoccupation with suicide.

During the past year, his school performance and mood were good (the 71–80 range), but his social functioning and avoidance of social groups always indicated moderate difficulty (51–60 range). Thus his highest rating in the past year could not be higher than 51–60.

3A.3. The Anxious Head Nurse

Specific functioning: Psychological: 51–60. **Social:** 81–90 or above. **Occupational:** 91–100.

Current GAF rating: 51–60. **GAF rating for the past year:** 91–100.

Explanation: His occupational functioning is superior (he is highly respected and sought out by others), which puts him in the 91–100 range. His social functioning is also very good (in the 81–90 range or higher), because conflicts are few and he is able to work through them well. However, his current symptoms of anxiety and occasional panic attacks place him in the 51–60 range. His current GAF rating (51–60) is based on the lowest of the three categories. In addition, there are several factors to consider about his alcohol problem. First, his history of drinking means he has had a problem with impulse control, which would be an additional concern for doing the uncovering and potentially destabilizing work of STDP. His sobriety for 2 years is a sign that he is in the process of developing better control. However, his current anxiety and panic attacks indicate that he is in a vulnerable period and needs to feel more stable before uncovering work in STDP can be done.

In contrast, for most of the past 2 years he demonstrated superior functioning in all areas, was sought out by others, and kept his problems in hand with the help of AA. Thus his GAF score for the past year, previous to this illness, would fall in the range of 91–100 for his superior functioning in all areas.

3A.4. The Irritable Stockbroker

Specific functioning: Psychological: 51–60. **Social:** 51–60. **Occupational:** 51–60.

Current GAF rating: GAF: 51–60. **GAF rating for the past year:** 51–60.

Explanation: The level of insomnia and irritability he's having would be rated in the 51–60 range, because it is intermittent and moderate in level (i.e., he still maintains his relationships, but he has conflicts). The relationships with moderate conflicts put him in the 51–60 range for social functioning. His occupational functioning is in the same range (51–60) because he maintains his job, but with moderate conflicts.

His GAF rating for the past year is the same as his current GAF rating, due to his sleeplessness and irritability, his chronic problems at work, and his inability to confide in friends all have been long standing.

EXERCISE 3B
Rate the Patient and
Choose a Predominant
Intervention Style

3B.1. The Divorced Secretary

Psychological functioning: 51. Her level of depression and the severity of her self-attacking defenses (e.g., her partner's unfaithfulness "proves" that she does not deserve to have someone reliable and successful) seem a little worse than "moderate" impairment. However, she does not have suicidal ideation or other indications of severe depression, so we rate her on the lower end of the moderate range.

Social functioning: 55. Although many aspects of her social functioning as a parent and friend could be rated higher, her social rating falls in the category of moderate impairment, due to her ongoing involvement in destructive relationships and occasionally lashing out at her children.

Occupational functioning: 85. She is a single mother of two children who has managed to complete a 2-year degree, obtain a good job, and become a very steady employee.

Current GAF rating: 51 (the lowest of the three ratings).

GAF rating for the past year: 58. Although in the past year the unfaithfulness had not become known, she had occasional conflicts with her partner, which would have placed her at the higher end of the 51–60 range. If moderate conflicts in relationships are 55 (54–56 range), then occasional conflicts would fall within 57–60. Frequent conflicts would fall in the 51–53 range. Ratings at this level of specificity are difficult to make, and absolute precision should not be expected. We try to estimate—depending on the severity of the problem(s)—whether the rating would fall in the high, medium, or low end of the range.

Would you use relatively more exploratory or supportive interventions? A careful balance of both, though given the severity of her self-attack, it may be necessary to use more **supportive** interventions and Self- and Other-Restructuring initially.

3B.2. The Estranged Architect

Psychological functioning: 41. This patient appears to be seriously depressed, based on her poor self-care, diminished appetite, and memory problems.

Social functioning: 51. She appears completely isolated from family, but has one close friend.

Occupational functioning: 41. Unable to hold a job. Her inability to work reflects serious, long-standing impairment that has seemed to worsen over several years' time.

Current GAF rating: 38. GAF rating for the past year: 45. Currently she has "major impairment in several areas." Therefore, according to the GAF Scale, her overall GAF rating should be lowered to the 31–40 category, even though her three scores range from 41 to 51. Because she does have one close friend, she is given a rating in the high 30s. During the past year she had a better appetite and better self-care, so her GAF rating is somewhat higher for that period.

Would you use relatively more exploratory or supportive interventions? Supportive. This patient should not be exposed to exploratory or uncovering interventions until she is functioning better. She would be better served by a supportive, cognitive-behavioral approach to treatment. A day treatment program that provides daily structure might be more beneficial initially than individual therapy.

3B.3. The Depressed Engineer

Psychological functioning: 55. This patient is experiencing significant self-blame, poor energy, dysphoria, and feelings of worthlessness and failure, putting him in the range of moderate symptoms.

Social functioning: 61. He is well liked by professors and by peers, and generally has had good relationships with them. But he does not experience much pleasure from these associations currently, because of feeling that he has to put on a happy face.

Occupational functioning: 65. He is generally doing well in school, but currently feels overwhelmed by pressures and is falling a little behind, which places him in the mild range.

Current GAF rating: 55. GAF rating for the past year: 65. Last year his functioning in all areas was fairly good with only mild difficulties noted, so he would fall in the middle of the 61–70 range.

Would you use relatively more exploratory or supportive interventions? A balance—but more supportive than exploratory, with careful attention to his urges for drug use. It would be important not to uncover a level of painful feelings that would worsen his already tenuous functioning.

CHAPTER 4

**EXERCISE 4A
How People Defend**

4A.1. *Anger can be defended against by:* Becoming passive and withdrawn (e.g., not speaking, going to sleep); attacking the self (e.g., feeling like a jerk, undeserving); intellectualizing (e.g., "I'm not mad, I'm just confused").

4A.2. *Enthusiasm can be defended against by:* Playing it cool; acting indifferent or uninterested; putting down others who show enthusiasm; leaving or avoiding the situation.

4A.3. *Closeness can be defended against by:* Doing the opposite (acting indifferent or as if there is no tenderness or attraction); acting gruff or angry; staying busy with other things; avoiding social situations.

4A.4. *Self Compassion can be defended against by:* Putting self down; giving someone else credit; denying compliments.

**EXERCISE 4B
Identify D-A-F-T-C-P**

4B.1. THERAPIST: It seems as though whenever you're in a situation where au-
  <u>C</u>   <u>A</u>   <u>D</u>
thority figures can evaluate you, you get <u>anxious</u> and <u>withdraw</u>, rather
       <u>F</u>
than <u>feel self-confident</u>. Do you see it that way?

4B.2. THERAPIST: Can you see how you may be using <u>anger</u> to <u>avoid</u> <u>closeness</u>
                                                    <u>D</u>   <u>C</u>   <u>D</u>   <u>D</u>   <u>F</u>
and to <u>push away</u> <u>your wife</u>?
                   <u>D</u>

4B.3. THERAPIST: So your tendency to <u>lighten up</u> seems to result from your
          <u>A</u>   <u>F</u>
feeling <u>ashamed</u> of showing your <u>sad feelings</u>. And this happens not
         <u>T</u>   <u>C or P</u>
only with <u>me</u>—but with <u>anyone</u>. Does that sound right to you?

4B.4. THERAPIST: Instead of allowing your tender feelings [F] to emerge, it seems as though you need to make yourself aloof [D] and distant [D] from people close to you [C or P] so you won't be hurt [A].

4B.5. THERAPIST: It seems like you deny [D] feeling proud [F] of yourself because of the discomfort [A] you feel about this emotion [F]. We have seen it with your parents [P] and your wife [C], and maybe in here with me [T] as well. What do you think?

<table>
<tr><td valign="top">

EXERCISE 4C
Formulate Core
Conflicts or Affect
Phobias

</td><td valign="top">

4C.1. The Worried Roommate

Defensive behaviors: Obsessive rumination, excessive worry, loss of sleep. Another defense is holding back from speaking up—passivity. However, if she spoke to her roommates about turning down the heat, it would only perpetuate her unnecessary guilt—which she admits is "crazy."

Inhibitory feelings: Guilt over self-gratification—whether it is spending money or having a warm apartment.

Adaptive activating feelings: Enjoyment/joy, or possibly care for self. This person is missing out on pleasurable experience. Healthy assertion is also a possible affect, because the student is not able to tell her roommate that she is upset. But the core issue is not only lack of assertion; it is the inability to enjoy her situation. It is important to keep in mind that assertion (though adaptive in other situations) could be a way, in this situation, to maintain her guilt and self-denial.

4C.2. The Distressed Virgin

Defensive behaviors: Finding fault with prospective boyfriends, perfectionism, pickiness, and excessive criticism. Also, loss of interest in the young men and loss of sexual attraction.

Inhibitory feelings: We don't have enough information yet. The inhibitory feeling could be shame over the self that is projected onto the men she dates, or possibly anxiety over being close, but at this point we would only be speculating.

Adaptive activating feelings: Closeness/tenderness, sexual desire, or possibly enjoyment in general. Again, we need more information.

4C.3. Top of the Class

Defensive behaviors: Anxiety or panic-like symptoms, avoidant behavior, inability to work.

Inhibitory feelings: Anxiety (possibly leading to the queasy stomach), dread over writing,

Adaptive activating feelings: Unclear from his report thus far, but feelings that are blocked might include (1) anger/assertion at parents, due to performance demands; (2) developmental issues related to graduating and taking on adult responsibilities (e.g., self-confidence and/or grief over lack of care).

</td></tr>
</table>

4C.4. The Blown Top

Defensive behaviors: Distancing (not talking); explosive, defensive anger (blowing his top); avoiding family (staying at office to avoid an explosion).

Inhibitory feelings: Possibly anxiety about closeness, or about appropriately asserting himself. There may also be guilt or shame about his sense of self, which makes him feel unentitled to closeness or assertion. Note that the fear of blowing his top and the guilt about doing so are associated with his "acting-out" defenses—they are **not** a block to activating feeling.

Adaptive activating feelings: Not clear yet, but may be closeness, or anger/assertion, or the lack of positive feelings about the self.

4C.5. The Wallflower

Defensive behaviors: Social withdrawal, sitting alone (acting like a wallflower), drinking to relax.

Inhibitory feelings: Anxiety and tension about saying the wrong thing.

Adaptive activating feelings: Self-acceptance, assertion and closeness/trust toward others, and enjoyment.

4C.6. The Overtime Worker

Defensive behaviors: Passivity (trouble asking for things, waiting for the boss to notice); overfunctioning (doing a lot of overtime).

Inhibitory feelings: Fear of rejection, fear of being turned down, possibly shame over self-worth.

Adaptive activating feelings: Assertion/anger, self-confidence.

4C.7. The Overspender

Defensive behaviors: Acting out (compulsive shopping, eating, and drinking—lack of impulse control); externalization (reliance on parents for limit setting); possibly defensive anger toward parents, acted out by spending their money.

Inhibitory feelings: Insufficient inhibitory affects to modulate behavior. Some adaptive levels of fear, guilt or shame are needed for self-control. However, there seem to be excessive shame-related feelings of inadequacy, due to lack of impulse control.

Adaptive activating feelings: Positive feelings toward self (self-care that leads to self-control through setting adaptive limits on own behavior).

4C.8. Her Mother's "Crutch"

Defensive behaviors: Numbing herself to emotional pain; distracting self and boosting self-image by caretaking for others; self-criticism for expressing emotions; externalization by acting as her mothers "crutch" to feel good about herself; defensive weepiness rather than a grief that is relieving.

Inhibitory feelings: Shame over expressing sadness or showing weakness. Shame over poor sense of self.

Adaptive activating feelings: Anger, grief, and positive feelings for the self. Anger may have been warded off in this case because she was doing so much for her mother. Her mother may have relied too heavily on her.

There is also some indication that her mother did not acknowledge feelings as a general rule, so the patient may not feel entitled to any of these feelings.

CHAPTER 5

EXERCISE 5A
Point Out Defenses

5A.1. **What the therapist might say to point out the defense:** Is it possible that you tense up [D] because of anxiety or shame [A] over your perfectly natural [anxiety regulation and supportive comment] sexual feelings [F]? [In this case, the Affect Phobia seems more likely to be about sexual feelings than about closeness, given her close and caring relationship with her husband.]

5A.2. **What the therapist might say to point out the defense:**

Possibility 1: I wonder if when you speak up you might be overly sensitive [A—pain] to people's reactions, and then shut down [D] too quickly, rather than saying what's on your mind [F—assertion]? What do you think?

Possibility 2: What proof is there that people never listen or are annoyed with you? Is that really happening, or could it be possible that you are expecting that to happen [D—projection] when it might not be so? Sometimes we can all imagine a situation as much more negative than it actually is. [Normalizing and supportive comment] Do you think that might be possible?

5A.3. **What the therapist might say to point out the defense:**

Possibility 1: It takes a lot of strength to grin and bear it to get through all you have, and that is admirable [supportive comment]. You say it's no big deal [D—denial or minimization], but I wonder if you avoid a lot of strong feelings [F] underneath that "grin and bear it" philosophy [D—excessive stoicism].

Possibility 2: It is true that bad things happen to everyone, but does that mean they have no feelings about it? I wonder if you might be rationalizing [D] as a way to avoid feeling? Of course, that is a very useful strategy when there is nothing else to be done, and it takes strength to do so [supportive comment]. But now here in therapy, there is the opportunity to experience things that you may not have been able to before.

5A.4. **What the therapist might say to point out the defense:** I notice that you nod and agree with me [D—compliance] a lot. I wonder if there is a silenced voice down inside you [D] that might not always agree [F—assertion]? What do you think? (*Later*) In this office, you are allowed to say whatever is on your mind [supportive comment]. Do you feel safe enough to try that?

EXERCISE 5B
Link Defenses, Feelings, and Anxieties

5B.1. *Patient speaks rarely*

Point out the defenses: You've been very silent [D]. I wonder what the silence might be doing?

Link defense to feeling: Could there be feelings [F] that you might be blocking with your silence [D]?

Explore anxieties: Is it difficult [A] or uncomfortable [A] for you to speak up [F] in here [T]?

5B.2. *Patient feels hopeless*

Point out the defenses: Have you considered that your hopelessness [D] might be protecting you from something?

Link defense to feeling: I wonder if that hopelessness [D] might be blocking something that is deeply wished for or longed for [F—interest/ excitement]? Or maybe you do not feel that you deserve to get what you want. Does either of these possibilities ring true to you? [Note: Hopelessness might also be a way to avoid assertion, which might also need to be explored.]

Explore anxieties: Could you be terrified [A] to let yourself hope [F] for anything?

5B.3. *Patient cries helplessly when focused on anger*

Point out the defenses: You know, when we were talking about anger, you quickly became weepy **[D]**.

Link defense to feeling: I wonder if the weepiness **[D]** might be blocking the anger **[F]**?

Explore anxieties: What is the most difficult thing **[A]** for you about feeling anger?

5B.4. *Patient avoids eye contact with the therapist*

Point out the defense: I have noticed that you look past me [D] when you speak. Are you aware of doing that?

Link defense to feeling: Do you think that by **not** making eye contact [D], you might be putting up a barrier to avoid [D] some feelings of closeness [F] here with me [T]?

Explore anxieties: I wonder if there is some anxiety [A] about looking at me? [And the therapist can add:] It's important that you feel safe and comfortable here. So can we explore these fears [A] so that you can begin to feel more at ease [F] with me [T] and able to do the work of therapy?

5B.5. *Patient changes subject away from self-esteem*

Point out the defenses: Did you notice that you just changed the subject [D]? Is there some reason that you might have done that?

Link defense to feeling: We were discussing how you felt about yourself [F] when that happened. Do you think there might be a connection to your changing the subject then [D]?

Explore anxieties: Did you notice any discomfort [A] related to feeling good about yourself [F]?

5B.6. *Patient lightens up to avoid sadness*

Point out the defense: You know, we were talking about your father's death, and now you seem very lighthearted [D] in the way you are speaking. Can you see that?

Link defense to feeling: Each time you seem to be on the verge of tears [F], you seem to back away and lighten up [D]. Do you think you avoid [D] your sadness [F] this way?

Explore anxieties: What's the hardest [A] thing about just staying with the sad feelings [F] for a while?

<table>
<tr>
<td valign="top">

EXERCISE 5C
Validate Defenses

</td>
<td valign="top">

5C.1. **What the therapist might say to validate the defense:** It's understandable [validation] that you would have become numb [D] when you need to cry [F] if it is has been so hard [A] to do for so many years. [The therapist could then explore the anxieties:] Can you remember the last time that you were able to cry [F]? What was the hardest [A] or most unbearable [A] part of it?

5C.2. **What the therapist might say to validate the defense:** It's no wonder [validation] you'd tend to express your anger indirectly [D] with your wife [C] if you think it will make the situation worse. [And, to explore this further the therapist might add:] Is this really the case? Has this happened before? What other way might you approach her?

5C.3. **What the therapist might say to validate the defense:** You know, grief [F] can feel overwhelming [A] at first, and people go through it at their own speed. It's not unusual [validation—normalizing] for people to shut their feelings off [D] immediately after a death. [To help regulate the anxiety, the therapist could say:] We can explore these feelings in doses you can bear, so that they do not become overwhelming for you.

5C.4. **What the therapist might say to validate the defense:** When subjects are so uncomfortable to even think about, it is not unusual to try to avoid them [validation]. So I can see [validation] why you might avoid talking [D]. [And to continue, the therapist might explore the anxieties:] What's the most uncomfortable part of talking about it?

5C.5. **What the therapist might say to validate the defense:** Of course you feel uncomfortable with joy [validation]. That was the whole message you got—first from your uptight parents [P], then from your very strict boarding school teachers [P]. What child wouldn't learn to devalue spontaneity [validation] if punishment was given for being playful [F—enjoyment] or spontaneous [F—interest or excitement]? [And the therapist might add, in trying to restructure the defenses:] Is that something you want to think differently about now and try to change?

</td>
</tr>
<tr>
<td valign="top">

EXERCISE 5D
Point Out Strengths

</td>
<td valign="top">

5D.1. **What the therapist might say to point out strengths:** Then doesn't it takes a lot of courage to come to therapy and bare your soul [strengths], when being close is so frightening [A] that you avoid people [D]?

5D.2. **What the therapist might say to point out strengths:** It sounds like you've been through really terrible times—yet you've kept going through it all [strengths]. When you're feeling that bad [D—depression or self-attack], it takes a lot of strength to get to work at all.

5D.3. **What the therapist might say to point out strengths:** But caring for an ill aunt does take up so much of your time [validation]. I wonder if you can put your disorganization [D] into more perspective when you consider all that you are handling at this point [strengths].

</td>
</tr>
</table>

CHAPTER 6

EXERCISE 6A
Identify the Benefits and Costs of Defenses

What might be possible gains or losses for each of the following defensive behaviors?

6A.1. Defensive behavior: Passivity and intermittent outbursts of temper.

Possible benefits: *Primary gain*: This teacher may be using passivity to avoid conflicts about angry/assertive feelings. *Secondary gain*: Sense of self as helpful and generous. The temper outbursts, though embarrassing, also may give him a secondary gain—a reward—of feeling some fleeting sense of power or dominance.

Possible costs: He ends up doing a lot of things he would rather not do, and missing out on opportunities to do enjoyable things. This leads to his feeling depressed. Another possible cost is becoming socially isolated because people tend to avoid those they perceive as "long-suffering" or unpredictably explosive.

6A.2. Defensive behavior: Taking care of others. Minimizing problems. Not speaking up.

Possible benefits: *Primary gain*: These defenses help her avoid feelings that she is probably uncomfortable with, such as anger and closeness with the therapist. *Secondary gain*: She can appear strong, not needy, and pleasant to be around—thus trying to preserve a positive connection to the therapist.

Possible costs: By minimizing problems, she deprives herself of her therapist's attention to important problem areas. She also deprives herself of one of the best ways for learning new, more adaptive interpersonal behavior: the relationship with the therapist.

6A.3. Defensive behavior: Inability to work productively. Possible denial of grief over losses.

Possible benefits: *Primary gain*: He may be avoiding pain of grieving his family's death. *Secondary gain*: Avoiding grieving may also help him preserve a sense of connection with the family. Not being successful can help him avoid "survivor guilt"—over succeeding when deceased loved ones have lost their opportunity to do so.

Possible costs: He feels "stuck" vocationally. There is a lack of enjoyment and satisfaction at work. He may be depressed. Also, lack of closeness to others is a possibility and will need to be considered.

6A.4. Defensive behavior: Irrationally picking fights with boyfriend.

Possible benefits: *Primary gain*: The therapist needs to spend some time going over their relationship and helping her sort it out. She could be avoiding closeness, intimacy, or commitment. On the other hand, it may be that she truly wants to break up, but her sense of self is not strong enough to do so in a mature, assertive manner. She may not be self-confident enough for her to disagree with her parents that he is not perfect for her, and her acting out and indirectness help her to avoid conflict over assertion and possibly sense of self. *Secondary gain*: This may be an opportunity for her to oppose her parents in an indirect way and thus not be controlled by them.

Possible costs: The acting out can prevent true closeness in an open, mutual relationship. In any case, it is generating a poor sense of self. She calls herself "a witch," and feels ashamed of her behavior.

6A.5. **Defensive behavior:** Inhibited sexual arousal possibly due to guilt from early life experiences with sisters.

Possible benefits: Primary gain: He may be avoiding conflict over sexual feelings, closeness, and/or assertion. *Secondary gain*: Lack of sexual arousal may help him avoid any behavior that might be construed as sexually exploitative in any way.

Possible costs: The sexual inhibition can cause problems with his relationship, and with self-confidence or self-esteem. He also prevents himself from having sexual pleasure.

EXERCISE 6B
Identify the Origins
and the Maintenance
of the Defenses

6B.1. **Defensive Behavior:** Doing projects and avoiding his family

What the therapist might say about origins of the defenses: It makes perfect sense that, growing up in your family, you would get the message that it's really not safe just to hang out with people you're close to.

What the therapist might say about maintenance of the defenses: But now it's keeping you so distant from your family. And the more your family members express their upset over your distance, the more flawed and unworthy you feel, so you wind up pulling away even more.

6B.2. **Defensive Behavior:** Making jokes. Changing the subject when dealing with grief-related issues.

What the therapist might say about origins of the defenses: That kind of grief is so painful, it can seem unbearable to go through it alone. When you were growing up, there were never any models of how to handle sad feelings. Also, you were given the strong message that crying was for "sissies," so there was never anyone to cry with. No wonder you avoid these feelings.

What the therapist might say about maintenance of the defenses: Your strength and your courage are important and admirable things about you. But in this case, you are continuing your family's overly stoic style, and you are carrying it into the future, with negative effects on you. Now you are in a situation where therapy can help you, and it would be a shame to maintain this avoidance when it is no longer necessary. What do you think?

6B.3. **Defensive Behavior:** Depressed feelings appear to block anger.

What the therapist might say about origins of the defenses: It makes sense; you were constantly told growing up that you could never fight, and had no right to get angry with people or assert any of your own needs.

What the therapist might say about maintenance of the defenses: So now any time an angry or assertive feeling starts to rear its head, you feel unentitled to it. And if you can never meet your own needs or set your own limits, the anger gets turned around on you, into self-attack, and you wind up feeling depressed. Even if you and your mother have a biological predisposition to depression, these self-attacking behaviors may be bringing it out. Does that fit with your understanding?

EXERCISE 6C
**Help Patients Grieve
the Costs of Defenses**

6C.1. Defensive Behavior: Numbing of feelings of grief

What the therapist might say to intensify: It's sad to see the way this numbness has robbed you of the enjoyment of life—for so many years now. It must have siphoned off so much richness in living.

What the therapist might say to lighten up: Many people numb themselves when in pain. [Support—normalization] You were so alone, it must have felt overwhelming to face those feelings all by yourself in the weeks and months after she died, and of course you would need to do something to dull the pain. [Validation] Despite this, it is impressive is how well you continued to function—working, caring for your wife and children. [Pointing out strengths/Putting defenses in perspective]

6C.2. Defensive Behavior: Lack of eye contact. Avoidance of closeness.

What the therapist might say to intensify: Averting your eyes may seem like a small thing, but you came into therapy talking about your difficulty finding a life partner, and you've been isolated and lonely for so many years. Your distance in here with me may be the "tip of the iceberg." You may have been inadvertently—and tragically—keeping people away who wanted to be close to you. You may have done this by not looking at them and thereby giving an impression of being disinterested. Does that seem possible?

What the therapist might say to lighten up: Eye contact is something that is often avoided in our culture. [Support] I think you may avoid eye contact to keep yourself feeling safe, and that is a way to protect yourself, when you cannot bear to be hurt. [Validation] Yet, in spite of keeping people at a distance, you've also managed to be a responsible and capable employee at your job. [Pointing out strengths/putting defenses in perspective] Can you give yourself credit for that?

6C.3. Defensive Behavior: Excessive house cleaning or "busy-ness" to avoid sexual pleasure.

What the therapist might say to intensify: Not only has this excessive cleaning robbed you of one of life's great pleasures, but it's threatening the whole fabric of your relationship with Elaine, and it sounds like it was a significant factor in a couple of other breakups. How tragic to diminish the amount of love in your life that way. Are you able to feel at all sad for yourself when you look at it this way?

What the therapist might say to lighten up: How sad to hear how you're struggling with this. [Support] You've had the "double whammy"—not just of the shame in your family around being a lesbian, but the shame there was around any kind of sexuality. I don't think there's a kid in the world who could come through that without some conflicted feelings about sexuality. [Validation] In spite of that, you've built some very strong relationships. There's genuine closeness between you and Elaine, and I'm touched by the very real kindness you show to one another. [Pointing out strengths/putting defenses in perspective]

EXERCISE 6D
**Identify the Hidden
Meanings of Defenses**

There can be many possible hidden or symbolic meanings behind these defensive thoughts and behaviors. We offer more than one example, but you may think of others.

6D.1. *I absolutely must look my best.* **Possible meanings:** (1) "People will laugh at me." (2) "I won't be liked." (3) "I'm unattractive and unappealing."

6D.2. *Those people are talking about me.* **Possible meanings:** (1) "Everyone hates me." (2) "At least someone is paying attention to me."

6D.3. *Why don't they realize how great I am?* **Possible meanings:** (1) "People should know how great I am without my having to tell them." (2) "I feel horrible about myself and keep hoping others will tell me differently." (3) "My parents loved every move I made; why doesn't everyone else?"

6D.4. *Inability to start tasks on one's own.* **Possible meanings:** (1) "I probably will fail, so why bother starting?" (2) "People will yell at me the way my mother did, so this way I won't get blamed." (3) "I am terrified that I might succeed. I couldn't handle the responsibility. I might not be able to keep it up."

6D.5. *Inability to throw things away.* **Possible meanings:** (1) "I am attached to where I came from and want to hold onto it". (2) "I do not feel secure with myself and it is safer to have all my things around me." (3) "If I change anything, it will only make things worse." (4) "If I didn't have these objects, then I would have nothing left [or I wouldn't have her love any more]." Note that this problem may be a different way of describing a problem about collecting things. Defenses can be described in many different ways.

6D.6. *Kicking the dog.* **Possible meanings:** (1) "At least I'm not just taking it all day long. I can dish it out too." (2) "I'm in so much pain that I want someone else to feel the same way with me." (3) "I hate anything or anyone that is dependent on me."

6D.7. *Sarcasm, Cynicism.* **Possible meanings:** (1) "I'm tough, and no one can hurt me." (2) "I refuse to let myself feel tender." (3) "I'll get you back, but I'll do it in an indirect or passive–aggressive way."

6D.8. *Stinginess.* **Possible meanings:** (1) "I'll never be taken advantage of." (2) "No one ever gave me anything, and I'll do the same." (3) "Whatever you give, it means you have less." (4) "I have to hold on to every dime, or I'll be poor again [or lose all my power]."

6D.9. *Mood swings.* **Possible meanings:** (1) "I'm a passionate person, not dried-out and dull like my mother." (2) "From one moment to the other, I don't know who I am or what I feel." (3) "My mood depends on the people I am with."

EXERCISE 6E
What Is the Hidden Reward (Secondary Gain) of the Defense?

6E.1. **What is the hidden reward of the defense?** Laughing off the unkindness (1) avoids conflict about anger and 2) avoids a hopeless feeling of moping when the patient feels unable to obtain a resolution with the other person. If the patient believes that any conflict would end the relationship, then maintaining pleasant feelings at all costs would keep the relationship (secondary gain 1), or prevent a devastating fear of aloneness (secondary gain 2), or maintain a fragile sense of being lovable (secondary gain 3).

What might the therapist say to point this out to the patient? Would you fear losing the relationship if you said something negative? [Costs]

6E.2. **What is the hidden reward of the defense?** A patient describing refusal to let someone get "something on me" suggests avoidance of anxiety about interpersonal closeness (primary gain 1) such as fear of vulnerability, pain of rejection, or anxiety over loss of autonomy. Secondary gain might include a self-image of invulnerability.

What might the therapist say to point this out to the patient? Maybe you really fear her criticism or her looking down on you [primary gain]. What do you think is the worst thing that might happen if she "had something on you"? [Anxiety regulation to elicit fears over, e.g., loss of respect, reprisal, etc.] I wonder if it's important for you to stay in a pleasant mood with her so you are protected from her retaliation [benefits or secondary gain 1], and you always stay in control [secondary gain 2]?

6E.3. **What is the hidden reward of the defense?** Avoidance of closeness that is terrifying by screaming at girlfriend, or, put another way, the angry outburst provides the blessed safety of distance.

What might the therapist say to point this out to the patient? I wonder if you are scared about getting really close to her (primary gain) and by screaming at her you were able to back her off and keep her at a safe distance (secondary gain 1). Also the temper outburst and irritability at her might give you a sense of autonomy (secondary gain 2). What do you think?

6E.4. **What is the hidden reward of the defense?** Not thinking about what to talk about in therapy may be avoiding the specific feelings that are coming up (primary gain). But it also can represent a way to sabotage therapy progress if change is greatly feared (secondary gain).

What might the therapist say to point this out to the patient? I wonder if there is some reason why you might not want to be moving along further in therapy? Are we coming up against some things you might want to avoid? It might not be on the tip of your tongue, but are you aware of any sense of this?

6E.5. **What is the hidden reward of the defense?** Being outraged at a therapist's confrontation of a hidden agenda suggests avoidance of shame about the self (primary gain). It also may reflect a lack of motivation for change (secondary gain).

What might the therapist say to point this out to the patient? I'm sorry that you feel so misunderstood. That must feel awful. What's the worst part of it for you? [Or:] Maybe I have been mistaken in how I understood what you said. Could you tell me more so I can understand you better? [Note: When a patient is extremely upset by a therapist's comment, it may reflect a narcissistic injury and a lack of capacity for exploratory methods. In such cases, it is better to make a frank apology and move to anxiety-regulating or supportive methods to correct the rupture in the alliance and assess the situation.]

CHAPTER 7

EXERCISE 7A
Identify Maladaptive versus Adaptive Versions of Specific Affects

7A.1. **Closeness/tenderness**

• Idealized, perfectionistic image of other	**Maladaptive**
• Self-absorption blocking empathy	**Maladaptive**
• "I–Thou"; other is cherished	**Adaptive**
• Envy	**Maladaptive**
• Acceptance of people's strengths and weaknesses, unexaggerated	**Adaptive**

- Comforting, hugging, and holding **Adaptive**
- Gratitude **Adaptive**
- Empathy for other **Adaptive**
- Anxiety or avoidance of eye contact **Maladaptive**

7A.2. Sexual desire

- Deeply satisfying sharing **Adaptive**
- Does not enhance closeness **Maladaptive**
- Addictive encounters **Maladaptive**
- Enhances closeness **Adaptive**
- Lust that objectifies partner **Maladaptive**
- Paired with love and care **Adaptive**

7A.3. Pain

- Signal of emotional harm **Adaptive**
- Leads to adaptive avoidance **Adaptive**
- Leads to depression/melancholia **Maladaptive**
- Chronic harm turned on self **Maladaptive**
- Feels unavoidable; "stuck" in it **Maladaptive**
- Leads to grieving for a loss **Adaptive**

7A.4. Enjoyment/joy

- Ignores the pain of others **Maladaptive**
- Vanishes quickly with loss of external stimulus **Maladaptive**
- Calming, soothing, quiet **Adaptive**
- Excessive urgency for it **Maladaptive**
- Lasting pleasure **Adaptive**
- Experienced deeply within **Adaptive**

7A.5. Shame/guilt

- Leads to self-recrimination **Maladaptive**
- Leads to genuine regret, remorse **Adaptive**

7A.6. Interest/excitement

- Compulsive attraction **Maladaptive**
- Deeply satisfying; care for subject **Adaptive**
- Intense and driven involvement **Maladaptive**
- Relaxed but deep attention **Adaptive**
- Excessive/manic energy **Maladaptive**
- Hope, optimism, looking forward to **Adaptive**

7A.7. Grief/sorrow

- Compassion for self **Adaptive**
- Crying that leads to feeling worse **Maladaptive**

• Tears shed with memories of loss, painful but relieving	**Adaptive**
• Self-blame, self-attack	**Maladaptive**
• Tears that cover up anger	**Maladaptive**

7A.8. **Anger**

• Conscious guiding of feelings	**Adaptive**
• Unreflective venting of feeling	**Maladaptive**
• Planning best course of action	**Adaptive**
• Little forethought of action	**Maladaptive**
• Loud swearing, yelling	**Maladaptive**
• Clear statement of wishes	**Adaptive**
• Frustration, hopelessness	**Maladaptive**
• Rush of energy to limbs, but well controlled	**Adaptive**

7A.9. **Fear**

• Actions to protect self	**Adaptive**
• Attacking, thwarting self	**Maladaptive**
• Paralyzed action, unable to cry out	**Maladaptive**
• Able to run, scream, freeze as needed	**Adaptive**

EXERCISE 7B
What's the Activating or Inhibitory Feeling under the Defense?

7B.1. *Patient: I feel butterflies in my stomach.*

Possible underlying affect(s): This behavior may indicate excitement (adaptive activation) or anxiety (inhibitory feeling) and needs to be further explored. Are the butterflies due to something good happening (suggesting activation of excitement), or due to something frightening (causing inner turmoil or suggesting anxiety or inhibition—e.g., feeling nervous about feeling angry, which is very common)?

7B.2. *Patient crosses legs and folds arms.*

Possible underlying affect(s): In some contexts, this behavior may suggest withdrawal or putting up barriers, which would imply that some type of inhibitory affect is involved, such as shame or anxiety. However, it is important to remember that the patient could also feel physically cold.

7B.3. *Patient sighs deeply.*

Possible underlying affect(s): Sighs can have many different meanings. Sighs can suggest a release of tension, and are often indicators of the emergence of deep feeling such as grief or anger. Sighs also can indicate that anxiety, shame, or pain is being raised because of the conflicts over the deep feelings that are being elicited. On the other hand, if the patient sighs deeply and rolls the eyes, this may indicate feelings of contempt or disgust toward the therapist.

7B.4. *Patient makes a fist.*

Possible underlying affect(s): A fist usually indicates that anger is building. But it can also indicate defensive self-attack, when patients feel angry at themselves. This should be explored to check whether the fist is turned toward others in affect-laden imagery (activation) or whether it is turned toward the self (inhibition).

7B.5. *Patient slowly and repeatedly strokes fingers through hair.*

Possible underlying affect(s): This sensual response suggests sexual feeling, which could be adaptive (if this is the affect being exposed) or defensive. Seductive behavior by the patient may be used to avoid a genuine closeness with the therapist or to avoid looking at painful topics.

7B.6. *Patient suddenly feels back pain during discussion of difficult topic.*

Possible underlying affect(s): If we rule out a back injury, this response suggests that the patient is tensing back muscles in a way that is painful. The question is this: What activating affect is being restrained? It could be that tension in the back is reining in anger or disgust. Another possibility is that the back tension/pain is tightening against feelings of grief or fear. You may be able to think of a number of other possibilities.

7B.7. *Patient covers eyes.*

Possible underlying affect(s): When patients cover their eyes or their faces, especially when crying, it is almost always a sign of conscious or unconscious shame—a signal that therapists should always be alert for.

EXERCISE 7C
Exposure—Experiencing Affect on Three Levels.

7C.1. **The Ungrateful Neighbor** (Affect Phobia: Closeness/Tenderness)

What therapist might say to label feeling: What would someone else be feeling for a neighbor who brought over chicken soup? [PATIENT: I guess warmly or grateful.] [Note: Feelings of warmth or gratitude are members of the closeness/tenderness family of feelings.]

What therapist might say to elicit physiological signs: If you let yourself imagine feeling some gratitude, how do you experience those grateful feelings in your body? [PATIENT: A softening in my chest and a warm glow. I can also feel some energy in my arms to reach out and hug her.]

What therapist might say to elicit imagined actions: If you had let yourself be moved by those warm feelings, what might those feelings have moved you to say or do. [PATIENT: I would have given her a big hug, and thanked her from the bottom of my heart.]

7C.2. **The Unhappy Painter** (Affect Phobia: Excitement)

What therapist might say to label feeling: What were you feeling just **before** you shut yourself off? [PATIENT: Excitement!]

What therapist might say to elicit physiological signs: How do you experience that excitement in your body? [PATIENT: A rush of good feeling—really good, filled up, like I wanted to do more.]

What therapist might say to elicit imagined actions: What would happen if you really allowed yourself to have all of that old rush? What would it make you want to do? [PATIENT: Oh, I'd want to paint for hours. I wouldn't want to stop!]

7C.3. **The Stressed Husband** (Affect Phobia: Joy or Closeness)

What therapist might say to label feeling: If you hadn't been in a bad mood, what might have you been feeling in reaction to the bath and the meal? [PATIENT: I guess I would have felt a lot of pleasure and love for my wife].

What therapist might say to elicit physiological signs: How would you experience each of those feelings in your body? [PATIENT: Well, pleasure would be a relaxed, comfortable feeling all over my body. Love would be a strong warm feeling in my heart. I don't indulge in either one of those feelings too often!]

What therapist might say to elicit imagined actions: How would you have acted if you had indulged yourself in those feelings and let them move you? [PATIENT: Maybe I would have just laid back in the bath and focused on all the good feelings. The same goes for dinner. I would have savored every bite, and my body would have been relaxed and comfortable all evening. If I let myself show my feelings for my wife, I would have been much more openly affectionate—like she always wants me to be.]

7C.4. **The Distressed Man Working Late** (Affect Phobia: Sexual Feelings)

What therapist might say to label feeling: People can have strong emotional reactions to people with whom they work, which doesn't mean the feelings have to be acted on. [Normalizing to reduce shame] Let's look at those feelings to see if we can understand them better. Tell me how were you feeling in those moments with your boss? [PATIENT: I was so turned on and aroused.]

What therapist might say to elicit physiological signs: How did you experience those sexual feelings in your body? [Patient: (*Blushing*) Actually, I'm starting to get an erection as I'm thinking about it.]

What therapist might say to elicit imagined actions: If you allowed yourself to have those sexual feelings—without judging them—what do you imagine you would be saying or doing? [Note: In addition to the three steps to affect exposure, repeated anxiety regulation will often be necessary to allow patients to experience conflicted affects and desensitize the inhibitory feelings fully.] It will be important to come to understand what you are longing for in this situation, to see if you can find something comparable in your marriage.

EXERCISE 7D
How to Deepen the Experience of the Affect

7D.1. **Sadness. B, C, D, and possibly A.** A is a simple invitation that sometimes can help to deepen the feeling but other times can make a patient feel self-conscious and thus more tense. By having her focus on her body, B and C are helpful ways to slip under the defense and loosen her restraint. D is also a standard way to deepen feeling; just talking about the sad event in specific detail can lead to deepening of the feeling.

7D.2. **Longing for closeness. A** focuses on her longing for touch, and is likely to bring out deep feeling by examining a specific recurring memory of being held. Although sex with this boyfriend was not enjoyable for her, sex can often be a means of obtaining much-longed-for touching and holding. B is an intellectual interpretation about the effect of the parents; it may evoke sadness, but it is not a direct way to deepen feeling. C is direct advice. It will probably generate disagreement, not a deepening of feeling. D is teaching. It may be useful, but it leads more to cognitive responding than to affective responding.

7D.3. **Feeling of care/closeness. C** is a self-disclosure that has the most potential to touch the patient. The issue is the patient's receptivity to closeness, and the patient has acknowledged the therapist's concern. The therapist models openness by repeating the concern, and also validates what the patient has said. Then the therapist deepens the experience by asking the patient to try to examine how that feels to her. (Note: This is said near the end of the session, and there is not time for extensive exploration of feeling. But if the patient were able to feel touched by the concern of the therapist even momentarily, that would be a step toward being more able to open and reach out to others.) A identifies the defense against the closeness, and could be a first step toward getting to the affect—but it is not a way to deepen feeling. Furthermore, the patient has just acknowledged some awareness of the therapist's concern, so it would be a mistake to confront her defensiveness rather than acknowledge the feeling. B acknowledges the concern, but minimizes it because it focuses on the therapist's beliefs rather than the patient's feelings. D is an invitation to call if needed and might be experienced warmly by the patient. But because it is given on an intellectual level, it is less likely than C to penetrate the patient's defenses against doing so. Also, the abrupt ending of the session in the next sentence could generate negative feelings toward the therapist.

7D.4. **Sadness. B and possibly C or A.** B is the most helpful thing, because it will deepen the patient's feeling to have her talk about specific sad memories. C takes an indirect step toward feeling by focusing on the blocks toward doing so. The goal is to reduce the inhibition of expressing sadness with therapist. A is encouragement to let go, which sometimes is helpful. But if the anxiety is too great, it can make some patients feel frustrated or inadequate. D is a supportive intervention. It will lighten the affective experience. This can be useful if it is at the end of the session, for example. Alternatively, it could indicate a therapist's collusion with the patient's defenses.

7D.5. **Anger/assertion. B or possibly C.** B would have the patient focus on his bodily signals. There is evidence of defensive frustration (i.e., self-attack or anger turned on the self), but the fist could also indicate some arousal of anger directed toward the father that could be explored. C is an empathic comment, and might also elicit some anger. A is a question that would lead toward intellectual exploration of the conflict with the father. Doing so might lead to an eventual building of feeling, but it is not a direct way to explore the feeling that is already present. D is an exploration of the father's motives; it might lead to more anger, but it could lead to squelching the patient's angry feelings through premature "compassion" before the patient's anger has been accessed.

7D.6. **Sexual desire. D and possibly A or C.** By getting into the details of what the patient finds sexually exciting, D moves toward direct exposure to feelings of sexual arousal. A is classic anxiety regulation, which may indirectly help to deepen the affect by allowing the patient to experience more sexual arousal before his inhibitions shut the experience down. C can also regulate the shame over his sexual desire by stressing the importance of healthy sexuality; it also encourages grieving over the losses due to the conflict. B focuses on a different affect, anger/assertion, which may or may not be a problem for this patient; a therapist who says this may be moving away from sexual issues because of his or her own discomfort.

EXERCISE 7E
How to Regulate
Anxieties about Feeling

7E.1. **What the therapist might say:** What's the hardest part about feeling so angry at your mother? [Cognitive technique] Do you think you are the first daughter who has ever felt anger at her mom? [Light humor to put her response in perspective; normalizing her response]

7E.2. **What the therapist might say:** Remember that these are just feelings we are exploring. You've been tormented by guilt about these sexual thoughts and feelings that you have been having. We're just allowing you a safe place to explore them in fantasy, where no one will get hurt [Reassurance, providing information]. What's most embarrassing for you?

7E.3. **What the therapist might say:** What has been the most difficult part about spending an hour here talking about yourself?

7E.4. **What the therapist might say:** Well, let's look at some of those fears about grieving. It is very common for people to feel as though their grief is so huge that if they start they will never stop crying [Normalizing]. Have you ever cried so much you couldn't stop? How long does it usually last? [Therapist can continue in this vein, providing information and reassurance that grief, when allowed full expression, is never unending, and often provides significant relief.]

7E.5. **What the therapist might say:** Heaven forbid that you should feel proud of yourself! [Light humor]. Seriously, it's sad to see how hard it is for you to receive my praise [Empathic response—self-disclosure]. What's the most uncomfortable thing about it for you? [Cognitive technique]

EXERCISE 7F
Systematic
Desensitization—
Response Prevention
and Exposure

7F.1. **Phobic affect:** Closeness.

What the therapist might say: See if you can imagine not hiding behind the newspaper [response prevention] and allow yourself to feel the warm feelings [exposure] that you've described having for her.

7F.2. **Phobic affect:** Grief.

What the therapist might say: If you could allow yourself not to be the strong one for once [response prevention]—here, where you don't have to take care of anyone [response prevention]—what might you be feeling (exposure)?

7F.3. **Phobic affect:** Pride in self.

What the therapist might say: If you didn't let your mind check out or drift to other thoughts [response prevention], what might you feel [exposure] about your promotion?

7F.4. **Phobic affect:** Anger/assertion. (Note: Interest/excitement is involved because she really wants the job, but this feeling is not conflicted. The patient acknowledges her interest, but has a conflict over asserting her wish for it.)

What the therapist might say: If you weren't avoiding asking for the job [response prevention], and if you allowed yourself to really ask for what you want [exposure] for a change, what would you be saying or doing? [This imagery would elicit the mix of assertive and anxious feeling.]

7F.5. **Phobic affect:** Interest/excitement. (This is the immediate affect being defended against, but anger toward the father may be another focus.)

What the therapist might say: Let's go back to that specific moment when you were feeling excited. If your father's voice didn't come in to dampen your enthusiasm about writing [response prevention], what would you be feeling about your writing [exposure]?

CHAPTER 8

EXERCISE 8A
Identify Inhibited,
Adaptive, and
Disinhibited Responses

8A.1. Excitement

A. **Inhibited.** Worries that friends will be wounded by her success.

B. **Disinhibited.** Tries to control and manipulate friends, presumably to celebrate with her.

C. **Adaptive.** Shares her good news.

8A.2 Anger/assertion

A. **Adaptive.** Assertive: Stands up for herself and asks to talk about it.

B. **Disinhibited.** Aggressive: Swearing and making threats are often immature and inappropriate.

C. **Inhibited.** Passive: Fakes a compliment and swallows the anger.

8A.3. Joy

A. **Adaptive.** Openly shares a moving experience.

B. **Inhibited.** Does not share his experience, and projects onto the others that they will be offended.

C. **Disinhibited.** Seems to need too much for others to participate in order to validate experience—and uses shame as a means of coercion.

8A.4. Sexual excitement

A. **Disinhibited.** Acts without connection to the other; may have initiated against the other's will.

B. **Inhibited.** Passively hopes that the other will initiate.

C. **Adaptive.** Both individuals are willing to initiate part of the way and wait for signals from the other to move closer.

8A.5 Grief

A. **Inhibited.** Numbs grief and does not acknowledge the loss.

B. **Adaptive.** Lets feelings show in a manner that is appropriate to the situation.

C. **Disinhibited.** Too strong an affective response for the setting; suggests poor modulation of feeling, which may be appropriate at home but not in a restaurant.

8A.6. Anger/assertion

A. **Inhibited.** Passive: Denies her irritation, and holds the tension and discomfort within.

B. **Adaptive.** Assertive: Tells the truth, but begins and ends with a positive statement. As noted in the explanation of the Exercise 8A example, this is what is referred to as a "positive sandwich"—a good formula for giving honest but compassionate feedback.

C. **Disinhibited.** Aggressive: Uses sarcasm as a "dig."

EXERCISE 8B

Help Integrate Feelings and Find the Missing Affect

8B.1. What affect is needed to balance the anger? Compassion/tenderness for the boss.

What might the therapist say to help elicit the compassion? I can understand your frustration about how you have had to pick up a lot of the slack since your boss's mother has been ill. But I wonder if there are other feelings that you might have toward her in addition to the anger.

8B.2. What affect is needed to balance the anger? Grief and/or tenderness.

What might the therapist say to help elicit the grief or tenderness? You've described lots of times that your father behaved terribly toward you, and I think anyone in your position might well feel relieved—and also furious. But you've also described some times when he was caring and apologetic for his actions. I wonder if there might be tender feelings or sad feelings that you might be somehow avoiding. I think it's important that we spend some time with those feelings, too. What do you think? [Note: Even when a parent has been predominantly abusive, it is helpful for a patient to experience sadness over the things missed and longing for things never received.]

8B.3. What affect is needed to balance the closeness? Anger.

What might the therapist say to help elicit the anger? Well, it does seem a little strange that there wouldn't be other feelings mixed in with your strong positive ones. If you consider her bad temper, what other feelings might you be having?

8B.4. What affect is needed to balance the assertion? Closeness/tenderness.

What might the therapist say to help elicit the closeness/tenderness? Well, I can see that it might not just be a joke. You've done really important work learning to stand up for yourself. Maybe now it's time to go back and practice mixing in some of the tender feelings you've told me you have for him. Can you think of a time recently when it was hard to express tender feelings?

EXERCISE 8C

Help the Patient with Interpersonal Expression

8C.1. What does the patient need help with? F. Conflict over closeness. Some obstacles to closeness are out of the way, but closeness is still missing, and the therapist must assess to what extent this is due to conflict on the part of the patient.

What might the therapist say? So it sounds like you're able to assert and protect yourself, but it's still hard to be close. Can you think of a time recently when you or your wife reached out to each other, or wanted to reach out, but it didn't work for some reason?

8C.2. What does the patient need help with? E. Conflict over assertion (remaining guilt).

What might the therapist say? Well, this is all so new to you that it's no wonder you would still have some guilty feelings about it. [Validation and support] Tell me, what felt the worst about it? [Anxiety regulation]

8C.3. What does the patient need help with? B. Mature expression of anger (possibly integrated with compassion). In certain instances, swearing can be appropriate; deciding whether it will take some judgment on the therapist's part.

What might the therapist say? You know, I think it's very important that you are able to set some limits with your boss, and I applaud your doing it. [Support] But I worry that the way you did it may make more problems for you. Can you think of some other ways you might have said what you needed to say, and then we can look at the pros and cons of each?

8C.4. **What does the patient need help with?** D. Information: The difference between grief and depression.

What might the therapist say? Well, we had been talking about your mother's death and you'd been feeling sad about that, so it's not surprising that you'd be tearful after the session. [Validation] But it can be hard to tell grief from depression. When you were crying, were you feeling sad about her? [PATIENT: Yes. I kept remembering things we'd done together.] That's more likely to be grief, and, remember, when you're grieving, there should be some relief after you cry. When people are depressed, they're more likely to be hopeless and think bad things about themselves when they cry. In such cases, tears don't provide relief, but make one feel as though things are getting worse. [Therapist is providing information and teaching.]

8C.5. **What does the patient need help with?** A. Addressing secondary gain.

What might the therapist say? Well, I think it's great that you were able to observe yourself while you were making an angry scene. That's a really important first step. But also you said there was some delight in blasting him, and right after that you said that your husband was really sweet to you. The way you've described him, that's not something that happens very often. Do you think there could be some connection between him being sweet and why you get so angry?

8C.6. **What does the patient need help with?** G. Blending of positive and negative feelings.

What might the therapist say? It's good that you were able to ask for quiet time. Sometimes if you're saying something that someone might see as negative, it helps to make it into a "positive sandwich"—putting something positive before and after the negative message. [Therapist is providing information and teaching.] It seems like you really appreciated her efforts in preparing dinner, and how good it was. Is there a way you could combine that with your request that she talk a little less?

CHAPTER 9

EXERCISE 9A
Assess Externalization of Needs or Excess Dependency on Others

9A.1. *Patient who has more to life than his job.*

How externalized are this patient's needs? Not overly dependent.

Why? This man is not desperately dependent on his job to validate his sense of self.

9A.2. *Man who feels miserable and lost when family is gone.*

How externalized are this patient's needs? Overly dependent.

Why? This father and husband "externalizes" or derives his sense of well-being from the physical presence of his wife and family. When his family is gone, he is unable to generate feelings of comfort or self-worth on his own (from his memories and feelings about his relationship with his family).

9A.3. *Patient who seeks therapist's reassurance.*

How externalized are this patient's needs? Overly dependent.

Why? This patient's ability to feel secure in her decisions are somewhat externalized because she is overly dependent on the therapist telling her that her decisions were valid. She is not yet able to generate a feeling of security in her judgment (i.e., pride, mastery) on her own, and this is reflected in her growing anxiety as she drives away from the therapist's office.

9A.4. *Patient who never feels good enough.*

How externalized are this patient's needs? Overly dependent.

Why? This patient is externalizing her need for self-respect by obtaining graduate degrees, but then realizes that even her accomplishments are not enough. She is unable to generate or sustain positive feelings about herself without aspiring to higher accomplishments.

9A.5. *Patient who is not agonizing about a breakup.*

How externalized are this patient's needs? Not overly dependent.

Why? This patient is able to reassure herself that her decision to leave her boyfriend was right, and to feel good about herself as well. She is not externalizing those needs (i.e., requiring a relationship to validate her sense of self-worth).

EXERCISE 9B
Help Build the Patient's Receptive Capacity

9B.1. **Yes.** This encourages compassion for self by recognizing compassion from another. (It is assumed that the mother is a benevolent person in the patient's life.)

9B.2. **No.** This is a confrontation that identifies a self-attacking or self-neglectful defensive behavior; it might lead to more self-compassion, but is not an active technique to build the patient's receptive capacity.

9B.3. **Yes.** This is a question that encourages the patient to be receptive or responsive to feelings of pride for self.

9B.4. **Yes.** This is an active technique that encourages the patient to "read," be receptive to, and "take in" the therapist's feeling toward him or her.

9B.5. **Yes.** This encourages feelings of pride or self-worth by heightening the patient's recognition and receptivity to the grandfather's fairly evident sense of pride in the patient.

9B.6. **No.** This is anxiety regulation, most likely aimed at helping reduce the inhibitions to receiving care from others. Of course, reducing the anxiety or shame about receiving care would be one step toward building the receptive capacity, but that is not the main thrust of the intervention.

EXERCISE 9C
Help Patients Grieve for What Was Missing

9C.1. **C.** This intervention encourages exposure to the care that is longed for. A is a supportive intervention that can ease the patient's frustration and support his trying again, but does not encourage more feeling. B encourages imaginal exposure to the care that he never got from his mother, but because it's a future "assignment," it takes the patient away from the immediate affect. D acknowledges the growth that the patient is making in at least letting his wife hold him, but it does not encourage further feeling.

9C.2. **A.** The patient is already experiencing the grief over never having been understood. A simply reflects the patient's grief, ideally facilitating a deepening of feeling. B, C, and D are more cognitive or informational interventions.

9C.3. **A, B, C, and D.** A is an intervention that uses imagery to deepen the feeling. The therapist could have the patient go through the return home step by step in memory, with much detail. This is often an excellent way to access feeling. B and C are empathic statements that might also lead to deepening the grief over what was missing. D focuses on the loneliness that is implied in the patient's description of growing up, and might deepen the sadness.

EXERCISE 9D

Address Domains of Self-Functioning

9D.1. *Patient who is working too hard and not sleeping.* **What the therapist might say:** It sounds pretty stressful. I'm wondering how much sleep you **do** get and whether you are eating regular meals at all. [Biological needs]

9D.2. *Overly self-reliant patient.* **What the therapist might say:** It's a real strength to be able to rely on yourself, but it sounds somewhat isolating. Have you met people to spend free time with? Do you have people you feel close to? [Social needs]

9D.3. *Patient who is bored with self.* **What the therapist might say:** Sounds like an awfully painful place to be. Are there things that you feel passionate about—now or in the past? What have been your strongest interests in life? What has given you the most pleasure? [Emotional needs—interest/excitement or enjoyment/joy]

9D.4. *Patient, turning 50, feels no purpose to life.* **What the Therapist Might Say:** Well, sometimes depression can cause that feeling but it may be more about existential or spiritual issues. I wonder if I can help you try to find what might be meaningful to you in your life right now, or what would give you a sense of purpose? Also, what it means for you to have turned 50 recently? [Spiritual needs]

EXERCISE 9E

Help Build Patients' Self-Image by "Changing Perspectives"

9E.1. *Patient who feels undeserving of therapy.*

What the therapist might say: It sounds as though you feel that you don't deserve the help you are getting here. If a good friend of yours had been telling you the story you've been telling me these past weeks, how would you feel about them spending an hour each week getting help for their problems?

Possible rationale: By imagining a compassionate response toward a good friend (which most patients are able to do), the patient may develop greater access to having compassion for himself.

9E.2. *Patient who has not cared for self since grandmother's death.*

What the therapist might say: If your grandmother were alive and heard you saying this, what do you think she would be saying to you right now?

Possible rationale: This intervention exposes patient to the memory of compassion from the loving grandmother. Allowing the patient to actively "take in" or be receptive to the love of a significant other (even in memory) can lead to increased self-compassion.

9E.3. *Patient who cannot relax with others.*

What the therapist might say: Well, can we look at what you feel in here with me? If you were sitting in my chair, could you view yourself differently?

Possible rationale: Encouraging the patient to imagine how she might view herself form the therapist's chair provides exposure to care or concern for herself. Asking the patient to generate the feeling within is a more powerful intervention than having the therapist tell the patient his view of her—which can easily be dismissed or defended against. This intervention can also identity the patient's self-critical judgments, which may be projected onto the therapist (e.g., "Oh, I'm just another clinical case to you, nothing more").

CHAPTER 10

EXERCISE 10A
Evaluate Patients'
Receptive Capacity

10A.1. **A.** Insufficiently receptive/attentive to secretary's biological needs; possibly lacks empathy for others and is overly attentive to self-needs, to the exclusion of others' needs.

10A.2. **B.** Appropriately attentive/receptive to secretary's biological needs; also attentive to own needs.

10A.3. **B.** Appropriately attentive/receptive to husband's hunger; not avoiding needs of self or other.

10A.4. **C.** Overly attentive/receptive to husband's hunger; inattentive to her own wants or needs.

10A.5. **C.** Overly attentive/receptive to kids' excitement; seems to avoid attending to self-needs or self-care.

10A.6. **A.** Insufficiently attentive/receptive to kids' excitement; avoiding empathy for their excitement (by not being willing to stay a few minutes longer) and overly attentive to her own (defensive?) needs to be on time or please others.

10A.7. **A.** Insufficiently attentive/receptive to wife's emotional need to grieve; possibly a way to avoid his own feelings of sadness.

10A.8. **B.** Appropriately attentive/receptive to wife's grief, and also to his relationship to his wife.

EXERCISE 10B
Help Patients Change
Inner Images of Others

10B.1. **B.** This response encourages the patient to allow him- or herself to have anger toward the therapist, and also encourages the patient to integrate positive and negative feelings toward others. Repetition of this kind of exposure will allow the patient to see that anger does not have to be stifled in order to preserve relationships. A points out a defense (holding in anger). C is a clarification or reflecting back to the patient. D validates the patient's feelings of frustration, but is also limit-setting. On the one hand, the patient might feel somewhat shamed rather than supported. It attends more to the therapist's boundaries than it does to exploring the patient's feelings. On the other hand, a patient who frequently oversteps boundaries might need this type of limit-setting response.

10B.2. **A.** This response allows the patient to start to evaluate whether her distrust is justified in the current relationship. B is supportive of the patient's need to be self-protective, which may or may not be appropriate, depending on the patient's history. C validates the patient's cautiousness—which may be overly defensive in this case, but may have been necessary when the patient was a child. D is exploration of her anxiety—which is helpful in finding the reality of her fears, or whether she is afraid of letting herself become close to him.

10B.3.   **B.** This response encourages the patient to imagine the father's feelings from a different perspective, and thereby begin to feel less bad about the self. A is similar in content, but the therapist is telling the patient what the father might feel, rather than encouraging the patient to discover an inner sense of the parent's love. This would be less likely to bring affective change to the patient than the patient's doing it independently would be. C is presenting reality or giving information that ideally would normalize the patient's negative feeling for the self. The patient probably is aware of this intellectually, but has not been able to change the feeling. D points out the defensive self-attack and its costs to the patient.

10B.4.   **D.** This response encourages the patient to explore his or her own reaction and begin to see that the patient might be the one viewing him- or herself with disgust, not the therapist. However, it also allows for exploring the therapist's behavior to see whether any critical or countertransferential response has been made by the therapist (i.e., therapist's issues that are being projected onto the patient). In such cases, it can be enormously healing to the patient for the therapist to take appropriate responsibility for his or her own behavior and/or give a frank apology if a mistake has been made. A normalizes the patient's response but does not explore it. B is supportive of the patient's disclosure, and begins exploration—but not specifically about the therapist's feelings. C is a confrontation of the defense of self-attack, but does not explore the feelings involved.

EXERCISE 10C
Identify and Adaptive and Addictive Attachments

10C.1.   **Addictive.** Mistakes being controlled in relationship for being taken care of, and stays "addicted" to it. Fits a pattern of relationships that is likely to become more abusive. This patient seems unable to assert her needs—or possibly feels unentitled or deserving enough to ask for more (lack of self-care).

10C.2.   **Addictive.** Longs for an idealized other—probably to resolve lack of esteem for the self (e.g., "someone who could make everything perfect"). He may also fear a deeper closeness with his wife.

10C.3.   **Addictive.** Devalues praise at hand, but longs for and stays addicted to what is unavailable and what is perceived as more difficult to attain (i.e., praise from the boss). This may be a way of avoiding being receptive to positive feelings from others—and also feeling better about the self.

10C.4.   **Addictive.** Addicted to relationships that break the rules or might be found out. This behavior could represent any of the following: (1) defensive avoidance of closeness to husband; (2) defensive and sadistic wish to hurt husband because of the inner pain she carries; (3) defensive acting out to protect against being hurt herself; or (4) poor self-esteem and acting in ways that thwart a positive sense of self.

10C.5.   **Adaptive.** Uses assertive behavior to protect himself from becoming more involved in relationship with unpredictable partner.

10C.6.   **Adaptive.** Able to have sexual fantasies without feeling compelled to act upon them and jeopardize the current relationship. The therapist might explore with her what the fantasies tell her she is longing for that she might be lacking in the relationship with her fiancée. This might uncover some sexual wishes—or other aspects of a relationship—that she has been hesitant to ask for.

References

Alexander, F., & French, T. (1946). *Psychoanalytic therapy: Principles and application.* New York: Ronald Press.

Alpert, M. (1996). Videotaping psychotherapy. *Journal of Psychotherapy Practice and Research, 5*(2), 93–105.

American Psychiatric Association. (2000). *Diagnostic and statistical manual of mental disorders* (4th ed., text rev.). Washington, DC: Author.

Balint, M. (1968). *The basic fault: Therapeutic aspects of regression.* London: Tavistock.

Basch, M. F. (1976). The concept of affect: A reexamination. *Journal of the American Psychoanalytic Association, 24,* 759–777.

Baxter, L. R. (1995). Neuroimaging studies of human anxiety disorders: Cutting paths of knowledge through the field of neurotic phenomena. In F. E. Bloom & D. J. Kupfer (Eds.), *Psychopharmacology: The fourth generation of progress* (pp. 1287–1299). New York: Raven Press.

Bramson, R. M. (1981). *Coping with difficult people.* New York: Anchor Press/ Doubleday.

Cautela, J. R. (1966). Treatment of compulsive behavior by covert sensitization. *Psychological Record, 16,* 33–41.

Cautela, J. R. (1973). Covert processes and behavior modification. *Journal of Nervous and Mental Disease, 1,* 157.

Cautela, J. R., & McCullough, L. (1978). Covert conditioning: A learning theory perspective on imagery. In J. L. Singer & K. S. Pope (Eds.), *The power of the human imagination* (pp. 227–254). New York: Plenum Press.

Damasio, A. (1994). *Descartes error.* New York: Harcourt Brace.

Damasio, A. (1999). *The feeling of what happens: Body and emotion in the making of consciousness.* New York: Harcourt Brace.

Davanloo, H. (1980). *Short-term dynamic psychotherapy.* New York: Jason Aronson.

Della Selva, P. C., (1996). *Intensive short-term dynamic psychotherapy: Theory and technique.* New York: Wiley.

Egner, T. (1955). *Folk og rovere i Kardemomme By.* Oslo, Norway: J. W. Cappelens.

Ekman, P. (1984). Expression and the nature of emotion. In K. Scherer & P. Ekman (Eds.), *Approaches to emotion* (pp. 319–340). Hillsdale, NJ: Erlbaum.

Ekman, P. (1992). Facial expressions of emotion: New findings, new questions. *Psychological Science, 3,* 34–38.

Ekman, P., & Davidson, R. J. (Eds.). (1994). *The nature of emotion: Fundamental questions.* New York: Oxford University Press.

Endicott, J., Spitzer, R. L., Fleiss, J. L., & Cohen, J. (1976). The Global Assessment Scale: A procedure for measuring overall severity of psychiatric disturbance. *Archives of General Psychiatry, 33,* 766–771.

Fensterheim, H., & Baer, J. (1975). *Don't say yes when you want to say no.* New York: McKay.

Forward, S., with Buck, C. (1989). *Toxic parents: Overcoming their hurtful legacy and reclaiming your life.* New York: Bantam.

Fosha, D. (2000). *The transforming power of affect: A model for accelerated change.* New York: Basic Behavioral Science.

Frijda, N. H. (2001). *The emotions.* Cambridge, England: Cambridge University Press.

Gustafson, J. P. (1986). *The complex secret of brief psychotherapy.* New York: Norton.

Hendrix, H. (1988). *Getting the love you want: A guide for singles.* New York: Holt.

Hendrix, H. (1992). *Keeping the love you find: A guide for couples.* New York: Pocket Books.

Izard, C. (1990). Facial expressions and the regulation of emotion. *Journal of Personality and Social Psychology, 58*(3), 487–498.

Kandel, E. R. (1998). A new intellectual framework for psychiatry. *American Journal of Psychiatry, 155*(4), 457–469.

Lazarus, R. S. (1991). *Emotion and adaptation.* New York: Oxford University Press.

LeDoux, J. (1996). *The emotional brain: The mysterious underpinnings of emotional life.* New York: Simon & Schuster.

Lemgruber, V. (2000). *O futuro da integracao: Desenvolvimentos em psicoterapia breve.* Porto Alegre: Artrned Editora.

Lerner, H. G. (1985). *The dance of anger: A woman's guide to changing the patterns of intimate relationships.* New York: Harper & Row.

Linehan, M. M. (1993). *Cognitive-behavioral treatment of borderline personality disorder.* New York: Guilford Press.

Luborsky, L. (1984). *Principles of psychoanalytic psychotherapy: A manual for supportive–expressive treatment.* New York: Basic Books.

Malan, D. M. (1976). *The frontier of brief psychotherapy.* New York: Plenum Press.

Malan, D. H. (1979). *Individual psychotherapy and the science of psychodynamics.* London: Butterworth.

Malan, D. M., & Osimo, F. (1992). *Psychodynamics, training, and outcome in brief psychotherapy.* London: Butterworth–Heinemann.

Mann, J. (1973). *Time-limited psychotherapy.* Cambridge, MA: Harvard University Press.

McCann, E. (1985). *The two-step: The dance toward intimacy.* New York: Grove Press.

McCullough, L. (1991). Davanloo's short-term dynamic psychotherapy: A cross-theoretical analysis of change mechanisms. In: R. Curtis & G. Stricker (Eds.), *How people change: Inside and outside of therapy* (pp. 59–79). New York: Plenum Press.

McCullough, L. (1993). An anxiety reduction modification of short-term dynamic psychotherapy (STDP): A theoretical "melting pot" of treatment techniques. In G. Stricker & J. Gold (Eds.), *Handbook of integrative psychotherapies* (pp. 139–150). New York: Plenum Press

McCullough, L. (1998). Short-term psychodynamic therapy as a form of desensitization: Treating Affect Phobias. *In Session: Psychotherapy in Practice, 4*(4), 35–53.

McCullough, L. (2000). Short term therapy for character change. In J. Carlson & L. Sperry (Eds.), *Brief therapy strategies with individuals and couples* (pp. 127–160). New York: Zieg/Tucker.

McCullough, L. (2002). Exploring change mechanisms in EMDR applied to "small t Trauma" in short term dynamic psychotherapy: Research questions and speculations. *Journal of Clinical Psychology, 58*(12), 1531–1544.

McCullough, L., & Andrews, S. (2001). Assimilative integration: Short-term dynamic psychotherapy for treating affect phobias. *Clinical Psychology: Research and Practice, 8*(1), 82–91.

McCullough, L., & Winston, A. (1991). The Beth Israel Psychotherapy Research Program. In L. Beutler & M. Crago (Eds.), *Psychotherapy research; An international review of programmatic studies* (pp. 15–23). Washington, DC: American Psychological Association Press

McCullough, L., Winston, A., Farber, B., Porter, F., Pollack, J., Laikin, M., Vingiano,

W., & Trujillo, M. (1991). The relationship of patient-therapist interaction to outcome in brief psychotherapy. *Psychotherapy, 28*(4), 525–533.

McCullough Vaillant, L. (1994). The next step in short-term dynamic psychotherapy: A clarification of objectives and techniques in an anxiety-regulating model. *Psychotherapy, 4,* 35–53.

McCullough Vaillant, L. (1997). *Changing character: Short-term anxiety-regulating psychotherapy for restructuring defenses.* New York: Basic Books.

Miller, A. (1990). *The drama of the gifted child and the search for the true self.* New York: Basic Books.

Miller, W. R., & Rollnick, S. (1991). *Motivational interviewing: Preparing people to change addictive behavior.* New York: Guilford Press.

Nathanson, D. L. (1992). *Shame and pride: Affect, sex, and the birth of the self.* New York: Norton.

Oatley, K., & Jenkins, J. M. (1996). *Understanding emotions.* Cambridge, MA: Blackwell.

Shapiro, F. (2001). *Eye movement desensitization and reprocessing (EMDR): Basic principles, protocols, and procedures* (2nd ed.). New York: Guilford Press.

Sifneos, P. E. (1972). *Short-term psychotherapy and emotional crisis.* Cambridge, MA: Harvard University Press.

Sifneos, P. E. (1973). The prevalence of "alexithymic" characteristics in psychosomatic patients. *Psychotherapy and Psychosomatics, 22,* 257–262.

Sifneos, P. E. (1979). *Short-term dynamic psychotherapy: Evaluation and technique.* New York: Plenum Press.

Solomon, M., Neborsky, R. J., McCullough, L., Alpert, M., Shapiro, & Malan, D. (2001). *Short-term therapy for long-term change.* New York: Norton.

Stern, D. (1985). *The interpersonal world of the infant.* New York: Basic Books.

Stickgold, L. (2002). EMDR: A putative neurobiological mechanism of action. *Journal of Clinical Psychology, 58,* 61–75.

Svartberg, M., Stiles, T., & Seltzer, M. H. (in press). The effectiveness of short-term dynamic psychotherapy and cognitive therapy for Cluster C personality disorders. *American Journal of Psychiatry.*

Tomkins, S. S. (1962). *Affect, imagery, consciousness: Vol. I. Positive affects.* New York: Springer.

Tomkins, S. S. (1963). *Affect, imagery, consciousness: Vol. II. Negative affects.* New York: Springer.

Tomkins, S. S. (1981). The quest for primary motives: The biography and autobiography of an idea. *Journal of Personality and Social Psychology, 41,* 306–329.

Tomkins, S. S. (1991). *Affect, imagery, consciousness: Vol. III. Negative affects anger and fear.* New York: Springer.

Tomkins, S. S. (1992). *Affect, imagery, consciousness: Vol. IV. Cognition.* New York: Springer.

Viorst, J. (1986). *Necessary losses: The loves, illusions, dependencies, and impossible expectations that all of us have to give up in order to grow.* New York: Simon & Schuster.

Wachtel, P. L. (1977). *Psychoanalysis and behavior therapy: Toward an integration.* New York: Basic Books.

Winston, A., Laikin, M., Pollack, J., Samstag, L., McCullough, L., & Muran, C. (1994). Short-term psychotherapy of personality disorders. *American Journal of Psychiatry, 151*(2), 190–194.

Winston, A., McCullough, L., Trujillo, M., Pollack, J., Laikin, M., Flegenheimer, W., & Kestenbaum, R. (1991). Brief psychotherapy of personality disorders. *Journal of Nervous and Mental Disease, 179*(4), 188–193.

Winston, A., & Winston, B. (2002). *Handbook of integrated short-term psychotherapy.* New York: Jason Aronson.

Wolpe, J. (1958). *Psychotherapy by reciprocal inhibition.* Stanford, CA: Stanford University Press.

Index